CANCER IN THE NECK

Evaluation and Treatment

EDITED BY

DAVID L. LARSON, M.D.
Formerly Associate Professor of Surgery, Surgeon
(Head and Neck, Plastic Surgery)
Department of Head and Neck Surgery
The University of Texas
M.D. Anderson Hospital and Tumor Institute
Houston, Texas

Currently Professor and Chairman
Department of Plastic and Reconstructive Surgery
Medical College of Wisconsin
Froedtert Memorial Lutheran Hospital
Milwaukee, Wisconsin

ALANDO J. BALLANTYNE, M.D.
Professor of Surgery, Surgeon
Department of Head and Neck Surgery
The University of Texas
M.D. Anderson Hospital and Tumor Institute
Houston, Texas

and

OSCAR M. GUILLAMONDEGUI, M.D.
Professor of Surgery, Surgeon
Department of Head and Neck Surgery
The University of Texas
M.D. Anderson Hospital and Tumor Institute
Houston, Texas

CANCER IN THE NECK

Evaluation and Treatment

Macmillan Publishing Company
NEW YORK

Collier Macmillan Canada, Inc.
TORONTO

Collier Macmillan Publishers
LONDON

Printed in the United States of America

Macmillan Publishing Company
866 Third Avenue, New York, New York 10022

Collier Macmillan Canada, Inc.
Collier Macmillan Publishers • London

Library of Congress Cataloging-in-Publication Data

Cancer in the neck.

Includes bibliographies and index.
1. Neck—Cancer. 2. Metastasis. I. Larson, David L. (David Lee), 1943- II. Ballantyne, Alando Jones, 1917- III. Guillamondegui, Oscar M. [DNLM: 1. Head and Neck Neoplasms—diagnosis. 2. Head and Neck Neoplasms—therapy. 3. Neoplasm Metastasis. WE 707 C2148]
RC280.N35C36 1986 616.99′493 86-12642
ISBN 0-02-367760-0

Printing: 1 2 3 4 5 6 7 8 Year: 6 7 8 9 0 1 2 3 4

This book is dedicated
to the memory of
Richard H. Jesse, M.D.
Head and Neck Surgeon,
teacher, leader, friend.

D.L.L.
A.J.B.
O.M.G.

Preface

Many books on cancer of the head and neck have been published recently. Perusal of these texts will show one very obvious fact—they portray the primary disease process as unquestionably the most important topic; in many tumor sites, it is the only topic addressed. The management of the neck, when mentioned, is relegated to a few paragraphs or a few pages. Yet patients with regional metastatic disease have half the chance of survival as those with cancers limited to the primary site.

Acknowledgment that the evaluation and treatment of cancer in the neck is a vital topic to the oncologist is only part of the story. Over the last 10 years there have been dramatic and exciting advances in the care of the cancer patient: on the diagnostic front, computerized tomography, nuclear magnetic resonance, and flow cytometry; in the reconstructive arena, musculocutaneous flaps and "customized" free-tissue transfer; and in treatment, refinement of radiation techniques and the still-unresolved topic of appropriate use of chemotherapeutic agents. Although the area of tumor ablation has seen the introduction of the highly specialized areas of craniofacial resection and middle fossa surgery, the most important advance for all head and neck surgical oncologists is related to the management of cancer in the neck. The role of modifications of the classical radical neck dissection (both less-than-radical and more-than-radical), their indications, and their correct uses with adjunctive treatment have been the topics of numerous articles. It would therefore seem only natural that a book be dedicated to such an important topic.

With this purpose in mind, we have attempted to provide the oncologist, in practice or in training, with a "state of the art" text. To this end, we have assembled leaders from all disciplines involved in head and neck cancer treatment. Because of the diversity of opinion, even among experts, we have attempted to give a balanced view, with objective data in areas of known controversy. Therefore, although the book was assembled under the direction of the members of the Department of Head and Neck Surgery at The University of Texas M.D. Anderson Hospital and Tumor Institute at Houston, it does not necessarily reflect only the "Anderson" approach to the treatment of cancer in the neck. Because the contributors are ecumenical and international, we believe we have produced a broad-based book with an equally broad-based appeal to the head and neck surgeon, the radiotherapist, and the clinical oncologist.

David L. Larson, M.D.
Alando J. Ballantyne, M.D.
Oscar M. Guillamondegui, M.D.

Foreword

Scientific revolution, a hallmark of the century, is opening innumerable doors and windows onto the secrets of nature and has given us a never-before-witnessed opportunity to look at biologic events and search for the truth. Coupled with this enormous leap in knowledge and as a necessary corollary to it, the therapeutic attempts to treat whatever illness afflicts humans have changed and are under constant evolution. Quantity of life and its quality are crucial issues in our existence and have a prevailing impact on how we treat our patients.

Cancer in the neck refers primarily, although not exclusively, to the growth of metastatic neoplasms in the regional lymph nodes. The proliferation of tumor cells in an environment distant from the site of origin is the morphologic representation of countless biologic events gradually being unveiled and understood. It is known that most of the frequent cancer sources of the head and neck have various potentials for dissemination to the regional lymph nodes, and the significance of such dissemination varies from one tumor to the other and from one host to the next. The simplistic approach to the management of cancer in the neck that prevailed yesterday is giving way to sophisticated management plans as we are gaining an understanding of the significance of such neoplastic growth in lymph nodes and tissues of the neck.

Our colleagues in the different disciplines of basic sciences are addressing important questions, and as nature gives out the answers to these queries, we will need to test the validity of their findings through proper clinical research. We can be certain that, in the near future, there are going to be important changes in the way we treat patients with cancer, achieving better survival and less treatment morbidity and sequelae. Better yet, we hope to find improved means of prevention beyond what we believe is important today.

As surgery for cancer in the neck is changing, so is the practice of radiation therapy. New sources of energy have been developed, and more sophisticated techniques are being tested. Medical oncology has gained access to new medications and has found better schedules and combinations to deliver chemotherapeutic agents. Tumor immunology has increased its knowledge of the biologic responses to the neoplastic process and pathologists are finding new ways to study and define the nature of the cancer cell. In this ever-changing environment, it is most important and befitting to have an update of the management of cancer in the neck. The editors of this book have assembled an impressive group of authors who have been chosen for their experience in each specific field. The collective knowledge assembled in this volume is the expression of a true "state of the art" of the management of cancer in the neck.

Helmuth Goepfert
Professor and Chariman
Department of Head and Neck Surgery
M.D. Anderson Hospital and Tumor Institute
Houston, Texas

Contributors

J. W. Arendse
Assistant Professor of Otolaryngology
Department of Otolaryngology/Head and Neck Surgery
Free University Hospital
Amsterdam, Netherlands

Charles M. Balch, M.D.
Professor and Chairman
Division of Surgery
The University of Texas
M.D. Anderson Hospital and Tumor Institute
Houston, Texas

Alando J. Ballantyne, M.D.
Professor of Surgery and Surgeon
Department of Head and Neck Surgery
The University of Texas
M.D. Anderson Hospital and Tumor Institute
Houston, Texas

A. J. M. Balm
Associate Professor of Otolaryngology
Department of Otolaryngology/Head and Neck Surgery
Free University Hospital
Amsterdam, Netherlands

Annabel Barber, M.D.
Department of General Surgery
New York Hospital
New York, New York

H. Bartelink, M.D.
Professor of Radiotherapy
Department of Radiotherapy
Netherlands Cancer Institute
Amsterdam, Netherlands

John G. Batsakis
Professor and Chairman
Division of Pathology
The University of Texas
M.D. Anderson Hospital and Tumor Institute
Houston, Texas

Robert Byers, M.D.
Professor of Surgery and Surgeon
Department of Head and Neck Surgery
The University of Texas
M.D. Anderson Hospital and Tumor Institute
Houston, Texas

Thomas E. Carey, Ph.D.
Cancer Research Laboratory
Department of Otolaryngology/Head and Neck Surgery
The University of Michigan
Ann Arbor, Michigan

William A. Cassel, Ph.D.
Department of Microbiology
Emory University School of Medicine
Atlanta, Georgia

Nicholas J. Cassisi
Professor and Chairman
Division of Otolaryngology
University of Florida College of Medicine
Gainesville, Florida

Isaiah W. Dimery
Assistant Professor of Medicine
Department of Medical Oncology (Head and Neck)
The University of Texas
M.D. Anderson Hospital and Tumor Institute
Houston, Texas

Isaiah J. Fidler, D.V.M., Ph.D.
Professor and Chairman
Department of Cell Biology
The University of Texas
M.D. Anderson Hospital and Tumor Institute
Houston, Texas

Helmuth Goepfert, M.D.
Professor and Chairman
Department of Head and Neck Surgery
The University of Texas
M.D. Anderson Hospital and Tumor Institute
Houston, Texas

Andrew Ralph Harwood, M.D.
Romagosa Radiation Oncology Center
Lafayette, Louisiana

Waun K. Hong
Professor of Medicine and Internist
Department of Medical Oncology
(Head and Neck)
The University of Texas
M.D. Anderson Hospital and Tumor Institute
Houston, Texas

Jerry L. Hudson, Ph.D.
Associate Professor of Pathology
Cell Identification Center
Department of Pathology
The University of Michigan
Ann Arbor, Michigan

Jonas T. Johnson, M.D.
Associate Professor of Surgery
Department of Otolaryngology
University of Pittsburgh School of Medicine
Pittsburgh, Pennsylvania

A. B. M. F. Karim, M.D.
Department of Radiotherapy
Free University Hospital
Amsterdam, Netherlands

Sewa S. Legha, M.D.
Associate Professor of Medicine
Department of Medical Oncology
The University of Texas
M.D. Anderson Hospital and Tumor Institute
Houston, Texas

Robert D. Lindberg, M.D.
Professor and Chairman
Department of Therapeutic Radiology
University of Louisville School of Medicine
Louisville, Kentucky

Jesus E. Medina, M.D.
Associate Professor of Surgery
Department of Otolaryngology
University of Oklahoma Hospitals
Oklahoma City, Oklahoma

William M. Mendenhall, M.D.
Associate Professor of Radiotherapy
Division of Radiation Therapy
University of Florida College of Medicine
Gainesville, Florida

Rodney R. Million, M.D.
Professor of Radiotherapy and Chairman
Division of Radiotherapy
University of Florida College of Medicine
Gainesville, Florida

Douglas R. Murray
Associate Professor of Surgery
Department of Surgery
Emory University School of Medicine
Atlanta, Georgia

Eugene N. Myers
Professor and Chairman
Department of Otolaryngology
Head and Neck Surgery
University of Pittsburgh School of Medicine
Pittsburgh, Pennsylvania

Garth L. Nicolson, Ph.D.
Professor of Tumor Biology and Chairman
Department of Tumor Biology
The University of Texas
M.D. Anderson Hospital and Tumor Institute
Houston, Texas

James T. Parsons, M.D.
Assistant Professor of Radiotherapy
Division of Radiation Therapy
University of Florida College of Medicine
Gainesville, Florida

Lester J. Peters
Professor of Radiotherapy and Head
Division of Radiotherapy
The University of Texas
M.D. Anderson Hospital and Tumor Institute
Houston, Texas

Janet E. Price, Ph.D.
Department of Cell Biology
The University of Texas
M.D. Anderson Hospital and Tumor Institute
Houston, Texas

Daniel Remmler, M.D.
Fellow/Instructor
Division of Facial Plastic and Reconstructive Surgery
Department of Otolaryngology—Head and Neck Surgery
Washington University Medical Center
St. Louis, Missouri

Jan Scheetz, P.T.
The University of Texas
M.D. Anderson Hospital and Tumor Institute
Houston, Texas

David E. Schuller
Professor of Surgery and Chairman
Head and Neck Oncology Program
Comprehensive Cancer Center
The Ohio State University
Columbus, Ohio

Jatin P. Shah, M.D.
Surgeon
Head and Neck Service
Memorial Sloan-Kettering Cancer Center
New York, New York

Rick Shallenberger, MPH
Assistant Epidemiologist
Department of Patient Studies
The University of Texas
M.D. Anderson Hospital and Tumor Institute
Houston, Texas

Barbara Shell, P.T.
Head, Department of Physical Therapy
The University of Texas
M.D. Anderson Hospital and Tumor Institute
Houston, Texas

Larry J. Sheman, M.D., F.A.C.S.(c)
Program Director
Manhattan Eye, Ear and Throat Hospital
Visiting Investigator, Head/Neck Surgery
Memorial Sloan-Kettering Hospital
New York, New York

G. B. Snow
Professor and Chairman
Department of Otolaryngology/Head and Neck Surgery
Free University Hospital
Amsterdam, Netherlands

Seng-jaw Soong, M.D.
Department of Biostatistics
University of Alabama at Birmingham
Birmingham, Alabama

Elliot W. Strong, M.D.
Surgeon and Chief
Head and Neck Service
Memorial Sloan-Kettering Cancer Center
New York, New York

R. M. Tiwari, M.D.
Department of Otolaryngology/Head and Neck Surgery
Free University Hospital
Amsterdam, Netherlands

Marshall M. Urist, M.D.
Assistant Professor of Surgery
Department of Surgery
University of Alabama at Birmingham
Birmingham, Alabama

I. van der Waal, M.D.
Department of Pathology
Free University Hospital
Amsterdam, Netherlands

Robert C. Wang, M.D.
Assistant Professor of Surgery
Division of Otolaryngology
Albany Medical College
Albany, New York

Georgia White, RN
The University of Texas
M.D. Anderson Hospital and Tumor Institute
Houston, Texas

Patricia F. Wolf, B.S.
Department of Head and Neck Surgery
The University of Texas
M.D. Anderson Hospital and Tumor Institute
Houston, Texas

Stuart Zimmerman, Ph.D.
Department of Biomathematics
The University of Texas
M.D. Anderson Hospital and Tumor Institute
Houston, Texas

Contents

Part Three: *RADIOTHERAPEUTIC CONSIDERATIONS*

Part Four: *NECK DISSECTION: ALTERNATIVES*

Part Five: *CHEMOTHERAPEUTIC CONSIDERATIONS*

Part Six: *MANAGEMENT OF THE NECK IN MELANOMA, THYROID, AND UNUSUAL TUMORS IN THE NECK*

PART ONE

BIOLOGIC BEHAVIOR OF NECK METASTASIS

CHAPTER 1

Properties of Metastatic Tumor Cells and the Generation of Tumor Phenotypic Diversity

Garth L. Nicolson

EDITORS' COMMENT

It is only fitting that the first two chapters of this book should be written by pioneers in the area of tumor biology. Both Dr. Nicolson and Dr. Fidler have done landmark work in identifying the characteristics of the metastatic tumor cell, the mechanism of its implantation into a receptor site, and the microenvironment in which it grows, reproduces, and engenders further metastasis. The next two chapters should be considered together when trying to develop a concept of the origin and evolution of the metastatic tumor cell. Dr. Nicolson concentrates on the diverse phenotypic properties of the metastatic tumor cell, while Dr. Fidler develops the influence of the microenvironment in which the tumor cell rests and the mechanisms of tumor-cell transport. These scientists demonstrate in their writings the ability to take basic tumor research and give it a practical meaning for the physician caring for the patient with metastatic carcinoma.

In this chapter, Dr. Nicolson focuses on human and experimental cancers and their use in defining the properties of the metastatic phenotype. After identifying the experimental considerations and limitations in the study of metastases, the author cautions that any animal models must be confirmed by using human tumors, preferably human tumor cells of varying metastatic potential isolated from the same patient.

As is well known, the tumor cell may spread by both hematogenous and lymphatic spread; most clinicians view the regional lymph nodes as acting as the first "barrier" to the spread of cancer from the primary tumor in the head and neck. This concept is only partially true because, as noted by Dr. Nicolson, the tumor cell may "proliferate, die, remain dormant, or enter the blood circulation through blood vessels in the node." These same cells may also have an affinity for becoming blood-borne and avoid the regional lymphatics altogether.

The author identifies a selection process by which a tumor implant may survive and proliferate at a specific site, as well as influence the extent and location of that metastasis. The very heterogeneity of a tumor cell secondary to its evolution and progression results in a phenotypic diversification that can lead to the characteristics that determine the inherent malignant potential of that cell. This results in a genetic instability that is associated with tumor changes that correlate directly with its metastatic potential. Dr. Nicolson believes that these may be related to specific regulatory gene sites that can also be responsible for instability in other properties such as chromosome markers, sensitivity to radiation, hyperthermia, and chemotherapeutic agents. The more phenotypic diversification within a tumor cell's makeup, the less effective antitumor agents become.

Add to this potpourri the microenvironment into which the metastatic tumor cell is thrust, as discussed in the following chapter by Dr. Fidler and Dr. Price, and we see another factor that can alter the phenotypic diversification of the tumor cell. Dr. Nicolson finishes the chapter with the question of what initiates this phenotypic diversification, but leaves us with the fact that this is the basis for further work at the molecular, genetic, and cellular level of the metastatic tumor cell.

INTRODUCTION

Neoplastic cells have particular alterations that make them distinct from normal cells, and these alterations are important in defining transformed and tumorigenic states (Nicolson, 1976). In addition, discrete cellular properties also define the highly malignant or metastatic states of tumor cells (Nicolson, 1982, 1984a; Nicolson and Poste, 1982, 1983a, b). These latter properties are associated with the clinical risk of advanced disease and account for the poor prognosis of most cancer patients. Certain cancers show high probabilities of metastatic spread, even at an early stage of the primary lesion, and it has been well documented that, in time, tumors can change in their phenotypic properties, giving rise to less stable, more metastatic cell progeny that are increasingly difficult to eradicate.

We now know that tumor metastasis occurs via a complex cascade of events, and it is thought that this process is the end result of several highly selective steps, whereby fewer and fewer malignant cells eventually survive to form metastatic colonies (Poste and Fidler, 1980; Fidler and Nicolson, 1981; Nicolson, 1982). This suggests that the tumor cells that are capable of forming metastatic lesions at near and distant sites are unique in their cellular properties, particularly those characteristics that are important for successful metastatic spread.

The process of metastasis is not a random phenomenon. Although random events are important in metastasis (Weiss, 1983), the secondary locations of many metastatic cancers cannot be explained by strictly random events. For example, most basal-cell carcinomas undergo extensive invasion at primary sites without evidence of distant metastases, and several types of cancers display unique organ colonization patterns that do not agree with random theories of cancer dissemination (Sugarbaker, 1981; Nicolson, 1982). To explain the apparent nonrandom nature of metastatic tumor spread, Paget (1889) proposed the "seed and soil" hypothesis, which states that the microenvironment of individual organs or tissues ("soils") influences cancer dissemination of particular tumor cells ("seeds"). We can now assign a variety of important properties to metastatic "seeds," as well as to the microenvironments of individual organs or tissues that allow metastatic implantation, invasion, survival, and growth (Table 1-1). The uniqueness of highly metastatic cells, as well as their target sites for survival and growth, are important parameters in the design of new therapeutic approaches against metastatic disease. If metastasis occurred by a strictly random process involving virtually any malignant cell, then specific therapeutic approaches could not be developed to prevent metastasis or selectively destroy metastatic cells.

Evidence has accumulated supporting the concept that metastasis is a nonrandom phenomenon. Histopathologic and anatomic observations have identified differences in the extent of invasion and tissue destruction produced by different human cancers and experimental tumors implanted at various sites in animals. These observations have focused on anatomic pathways of cancer invasion and dis-

Table 1-1. Factors Affecting the Phenotypic Diversities and Metastatic Behaviors of Malignant Tumor Cells

SOURCE	FACTOR OR CHARACTERISTIC
Tumor cell ("seed")	Cell growth/dormancy Chemotaxis and locomotion Immunologic properties Metabolic/nutritional responses Hormone/growth factor receptors Mutability/DNA repair Nongenetic DNA alterations Chromosome structural alterations Oncogenes/protoconcogenes Cell-cell interactions/adhesion Therapeutic sensitivities Cell fusion Gene transcriptional/posttranscriptional controls
Host environment ("soil")	Tissue and stromal environment/matrix Hormones/growth factor concentration Chemotactic factors Vascularization/neovascularization Inflammatory/noninflammatory responses Natural/immunologic responses Fibroblastic/stromal responses Differentiation inducers/inhibitors Mutagenic/antimutagenic processes Oxygen, CO_2, nutrients

semination; the resistance of certain tissues to tumor infiltration and tissue destruction; and host stromal, inflammatory, and immune responses to tumors (Nicolson, 1982; Nicolson and Poste, 1982, 1983a, b). Although the mechanisms underlying these phenomena have not been elucidated by classical anatomic and pathologic examination, they have been approached by techniques of experimental pathology and tumor biology. This review will focus on human and experimental cancers and their use in answering basic questions on the properties that define the metastatic phenotype.

EXPERIMENTAL CONSIDERATIONS IN STUDYING METASTASIS

The Models

To study the tumor-cell properties that are important in invasion and metastasis, most investigators have used animal tumor models that mimic human metastatic cancer (Nicolson, 1982; Nicolson and Poste, 1982, 1983b). Some of these models are probably of limited value in answering only certain questions on particular steps of the metastatic process, whereas others appear to be useful in answering a wide range of questions on metastatic spread. For example, tumor-cell invasion and dissemination in vivo have been assessed by inoculating tumor cells into experimental animals and studying their routes of invasion and dissemination.

Although these approaches have their limitations, such as the simultaneous introduction of large numbers of tumor cells into non-tumor-bearing animals, they have been useful for studying the role of cellular properties in metastatic processes. Another limitation of these approaches is that most investigators have used rapidly proliferating transplantable tumors, which are quite unlike their slow-growing, spontaneously arising human counterparts in their vascular responses, hypoxic fractions, and cellular and stromal organizations (Nicolson and Poste, 1982, 1983b). Most of the animal tumor models now in use to study metastatic phenomena are based on selection techniques that obtain highly metastatic subpopulations of tumor cells so that these can be directly compared with equivalent nonmetastatic cells or tumor cells of low metastatic potential.

Selection

Once a suitable animal tumor model is established, various techniques are used in vivo to select variant malignant cells for particular properties, such as colonization of lymph nodes, blood-borne organ implantation, and survival and growth at particular sites (Hart and Fidler, 1981; Nicolson, 1982; Nicolson and Poste, 1982, 1983b). Alternatively, completely in vitro approaches have been used to obtain metastatic variant cells, such as cell cloning or selection for resistance to lymphocyte-, natural killer cell-, or antibody complement-mediated cytoxocity; decreased sensitivity to lectin toxicity; binding to immobilized lectins; or selective invasion of tissues, blood vessels, or endothelial cells (reviewed in Nicolson, 1982; Nicolson and Poste, 1983b). Although most of these studies have been conducted with animal tumors, there appear to be close similarities in the behavior of some animal and human malignant tumors.

Assays

A major problem in examining human tumors for their invasive and metastatic properties has been the lack of an appropriate assay system. In many experiments, immunosuppressed animals have been used as recipients for human tumor xenografts, or human tumor cells have been implanted at immunologically privileged sites in specific species of animals. In addition to the difficulties of maintaining large numbers of immunosuppressed animals for such experiments, the grafting of human tumor cells to such recipients usually does not correspond to the microenvironmental conditions at the sites of origin of the human tumors.

The Recipients

The athymic nude mouse has been the most popular experimental recipient for studying the in vivo growth behaviors of human tumors (Table 1-2). However, if a particular human tumor can be grown in nude mice, a major problem is that most malignant human tumors are rarely metastatic in these animals. Indeed, highly metastatic murine tumor cells also show lower incidences of metastasis or blood-borne implantation, survival, and growth in nude mice (Fidler and Nicolson, 1978; Hanna, 1980). In some cases, malignant tumors that are nonmetastatic in adult nude mice are fully capable of metastasizing at high frequencies in newborn or 2- to 3-week-old nude mice, or in nude mice that have received X-irradiation (Hanna and Fidler, 1981). These results suggest that the immune systems of young nude mice must undergo further maturation before they are fully competent in suppressing metastatic cells. In older nude mice, natural killer systems appear to inhibit the spread of most metastatic tumor cells (Hanna and Fidler, 1981; Hanna, 1982). Thus, the young or newborn nude mouse is a more suitable recipient for evaluating the metastatic potential of human tumors; however, even in the newborn nude mouse, some metastatic human tumors are rarely malignant. This could be due in part to differences in tissue stroma at the implant site, since most human tumor cells are implanted subcutaneously and are not returned to their comparable tissue of origin.

Table 1-2. Use of Nude Mice to Study the Biology of Human Tumor Cells

1. The majority of human tumors do not grow in nude mice
2. Few human tumors metastasize in nude mice
3. Natural immune responses against human tumor cells exist in nude mice
4. Stromal requirements for growth of human tumor cells may be different
5. Environmental factors may modify the biologic properties of human tumor cells
6. Selection of variant human tumor-cell subpopulations can occur
7. Cell fusion can result in mouse-human heterokaryons

These findings have raised concerns that nude mice mount at least feeble responses against tumor xenografts, suggesting that immunoselection may occur during the transplantation of human tumor cells in such recipients. Other potential problems are that changes in tumor-stromal requirements may result in the selective survival of human tumor cells with particular properties, and that the cellular diversity present in the original human tumors is altered when these tumors are grown in nude mice as xenografts.

For the most part, the establishment of various cell lines or strains from solid human tumors obtained from both primary and metastatic lesions of the same patient has not been successful using in vitro techniques or nude mouse xenografts. Often, this failure is due to the difficulties encountered in obtaining enough fresh tissue and the lack of appropriate facilities for their culture, which is usually done under suboptimal conditions. One potential problem during the transplantation of human tumor cells into nude mice is the possibility that these cells can fuse with normal surrounding mouse cells, resulting in the formation of heterokaryons. It is not uncommon that the karyotypes of tumor cells obtained from nude mouse xenografts are hybrids of human and mouse cells; in some cases, they are almost entirely mouse. In the past, these events have also been responsible to some degree for the incorrect classification of nonhuman tumor viruses as viruses of human origin. However, the main problem remains the lack of directly comparable primary and secondary tumor-derived cells that can be directly examined. This has resulted in the widespread use of animal tumor models to study various aspects of cancer invasion and dissemination. In most cases, this approach appears to be reasonable and highly relevant to human cancer; however, any data obtained using animal tumor models must be confirmed using human tumors, preferably human tumor cells of varying metastatic potentials isolated from the same patient.

LYMPHATIC VERSUS HEMATOGENOUS TUMOR SPREAD

A common mode of invasion and metastasis of cancer cells is through lymphatic channels (Del Regato, 1977; Van de Velde and Carr, 1977). The release of malignant cells from the primary tumor into the lymph fluid and their invasion of lymphatic vessels with their multiple endothelial fenestrations can result in the passive entry of cancer cells into the lymph (Carr and Carr, 1982). Since lymphatic vessels are not surrounded by a thick basal lamina or basement membrane, modifications in fluid pressure can open the lymphatic vessel walls, allowing entry of malignant cells. In addition, since the sites of tumor growth are commonly centers of inflammation and high interstitial fluid pressures, increased numbers of malignant cells may be forced through lymphatic junctions (Casley-Smith, 1977). Carr et al. (1976) have examined the passage of metastatic tumor cells into lymphatic vessels by electron microscopy and have concluded that single migrating tumor cells can easily penetrate into the lymphatics by the protrusion of tumor cell processes through gaps between lymphatic endothelial cells (Van de Velde and Carr, 1977).

Once inside the lymph, cancer cells are transported passively to the first draining lymph node. The draining lymph nodes of tumors have been proposed to act as "barriers" to the spread of cancer (Van de Velde and Carr, 1977). However, investigators now consider that such a barrier, if it exists, is at best temporary, since some tumor cells can quickly pass through the first lymph node they encounter (Zeidman and Buss, 1954; Fisher and Fisher, 1965). Once tumor cells arrive at a draining lymph node, they can proliferate, die, remain dormant, or enter the blood circulation through blood vessels in the node.

The killing of tumor cells in lymph nodes by host mechanisms has been studied in animal tumor models, although the findings may not be relevant to human tumors in lymph nodes. Hermann et al. (1976) demonstrated that lymph nodes possess transplantation immunity and are capable of tumor-cell destruction. In some cases, antitumor responses can occur in the draining lymph nodes, but in time these responses are circumvented, probably by selection of immunoresistant tumor-cell subpopulations or stimulation of suppressor immune cells, which turn off host response mechanisms (Alexander et al., 1967). For example, the kinetics of spontaneous spread of squamous cell carcinoma to regional lymph nodes in mice has been studied by transplantation techniques (Hewitt and Blake, 1975, 1977). In these studies, the growth of tumor cells in regional lymph nodes did not parallel the growth of the primary tumor, suggesting that many of the tumor cells that are capable of reaching lymph nodes do not survive. However, Hewitt and Blake (1977) could not detect immunologic responses against tumor cells, suggesting that the lymph-node environment, rather than host immune cells, plays a more important role in determining whether lymphatic metastasis occurs.

Metastasis via hematologic mechanisms can occur by direct invasion into blood vessels or by spread to regional lymphatic nodes and entry into the circulation at that point. Once vascularization of tumors has occurred, usually when they are greater than 0.1 to 1 mm in size, rapid rates of neoplastic growth and increased rates of intravasation can occur. Willis (1973) examined 500 necropsy samples from all types of cancer and found that blood-vessel invasion was extensive in 143 patients. Once inside blood vessels, some cancers can extend for long distances within the unoccluded vessels, whereas others detach and circulate as single cells or cell emboli without apparent growth at the site of intravasation.

The rates at which malignant cells are shed into the circulation have been determined in at least a few animal tumor systems. Tumor-cell shedding into the afferent venous circulation has been measured by Butler and Gullino (1975) using rat mammary carcinoma transplants into rat ovaries, which were in turn grafted at subcutaneous sites in rats. Tumors in the range of 2 to 4 g released up to 4×10^6 cells/g of tumor tissue per day. In some tumor systems, the rates of malignant-cell release into the blood correlate with the size of the primary tumor, whereas in other systems they do not. In tumors such as melanomas, there is apparently a greater chance of tumor-cell intravasation, but there are wide differences in the degrees of survival of tumor cells in the blood.

Circulating tumor cells are rapidly eliminated in the circulation, mostly by nonspecific mechanisms (Butler and Gullino, 1975; Fidler, 1976). Salsburg (1975) has concluded that the mere presence of tumor cells in the circulation is not of prognostic significance, since most of these tumor cells fail to form metastases at distant sites, and Malmgren (1967) found that the incidence of metastasis in patients did not correlate with the presence of tumor cells in blood samples.

The success of lymphatic or blood-borne metastasis appears to be determined by both tumor and host factors, some of which are listed in Table 1–1. Certain tumor cells are apparently capable of producing both lymphatic and distant blood-borne metastases, suggesting that they have all the properties necessary for detachment, penetration into lymph or blood, implantation, and survival and growth at these secondary sites, whereas other malignant cells appear to colonize the lymphatics exclusively (Table 1–3). To explain why some tumor cells are predominantly capable of lymphatic metastasis and others preferentially form blood-borne metastases, we used an experimental adenocarcinoma that arose in syngeneic Fischer 344 rats (Neri et al., 1982). In this system, we have obtained cell clones of varying metastatic potentials and other properties, including the ability to colonize regional lymph nodes and distant organs, such as lung. We have examined experimentally the question of whether metastasis to distant sites occurs by direct entry into the circulation or by entry into lymphatic vessels prior to blood-borne spread (Table 1–3).

Table 1–3. Situations in Which Observable Lymphatic Metastasis Occurs Exclusively or Before Distant Metastasis

1. Tumor cells are shed into surrounding fluid at high rates
2. Tumor cells invade blood vessels at low rates and lymph vessels at high rates
3. Tumor cells are stimulated or are not growth-inhibited in lymph nodes
4. Tumor cells die quickly in blood circulation
5. Tumor cells fail to implant in microcirculation
6. Tumor cells implant and invade but fail to grow at distant organ sites

In our experiments, various cell sublines and cell clones were implanted subcutaneously into Fischer 344 rats. At various times, the presence of lymph node and distant metastases was determined, and the cells from these deposits were placed into tissue culture for karyotyping and cell-surface analysis. Tumor-cell clones that spread predominantly to regional lymph nodes or to distant organs possessed different cell-surface properties and different marker chromosomes after Giemsa (G) banding, suggesting that the particular tumor cells that colonize regional lymph nodes (as opposed to lungs) are different subpopulations derived from the same parental tumor. Most of the cell clones and cell lines, however, metastasized to both regional lymph nodes *and* lungs. For example, implantation of the parental tumor-cell line of low spontaneous metastatic potential into rats resulted in a few animals having both regional lymph node and lung tumor involvement.

At this point, all tumors were placed into tissue culture and their kayotypes and chromosomal markers examined (Table 1–4) (Pearce et al., 1984). The results of G-banding suggested that the lymph node-metastasizing cells were a subpopulation of the original tumor, because these cells carried only some of the chromosome markers present in cells obtained from the original tumor. However, the lung metastasis-derived cells possessed some of the marker chromosomes found in the lymph node-metastasizing cells, suggesting

Table 1–4. 13762NF Adenocarcinoma Marker Chromosomes Shared by Primary, RLN, and Lung Metastases

CHROMOSOME MARKER	NO. OF CELLS/100 CELLS WITH MARKER		
	Primary	*RLN*	*Lung*
M1	4	96	0
M2	2	100	75
M3	1	100	63
M5	4	4	0
M14	1	94	80
M17	0	90	100
M25	0	92	75
M32	6	6	0
M34	0	92	90

For identification of marker chromosomes, see Pearce et al. (1984).

that the lung-colonizing tumor cells are derived from a subpopulation that first colonized the lymph node. Cloning the cell line obtained from the lymph-node metastasis and examining the spontaneous metastatic properties of each cell clone revealed that some cells are capable of lymphatic metastasis and some are capable of both lymphatic and hematogenous metastasis.

To determine whether lymph-node colonization is a necessary prelude to distant metastasis, we performed another experiment in which the primary tumor or regional lymph nodes were surgically excised at various times (Figure 1–1). Excision of the subcutaneous tumor implant within 6 days after inoculation of 10^6 tumor cells prevented metastasis to either lymph nodes or lungs, but excision after 6 days did not prevent metastasis via lymphatics or blood circulation. By contrast, excision of regional lymph nodes before or after tumor-cell inoculation prevented extensive metastasis to the lungs and delayed the appearance of any metastases compared with animals that underwent sham lymphoidectomies (North and Nicolson, 1985). These experiments suggest that in this system, lymphatic metastasis occurs before blood-borne metastasis and metastatic cells probably enter the circulation from regional lymph nodes.

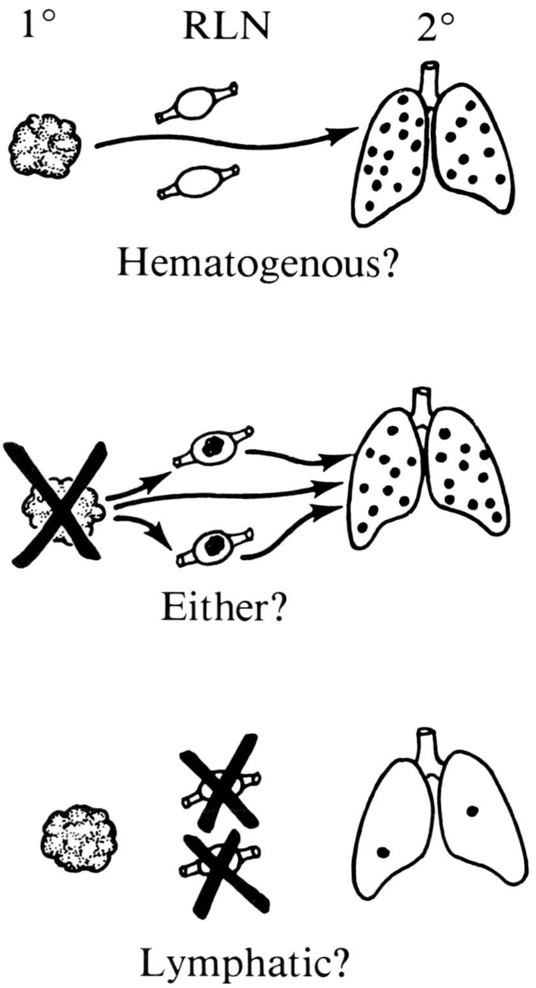

Figure 1–1. Experiments to determine whether tumors metastasize from primary (1°) to secondary (2°) sites via regional lymph nodes (RLN). In tumors where distant metastases are found without RLN involvement, metastasis probably occurs via a hematogenous mechanism. In tumors where both RLN and distant metastases are found, distant metastasis could occur directly from a primary tumor or via RLN. In tumors where RLN are removed surgically and few or no distant metastases form (but do so when RLN are not excised), metastasis probably occurs first to RLN, then to distant sites from the RLN.

ADAPTATION VERSUS SELECTION AND THE ORIGIN OF METASTATIC VARIANTS

Metastasis appears to be the result of nonrandom detachment, transport, implantation, survival, and growth of tumor cells in regional lymph nodes or at distant organ sites. Additional support for this concept is that variant sublines of tumor cells possessing quite different patterns of metastatic colonization have been selected in vivo (reviewed in: Nicolson, 1982; Nicolson and Poste, 1982, 1983b). In the murine B16 melanoma system, the ability to select variant sublines of B16 melanoma that show quite different metastatic patterns (preferential organ colonization of brain, lung, ovary, or liver) argues against theories based entirely on the random arrest and survival of circulating malignant cells. In fact, the same colonization patterns have been obtained after introducing tumor cells into the blood via different injection routes (Fidler and Nicolson, 1976) or by use of parabionts, surgically joined so that tumor cells can recirculate from an injected parabiont to an uninjected parabiont to form tumor colonies in particular organs (Fidler and Nicolson, 1977).

Compelling data indicating that nonrandom, blood-borne tumor-cell colonization occurs have also been obtained using animals with ectopically implanted organ fragments (Kinsey, 1960; Sugarbaker et al., 1971; Hart and Fidler, 1980). Using transplanted lung grafts, Hart and Fidler (1980) injected animals with lung-colonizing B16 melanoma cells and found formation of tumors in the lungs and in the ectopic lung grafts. In control experiments, nontarget organ grafts in mice were not colonized by the lung-colonizing blood-borne tumor cells. Thus, mere surgical trauma or the presence of engrafted tissue was insufficient for melanoma metastasis formation.

To explain the unique organ colonization properties of metastatic tumor cells, Weiss (1980) has proposed that adaptation of tumor cells to specific tissue or organ microenvironments occurs, and that metastatic cells possess transient properties that are also important in determining their metastatic phenotypes. The role of adaptation versus selection in the formation of metastasis has been approached in experiments that have attempted to select sequentially melanoma cells for their abilities to "adapt" or grow at various organ sites (Brunson and Nicolson, 1980). In these experiments, B16 melanoma cells were sequentially implanted in brain parenchyma by direct intracerebral injection, and the tumors that formed were removed and cultured in vitro, then reinjected back into other animals for "readaptation" in vivo. After 10 cycles of adaptation for brain survival and growth, the final melanoma tumor was placed in culture, and the resulting cell subline was examined for its ability to metastasize from subcutaneous implants to brain or undergo blood-borne implantation, survival, and growth in the brain after intraveneous injection.

The 10-times brain-adapted B16 subline did not differ in its brain implantation and survival properties from the original B16 parent line. This was in marked contrast to the results obtained from the in vivo selections in which the heterogeneous parental tumor-cell population was selected for the ability of single-cell suspensions of B16 cells to implant, survive, invade, and grow to form macroscopic tumor colonies in the brain after intravenous injection (Brunson et al., 1978; Miner et al., 1982). In these experiments, only the sublines selected sequentially 10 to 14 times for blood-borne brain colonization formed significantly more brain tumor colonies than parental tumor cells or cells sequentially "adapted" for brain survival and growth.

We have also approached this problem by injection of parental B16 melanoma cells attached to Bio-Carrier beads, which were then injected intravenously into syngeneic mice. The cell-coated beads, which are too large to pass through the microcirculation, lodge mechanically in the lungs (Nicolson and Custead, 1982). The B16 cells on the mechanically arrested beads grew to form gross lung-tumor nodules, which were excised and established in tissue culture. The cultured B16 cells were then reattached to new beads, which were then injected into mice to repeat the in vivo adaptation sequence. After this sequence was repeated nine times, the resulting lung-adapted B16 cells were tested for their metastatic properties after intravenous or subcutaneous injection. They were found to be low in their metastatic potential, similar to parental cells, in contrast to B16 cells selected for blood-borne implantation, invasion, survival, and growth by intravenous injection of single-cell suspensions (Nicolson and Custead, 1982). These negative results and the ones described earlier collectively argue against an important role for adaptation in metastatic colonization, and are more consistent with the alternative possibility that metastasis involves a selection process—the result of selection of subpopulations of tumor cells with enhanced metastatic potentials and increased abilities to implant, survive, and proliferate at specific sites.

If the formation of distant metastases is a nonrandom selection process, then subpopulations of tumor cells able to colonize specific sites should show unique characteristics important in such processes. This question has been approached experimentally by using small fragments of organ tissue as target sites for the attachment and invasion of organ-colonizing subpopulations of melanoma cells in vitro (Nicolson et al., 1985). These tissue adhesion and invasion experiments were performed using adult syngeneic organ tissues as substrates for the binding and invasion of B16 melanoma sublines that differ in their patterns of colonization. Very small (0.1 to 0.5 mm^3) pieces of organ tissue from newborn syngeneic mice can be maintained for a 24- to 48- hour incubation period in culture without evidence of necrosis or tissue degeneration.

Three sources of tissue were used for these studies: lung, ovary, and heart muscle. Although these tissues basically maintain their normal histiotypic organization during the culture period, other tissues from newborn mice, such as brain tissue, undergo dramatic rearrangements during culture in vitro (Wang and Nicolson, 1983). B16 melanoma sublines selected for their abilities to colonize lung (B16-F10), ovary (B16-O10), or brain (B16-B14b), and a series of sublines selected for enhanced tissue invasion (B16-BL6), were used to examine the ability of tumor-cell suspensions to attach to and invade syngeneic host tissues within 48 hours. In these experiments we found differential attachment (Table 1–5) and invasion (Table 1–6) of various melanoma sublines. For example, high lung-colonizing B16-F10 cells attached more rapidly to lung tissue and invaded lung tissue more rapidly in vitro than any of the other B16 melanoma sublines. In contrast, high ovary-colonizing B16-O10 cells attached more rapidly to ovary tissue and invaded ovary tissue in vitro more rapidly than any of the other B16 melanoma sublines (Tables 1–5, 1–6). In general, the specificity of tumor-cell attachment and subsequent invasion into the different syngeneic tissues mimicked their preferential in vivo colonization properties (Nicolson et al., 1985). Thus, specific properties of tumor cells, as well as those of the secondary site, influence the extent and location of metastasis.

Metastatic cells are known to be characterized by quantitative alterations in the amount of specific cell-surface glycoproteins that are involved in various steps of the metastatic sequence (Nicolson, 1982, 1984a). For example, the displays of particular sialoglycoproteins have been related to blood-borne metastasis formation at specific sites of murine melanoma (Irimura et al., 1981; Miner et al., 1982; Irimura and Nicolson, 1984), mammary carci-

Table 1–5. Attachment of B16 Melanoma Cells to Syngeneic Organ Tissue *In Vitro**

TIME (HR)	DEGREE OF ATTACHMENT OF B16 SUBLINE†				
	F1	*F10*	*O10*	*B14b*	*BL6*
Lung					
0.5	3.3 ± 1	12.0§ ± 1.5	0.3 ± 0.7	2.5 ± 0.5	3.0 ± 0.5
1	7.5 ± 1.5	14.0§ ± 2	6.5 ± 1.5	3.0 ± 1	4.3 ± 2.2
3	10.8 ± 2	24.0§ ± 3.5	7.5 ± 2	7.0 ± 2.3	8.0 ± 3
6	17.5 ± 5	31.0§ ± 3	9.5 ± 2.4	8.7 ± 2.5	9.6 ± 3.5
Ovary					
0.5	1.5 ± 1.6	1.2 ± 1.5	2.5‡ ± 1	0.5 ± 0.7	0.2 ± 0.4
1	3.5 ± 1.5	3.5 ± 1.5	7.0‡ ± 2	2.1 ± 1.7	2.0 ± 1.5
3	4.6 ± 2	4.0 ± 1.6	18.3§ ± 3.5	3.8 ± 2.2	9.0 ± 1.5
6	5.6 ± 1.5	5.0 ± 1	19.5§ ± 4	4.2 ± 2	9.1 ± 3
Heart					
0.5	0.6 ± 0.7	0.8 ± 1.1	0.6 ± 0.5	1.0 ± 0.5	1.7 ± 1.4
1	2.1 ± 1	3.4 ± 1.2	3.6 ± 1.6	3.5 ± 2	3.7 ± 1.5
3	2.3 ± 1	3.9 ± 1.7	7.7 ± 2.5	6.1 ± 1.5	6.4 ± 2
6	4.7 ± 1.5	9.7 ± 2	10.8 ± 2.5	8.6 ± 3	12.3 ± 2

*Data are from Nicolson et al., 1985a.
†Number of melanoma cells attached to tissue edge ± SD per 10 X power field. At least 50 fields were examined.
‡$p < 0.01$ compared with all other sublines.
§$p < 0.001$ compared with all other sublines.

Table 1-6. Invasion of B16 Melanoma Cells into Syngeneic Organ Tissue *In Vitro**

TIME (HR)	DEGREE OF INVASION OF B16 SUBLINE†				
	F1	*F10*	*O10*	*B14b*	*BL6*
Lung					
6	0	10.3§ ± 3	0	0	1.1 ± 1
12	1.6 ± 1.5	13.3§ ± 3	0.5 ± 0.8	1.0 ± 8	3.5 ± 1
18	5.3 ± 1.5	16.0§ ± 3.3	4.0 ± 1.5	6.1 ± 1.5	9.6 ± 2
24	9.2 ± 2	18.5§ ± 2.5	4.5 ± 2	11.1 ± 2	11.5 ± 2.2
36	11.0 ± 3	22.0§ ± 3	5.0 ± 1.7	12.9 ± 3	12.5 ± 3
Ovary					
6	0	0	0	0	0
12	0.9 ± 0.6	0.9 ± 1	4.3§ ± 1	0	0
18	2.3 ± 0.8	3.7 ± 1.3	5.8‡ ± 1.5	0	0
24	4.5 ± 1.5	3.5 ± 1	9.3§ ± 1.5	0	0
36	6.6 ± 1.7	4.6 ± 2	11.7‡ ± 2	1.1 ± 1	6.1 ± 2
48	7.1 ± 2	9.7 ± 2.5	18.5‡ ± 2	3.9 ± 1.5	9.2 ± 2.4
Heart					
6	0	0	0	0	0
12	0	0	0	0	0
18	1.1 ± 0.8	0.7 ± 0.5	1.5 ± 1.2	0	4.5‡ ± 1
24	2.3 ± 1	2.5 ± 1.5	2.9 ± 1	0	5.6‡ ± 1
36	3.6 ± 1.8	3.5 ± 1.2	5.6 ± 2	0.4 ± 0.5	6.9 ± 1.5
48	5.8 ± 3	3.8 ± 1.5	9.1 ± 2	3.1 ± 1	10.1 ± 2

*Data are from Nicolson et al., 1985a.
†Number of melanoma cells invading tissue ± SD per 10 X field. At least 50 fields were examined.
‡p < 0.01 compared with all other sublines.
§p < 0.001 compared with all other sublines.

noma (Steck and Nicolson, 1983), and lymphoma (Schirmacher et al., 1982; Nicolson et al., 1982). Specifically blocking the biosynthesis of these cell-surface glycoconjugates by use of agents such as tunicamycin was found to reversibly alter metastatic properties, confirming their importance in distant tumor spread (Irimura et al., 1981).

TUMOR CELL HETEROGENEITY AND THE EVOLUTION OF METASTATIC PHENOTYPIC DIVERSITY

Differences in the properties of particular subpopulations of tumor cells that are important in determining their sites of secondary colonization have been discussed. In addition, a number of other cellular properties are heterogeneously expressed in cells within tumors of the same histiotypic class, such as cell morphology, cell-surface antigens, glycolipids, glycoproteins, cell adhesion and recognition components, hydrolytic and synthetic enzymes, cell locomotion, and the abilities to invade and metastasize. There is also heterogeneity in the sensitivities of individual cells to therapeutic agents, such as drugs, radiation, hyperthermia, and host response mechanisms (reviewed in Heppner, 1984; Nicolson, 1982, 1984a; Nicolson and Poste, 1982, 1983a, b).

The cellular heterogeneity of malignant tumors has been explained by a process of tumor evolution or progression (Foulds, 1975; Nowell, 1976, 1983). Since it is well established that most, if not all, spontaneous and induced neoplasms develop from single cells, the progeny of such single cells must have diversified to multiple cellular phenotypes in order to form heterogeneous tumors (Nowell, 1976; Fialkow, 1979). Tumor evolution or progression is thought to occur by a process of cellular phenotypic diversification, which leads to heterogeneous cell populations and sequential host selection, which in turn results in the emergence of tumor cells possessing enhanced autonomy, survival, growth, and malignant properties (Figure 1-2) (Foulds, 1975; Nowell, 1976, 1983). In addition, the microenvironments of proliferating tumor cells may also be important in generating phenotypic diversity, as well as in selecting variant cells for enhanced survival and growth characteristics in a competitive cell population (Nicolson, 1984

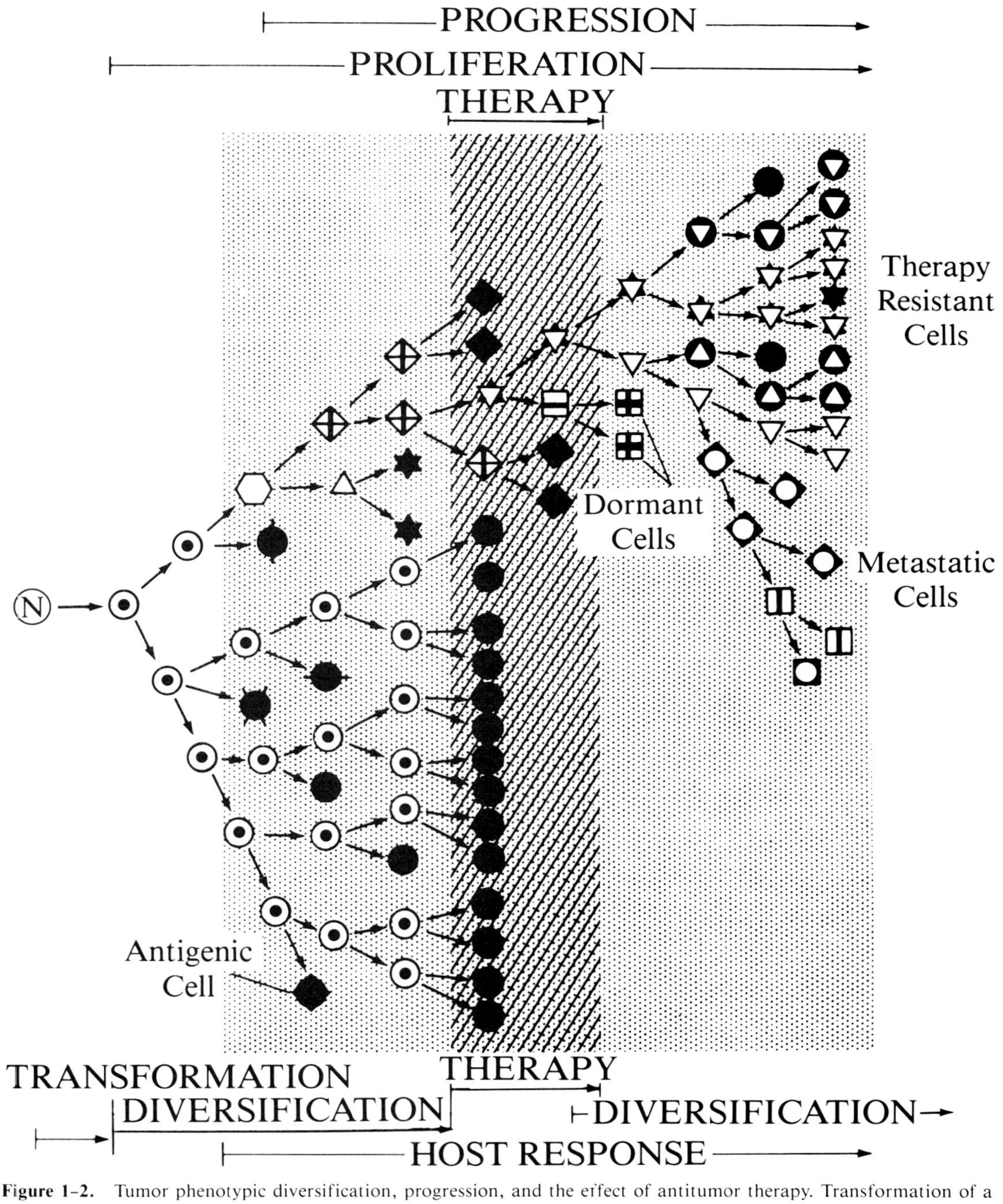

Figure 1-2. Tumor phenotypic diversification, progression, and the effect of antitumor therapy. Transformation of a normal cell (N) to a tumor cell (O) can lead to cellular diversification in malignant neoplasms. Some of these variant tumor cells die (solid symbols) because of lethal mutations or host responses, or they fail to grow and so become dormant; other tumor cells become more competitive and malignant as they undergo phenotypic diversification. Cytotoxic therapy results in the death of most tumor cells (solid symbols) and restriction of phenotypic diversity. However, some malignant cells escape randomly, or are resistant to therapy and continue to diversify phenotypically. Eventually, a malignant subpopulation arises that possesses the correct phenotypic properties for metastasis. (Reproduced from Nicolson, 1984b, with permission of Martinus Nijhoff).

b, c). Tumor cells not inhibited by host defenses and responsive to microenvironmental signals possess competitive advantages over neighboring cells, and these more competitive cells eventually become the dominant subpopulations within a tumor, evolving with particular phenotypic characteristics (Nicolson, 1984a, b, c).

One aspect of tumor-cell behavior that may determine to a large degree the malignant phenotype is the rate at which tumor-cell phenotypic diversification occurs (Nicolson, 1984b, c). In this scheme, benign tumors would be expected to show minimal rates of phenotypic diversity compared with malignant neoplasms, which are expected to diversify phenotypically at various rates. In addition, tumors and individual tumor cells can change their rates of phenotypic diversification in response to changes in host microenvironments or to cell-cell interactions. These interactions may be important in "stabilizing" or "destabilizing" rates of phenotypic diversification (Poste et al., 1981; Miner et al., 1982; Miller, 1983).

Not all the differences found in malignant tumor cells appear to be related to states of progression or malignancy. For example, properties that are unimportant in tumor-cell survival and malignant behavior may diminish in importance or disappear at certain stages during tumor evolution and progression. In particular tumors, the loss or reduction of certain components or their activities has been termed "loss of differentiation"; however, the relationship between such changes and cellular morphologic differentiation, tumor progression, and malignancy have not been established (Nicolson, 1984b, c).

The model of tumor progression of Foulds (1975) and Nowell (1976) states that increasing genetic alterations are generated by random somatic mutational events. These then allow the eventual progression of emergent tumor cell subpopulations with particular malignant and other phenotypic properties (Figure 1–2). The tumor-cell subpopulations that diversify rapidly should display enhanced genetic instability, as well as changes in those properties important for their survival, growth, and malignancy in differing microenvironments and under changing host selection pressures.

TUMOR-CELL INSTABILITY AND TUMOR PROGRESSION

The hypothesis first discussed—that malignant neoplasms undergoing progressive growth and changes in malignant properties should display increased genetic instability—is supported by experimental data. Examination of the rates of acquisition of gross chromosomal alterations, mitotic errors, and the rates of spontaneous mutations in highly malignant cells compared with counterpart nonmalignant or low malignant cells indicates that highly malignant cells are genetically less stable (Nowell, 1983; Wolman, 1983). When tumor cells evolve into more malignant cells, chromosomal abnormalities or alterations in the morphologies or banding patterns of specific chromosomes invariably increase in frequency (Wolman, 1983). Similar changes have been found in malignant animal tumors, such as the rat adenocarcinoma system described earlier (Pearce et al., 1984). In some instances, changes in cell ploidy are related to increased states of neoplastic progression (Wolman, 1983) and poor prognosis (Barlogie et al., 1982), but this is not an absolute requirement for metastatic cells.

The instability of tumors has been estimated on a cellular level by determining the rates of spontaneous gene mutation in individual cells. Cifone and Fidler (1981) have examined the rates of spontaneous mutation to drug resistance in murine melanomas and fibrosarcomas that possess differing metastatic potentials. They found that the cells of highest metastatic potential possessed the highest rates of spontaneous mutation, rates approximately six to seven times the spontaneous mutation rates found in nonmetastatic cells or cells of low metastatic potential.

There appear to be a number of different possible mechanisms for generating increased genetic instability, including inherited defects in DNA repair or maintenance genes; acquired defects in specialized genes, such as "mutator" genes or genes involved in synthesizing DNA; chromosomal alterations, such as aneuploidy, transpositions, abnormal sister-chromatid exchanges, and chromosome amplification regions; gross chromosomal abnormalities, such as double minutes; integrated virus sequences or oncogenes, mutagenic agents, such as radiation or chemotherapeutic drugs; and microenvironmental alterations, such as nutritional and gas differences (Nowell, 1983; Nicolson, 1984b, c).

Phenotypic Instability and Its Modulation

To explain the rates of neoplastic progression and tumor diversification in many systems, mechanisms other than host selection and phenotypic instability are required (Nicolson, 1984b, c). Certainly genotypic instability alone cannot explain the extremely high rates of phenotypic change (as high as 10^{-2}/cell/generation), because the highest known rates of spontaneous gene mutation in metastatic cells (approximately 7×10^{-5}/cell/generation) are orders of magnitude lower than the rates of phenotypic variation. Thus, it has been proposed that gene mutations occur at specific DNA sites, such as regulatory gene sites, and these changes are responsible for generating the rapid cellular heterogeneity seen in highly malignant neoplasms (Nicolson, 1984b, c). The hypothesis that modifications in regulatory genes occur in malignant neoplasms is not unreasonable, since the changes in gene products associated with the malignant phenotype appear to be quantitative rather than qualitative (Nicolson, 1984a, b, c). For example, we have recently examined differences in gene expression between metastatic large-cell lymphoma sublines of very high and extremely low metastatic potentials, and have found less than 100 statistically significant qualitative differences in gene expression using a genome library of greater than 17,000 cDNA clones (Nicolson et al., 1985b).

Rates of phenotypic diversification in a limited number of animal and human tumors have been calculated. For example, Peterson et al. (1983) have estimated that the rates of formation of variants with highly significant quantitative differences in the expression of a cell-surface glycoprotein on normal breast epithelial cells and on primary and metastatic breast cancer cells are different. They found that the rate of variant formation in the tumor-cell population of malignant breast cancer was approximately six times higher (2.2×10^{-2}/cell/generation) than in normal breast epithelial cells (0.36×10^{-2}/cell/generation). Extremely rapid rates of phenotypic diversification have also been observed in various animal tumor systems (Stackpole, 1983; Talmadge et al., 1979; Nicolson et al., 1982; Bosslet and Schirrmacher, 1982).

Such high rates of phenotypic change in tumor-cell subpopulations can result in a rapid loss, as well as gain, in metastatic properties (Fidler and Nicolson, 1981; Kerbel, 1979; Dennis et al., 1981; Neri and Nicolson, 1981; Nicolson et al., 1982; Poste et al., 1981, 1982; Welch et al., 1984a,b). Highly malignant cells that revert to a more benign phenotype should be more susceptible to host immune or nonimmune surveillance mechanisms, as well as host microenvironment. Thus, these cells should diminish with time in the tumor-cell population, and eventually be dominated by more malignant cell phenotypes within the tumor. This phenomenon has been found in an experimental animal tumor by Dennis et al. (1981). In this system, low malignant-potential variants of the tumor were rapidly generated; however, these cells just as rapidly generated cells of highly malignant phenotypes in vivo, which then metastasized. From these experiments, rates of spontaneous reversion to the highly malignant phenotype were estimated at approximately 2×10^{-5}/cell/generation, a rate much higher than the estimated rate of spontaneous mutation.

In addition to instability of the malignant phenotype, highly metastatic cells are also phenotypically unstable in a variety of other properties. Using the rat adenocarcinoma system described previously, we found that tumor-cell clones can reproducibly vary in their metastatic properties during in vitro growth (Neri et al., 1982; Welch et al., 1984a), and these changes in malignant properties occurred concomitant with changes in a variety of other cellular characteristics, such as expression of particular cell-surface glycoproteins (Neri et al., 1981; Steck and Nicolson, 1983), cell and tissue morphologies (Neri et al., 1982; Welch et al., 1984a), chromosome markers (Pearce et al., 1984), and sensitivities to gamma radiation (Welch et al., 1983, 1984b), hyperthermia (Tomasovic et al., 1982; Welch et al., 1984b), and chemotherapeutic drugs (Welch and Nicolson, 1983; Welch et al., 1984b). Since the phenotypic changes, if they occurred, did so at predictable times, the generation of phenotypic diversity is not random in this system. In addition, phenotypic change did not occur at similar rates for all cellular properties and, as mentioned, some properties did not change, indicating that phenotypic variation can occur at different specific rates.

Other procedures, such as subcloning in semisolid media (''clonogenic'' or ''stem-cell cloning'' assay), have been used to demonstrate the rapid generation of phenotypic cell variants in tumor cell populations. Raz (1982) described the rapid emergence of metastatic variants in clonal B16 melanoma cells during their growth in semisolid medium, and Nicolson et al. (1983) noted the rapid emergence of adenocarcinoma cell colonies with differing phenotypes in a clonogenic assay. In this experiment, the spontaneous metastatic properties of subclones derived from colonies, themselves derived from a clonal population of tumor cells at low passage, rapidly changed during growth in semisolid agarose, as did their sensitivities to chemotherapeutic drugs.

The high rates of phenotypic variability seen in sublines, clones, and subclones derived from malignant tumors can also change with time. In one of the first examples of this phenomenon, Poste et al. (1981) found that mixing several B16 melanoma cell clones in vitro stabilized the characteristics of individual cell clones and reduced their normally rapid rates of phenotypic change. Similarly, B16 cell sublines repeatedly selected for organ colonization were found to be stable for long periods of time in culture, but became unstable after single-cell cloning. In these latter experiments, the brain-colonizing subline B16-B14b was found to be stable in its brain colonization and cell-surface properties for more than a year in tissue culture (Nicolson, 1983); however, clonal derivatives of this subline were quite unstable during growth (Figure 1-3). By allowing three B16-B14b cell clones to grow together as a triclonal mixture, phenotypic stabilization occurred, and the metastatic properties of the co-culture were stabilized compared with

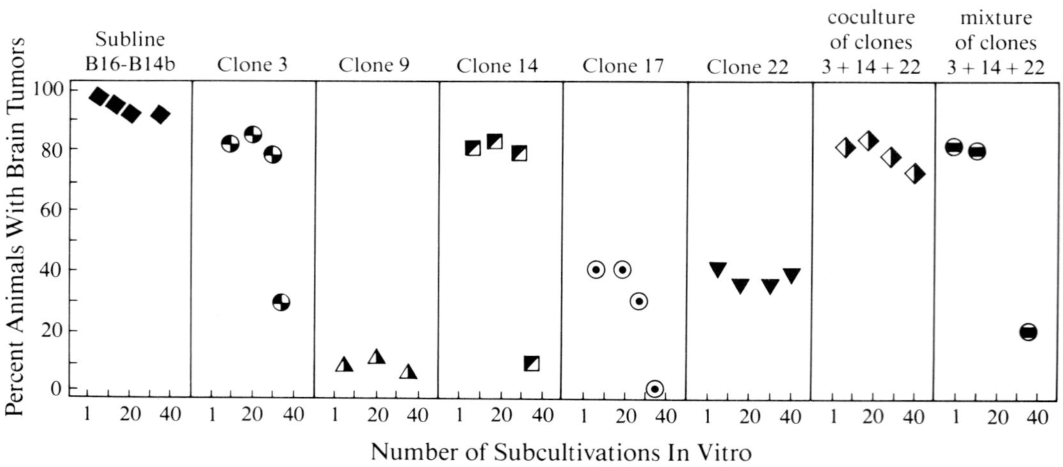

Figure 1-3. The instability of individual brain-colonizing B16 melanoma cell clones and their polyclonal stabilization. Cell clones were derived from the murine B16-B14b melanoma subline and cultured for various intervals in vitro after being assayed for their metastatic properties according to Miner et al. (1982). Some cultures were established with equal numbers of cells from three different clones (coculture of clones), and these were subcultured for various intervals and tested for their biologic properties. As a control for this type of experiment, equal numbers of cells from the three clones grown separately were combined (mixture of clones) immediately before the in vivo assays. Experimental metastatic brain colonization was assessed by intravenous injection of 2×10^4 singly suspended melanoma cells and determination of brain colonization 5 to 8 weeks later. (Data are from Miner et al., 1982; figure reproduced from Nicolson and Poste, 1983b, with permission of Academic Press).

growth of the three cell clones grown separately and mixed just prior to injection into animals (Figure 1-3). In this system, the expression of a particular cell-surface glycoprotein (gp90) correlated with the phenotypic changes and brain colonization properties. Sialoglycoprotein gp90 was found to be expressed in higher amounts on the high brain-colonizing clones than on the low brain-colonizing clones, and as the high brain-colonizing clones lost their potential to implant and grow in the brain meninges, the amounts of gp90 decreased concomitantly with a decrease in metastatic properties (Miner et al., 1982).

Modulation of phenotypic stability in vitro can also be achieved by the fusion of neoplastic cells with normal cells. The fusion of neoplastic cells in vivo with normal host cells to form hybrids has been shown by Goldenberg et al. (1974) to change their phenotypic properties. Cell fusion could also lead to progression and to the emergence of more-malignant cell phenotypes, as found by De Baetselier et al. (1981) when they fused nonmetastatic plasmocytoma cells with normal B-lymphocytes. This particular cell fusion results in hybrid cells that are more metastatic to liver and spleen. Lagarde et al. (1983) have proposed that the emergence of highly metastatic cells in a low malignant tumor line during growth in vivo can occur with the hybridization of nonmetastatic cells with a normal host cell, resulting in a cell hybrid that eventually evolves to the metastatic phenotype. This could be an important mechanism for generating increased ploidy in tumor cells, as well as genomic instability.

THE GENERATION OF TUMOR-CELL PHENOTYPIC DIVERSIFICATION

The ability of tumor cells to undergo rapid phenotypic change and diversify into heterogeneous cell populations has important implications for cancer therapy. Malignant tumors possess heterogeneous sensitivities to ionizing radiation, cytotoxic and cytostatic drugs, hyperthermia, and host immune mechanisms (reviewed in Nicolson, 1982; Nicolson and Poste, 1983a, b). As phenotypic diversification occurs, the ability of antitumor agents to eliminate all tumor cells diminishes, and variants arise in the tumor-cell population that account for recurrence or resistance to continued therapy. Interactions between tumor-cell subpopulations can also affect sensitivity to therapy. Miller et al. (1981) found that certain mammary tumor-cell subpopulations can influence the drug sensitivities of other subpopulations, even when present at sites distant from one another.

Therapeutic destruction of malignant tumors can also stimulate diversification of the surviving tumor-cell subpopulations. For example, Poste et al. (1981) found that cytotoxic drugs can deplete polyclonal tumor-cell populations of drug-sensitive cells, yielding a few cell clones that are drug resistant but highly unstable in their biologic properties. These unstable subclones quickly generated a new panel of cell subpopulations with widely different metastatic and other phenotypic properties. These results suggest that the tumor-cell subpopulations that survive therapy are not under the same type of polyclonal "interactions" as described earlier in the experiment with different brain-colonizing B16 melanoma cells, and the therapy itself, although depleting the number of tumor cells, can stimulate the diversification of the surviving tumor cells, leading to a new set of heterogeneous cell subpopulations with differing properties. Thus, the success of antitumor therapies could well depend on the ability of these therapies to eliminate the rare, highly malignant cells, and also the highly unstable tumor-cell subpopulations that have the potential to diversify rapidly (Nicolson, 1984b, c).

The rates of cellular phenotypic diversification of malignant tumor cells has not been easily explained by the sole mechanisms of genetic mutation and host selection (Nicolson, 1984b, c). Therefore, additional mechanisms involving gene rearrangements and epigenetic changes have been invoked. These mechanisms could involve nommutational modifications in regulatory genes, alterations in gene arrangements, integration of viral gene sequences or oncogenes, and nomutational modifications in DNA, such as methylation.

These modifications can alter gene expression without causing detectable mutational changes in cells. For example, modifications in DNA methylation can lead to phenotypic changes that persist for a few generations. Using the nucleoside analog 5-aza-cytidine, Kerbel et al. (1984) modulated the tumorigenic and metastatic phenotypes of several tumor-cell lines. However, the modified cells reverted to their original phenotypes within a few generations, concomitant with restoration of the normal levels of DNA methylation.

Another major factor in determining the rates of phenotypic diversification may reside in the microenvironments around tumor cells, which can influence transcriptional activities. Individual cells within a tumor have unique environments because of variations in the concentrations of nutrients, oxygen, growth hormones, enzymes, ions, inducers, and other regulatory molecules (Figure 1-4). For example, tumor-cell interactions with extracellular matrix or stromal components can result in differential activation of specific genes (Bissel et al., 1983), and tumor cells may respond in varying degrees to microenvironmental signals that control normal cellular differentiation (Nicolson, 1984c). Other examples of microenvironmental influences on tumor-cell diversification are those mediated by normal host cells, such as stromal cells, lymphocytes, granulocytes, and macrophages. When these cells are in close proximity to tumor cells, they can have profound effects on tumor-cell phenotype (Heppner et al., 1984). For example, macrophages are able to release mutagenic substances that can modulate the spontaneous mutation frequencies in tumor cells. Thus, the

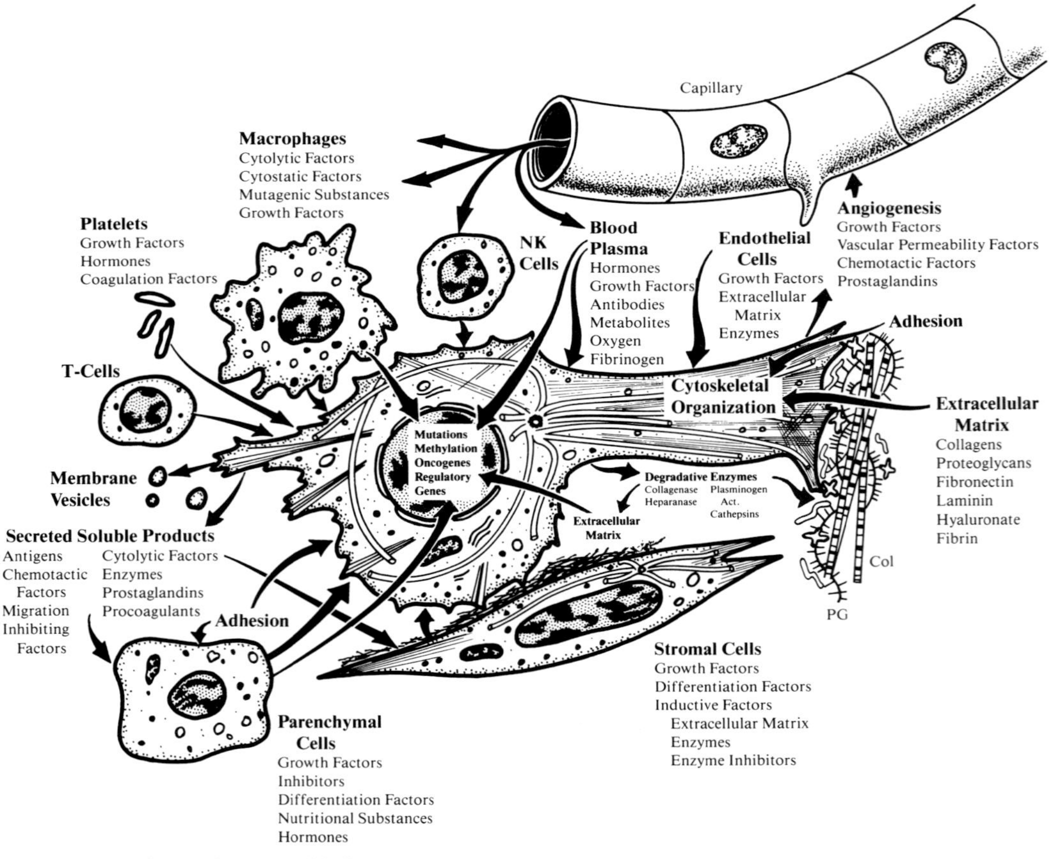

Figure 1-4. Microenvironmental influences on malignant tumor cells. Soluble components, cells, extracellular matrix, and other factors affect individual tumor cells differentially. (Reproduced from Nicolson, 1984b, with permission of Martinus Nijhoff).

proximity of particular normal cells to tumor cells within a tumor can result in modulation of phenotypic properties.

Because of differences in tumor-cell mutational events, host selection, and microenvironment, generation of phenotypic diversity will undoubtedly be different for each cell within a tumor, as well as for each cell within different tumors. One could now reasonably ask, what initiates phenotypic diversification of tumor cells? Unfortunately, the answer to this important question remains elusive. It may be profitable to examine several biologic systems for similarities to the phenotypic diversification seen in malignant cells. There are good examples in normal cells for phenotypic diversification, such as the somatic diversification of lymphocyte stem cells, resulting in a large number of different mature immunoglobulin-producing B-cells, each of which synthesizes unique immunoglobulin molecules. In this system, diversification depends on the generation of molecular diversity at two levels. At the genetic level, hypermutable regions of the genome yield diversified DNA sequences; at another level, different joining combinations of several genes yield diversification of the final immunoglobulin gene sequence. Using this as a model, we have postulated that phenotypic diversification might be initiated by the insertion of transcriptional promotor or enhancer elements that are adjacent to oncogenes at the appropriate DNA sites. Once initiated, diversification could proceed similar to normal lymphocyte diversification, using hypermutable regions of the genome and different joining mechanisms to create widely diverse gene products.

The misuse of developmentally regulated cellular enhancer or promotor elements, resulting in activitation of cellular genes and multigene families, might set in motion the generation of quantitative alterations in regulatory genes or their promotors, which could in turn control the differential activation of a number of different genes (Nicolson, 1984b, c). The differential control of multigene families in individual cells could also depend in part on a cell microenvironment similar to normal lymphocytes, which are triggered by factors from the environment, as well as from other cells. Since each tumor cell is in a slightly different microenvironment (Figure 1-4), the external signals received by each cell and their internal processing could stimulate individual cells to proceed down different pathways of differential gene regulation. Since the progeny of each tumor cell would be continually exposed to changing host microenvironment and selection pressures, the evolution of specific variant subpopulations with unique properties to be highly metastatic would be expected, given enough time for diversification and continued host selection.

REFERENCES

Alexander, P., Bensted, J., Delorme, E. J., and Hodgett, J.: The cellular immune response to primary sarcomata in rats. II. Abnormal responses of nodes draining the tumour. *Proc. Royal Soc. (Lond. Ser. B.)*, 174(35):237-51, 1969.

Barlogie, B., Johnston, D. A., and Smallwood, L.: Prognostic implications of ploidy and proliferative activity in human solid tumors. *Cancer Genet. Cytogenet.*, 6:17-28, 1982.

Bissel, M. J., Hall, H. G., and Parry, G.: How does the extracellular matrix direct gene expression? *J. Theoret. Biol.*, 99:31-68, 1983.

Bosslet, K., and Schirrmacher, V.: High-frequency generation of new immunoresistant tumor variants during metastasis of a clone murine tumor line (ESb). *Int. J. Cancer*, 29:195-202, 1982.

Brunson, K. W., and Nicolson, G. L.: Experimental brain metastasis. In Weiss, L., Gilber, H., Posner, J. B. (eds.).: *Brain Metastasis*, pp. 50-65, G. K. Hall, Boston, 1980.

Brunson, K. W., Beattie, G., and Nicolson, G. L.: Selection and altered tumour cell properties of brain-colonising metastatic melanoma. *Nature*, 272:543-5, 1978.

Butler, T. P., and Gullino, P. M.: Bulk transfer of fluid in the interstitial compartment of mammary tumors. *Cancer Res.*, 35:3084-8, 1975.

Carr, I., and Carr, J.: Experimental models of lymphatic metastasis. In Liotta, L. A., Hart, I. R. (eds.): *Tumor Invasion and Metastasis*, pp. 189-205, Martinus Nijhoff Publishers, The Hague, Netherlands, 1982.

Carr, I., Mc Ginty, F., and Norris, P.: The fine structure of neoplastic invasion: Invasion of liver, skeletal muscle and lymphatic vessels by the Rd/3 tumour. *J. Pathol.*, 118:91-9, 1976.

Casley-Smith, J. R.: Lymph and lymphatics. In Kaley, G., Altura, B. (eds.): *Microcirculation*, Vol. 1, pp. 423-502, University Park Press, Baltimore, 1977.

Cifone, M. A., and Fidler, I. J.: Increasing metastatic potential is associated with increased genetic instability of clones isolated from murine neoplasms. *Proc. Natl. Acad. Sci. U.S.A.*, 78:6949-52, 1981.

DeBaetselier, P., Gorelik, E., Eshhar, Z., Ron, Y., Katzav, S., Feldman, M., and Segal, S.: Metastatic properties conferred on nonmetastatic tumors by hybridization of spleen β-lymphocytes with plasmocytoma cells. *J. Natl. Cancer Inst.,* 67:1079–87, 1981.

Del Regato, J. A.: Pathways of metastatic spread of malignant tumors. *Semin. Oncol.,* 4:33–8, 1977.

Dennis, J. W., Donaghue, T. P., and Kerbel, R. S.: An examination of tumor antigen loss in spontaneous metastasis. *Invasion Metastasis,* 1:111–25, 1981.

Fialkow, P. J.: Clonal origin of human tumors. *Ann. Rev. Med.,* 30:135–76, 1979.

Fidler, I. J.: Patterns of tumor cell arrest and development. In Weiss, L. (ed.) *Fundamental Aspects of Metastasis,* pp. 275–89, North-Holland, Amsterdam, 1976.

Fidler, I. J., and Nicolson, G. L.: Organ selectivity for implantation, survival and growth of B16 melanoma variant tumor lines. *J. Natl. Cancer Inst.,* 57:1199–202, 1976.

Fidler, I. J., and Nicolson, G. L.: Fate of recirculating B16 melanoma metastatic variant cells in parabiotic syngeneic recipients. *J. Natl. Cancer Inst.,* 58:1867–72, 1977.

Fidler, I. J., and Nicolson, G. L.: Tumor cell and host properties affecting the implantation and survival of blood-borne metastatic variants of B16 melanoma. *Isr. J. Med. Sci.,* 14:38–50, 1978.

Fidler, I. J., and Nicolson, G. L.: Immunobiology of experimental metastatic melanoma. *Cancer Biol. Rev.,* 2:171–234, 1981.

Fisher, E. R., and Fisher, B.: Experimental study of factors influencing the development of hepatic metastases from circulating tumor cells. *Acta Cytol.,* 9:146–58, 1965.

Foulds, L. (ed.): *Neoplastic Development,* Academic Press, New York, 1975.

Goldenberg, D. M., Pavia, R. A., and Tsao, M. C.: *In vivo* hybridization of human tumor and normal hamster cells. *Nature,* 250:649–51, 1974.

Hanna, N.: Expression of metastatic potential of tumor cells in young nude mice is correlated with low levels of natural killer cell-mediated cytotoxicity. *Int. J. Cancer,* 26:675–80, 1980.

Hanna, N.: Inhibition of experimental tumor metastasis by selective activation of natural killer cells. *Cancer Res.,* 42:1337–42, 1982.

Hanna, N., and Fidler, I. J.: Expression of metastatic potential of allogeneic and xenogeneic neoplasms in young nude mice. *Cancer Res.,* 41:438–44, 1981.

Hart, I. R., and Fidler, I. J.: Role of organ selectivity in the determination of metastatic patterns of B16 melanoma. *Cancer Res.,* 40:2281–87, 1980.

Hart, I. R., and Fidler, I. J.: The implications of tumor heterogeneity for studies on the biology and therapy of cancer metastasis. *Biochim. Biophys. Acta,* 651:37–50, 1981.

Heppner, G. H.: Tumor heterogeneity. *Cancer Res.,* 44:2259–65, 1984.

Heppner, G. H., Loveless, S. E., Miller, M. F. R., Mahoney, K. H., and Fulton, A. M.: Mammary tumor heterogeneity. In Nicolson, G. L.; Milas, L. (eds.): *Cancer Invasion and Metastasis,* pp. 209–21, Raven Press, New York, 1984.

Hermann, P. G., Lyonnet, D., Fingerhut, R., and Tuttle, R. N.: Regional bloodflow to the lymph node during the immune response. *Lymphology,* 9:101–4, 1976.

Hewitt, H. B., and Blake, E.: Quantitative studies of trans lymph-node passage of tumour cells naturally disseminated from a non-immunogenic murine squamous carcinoma. *Br. J. Cancer,* 31:25–35, 1975.

Hewitt, H. B., and Blake, E. R.: Further studies of the relationship between lymphatic dissemination and lymph nodal metastasis in nonimmunogenic murine tumours. *Br. J. Cancer,* 35:415–19, 1977.

Irimura, T., and Nicolson, G. L.: Carbohydrate chain analysis by lectin binding to electrophoretically separated glycoproteins from murine B16 melanoma sublines of various metastatic properties. *Cancer Res.,* 44:791–98, 1984.

Irimura, T., Gonzalez, R., and Nicolson, G. L.: Effects of tunicamycin on B16 metastatic melanoma cell-surface glycoproteins and blood-borne arrest and survival properties. *Cancer Res.,* 41:3411–18, 1981.

Kinsey, D. L.: An experimental study of preferential metastasis. *Cancer,* 13:674–76, 1960.

Kerbel, R. S.: Immunologic studies of membrane mutants of a highly metastatic murine tumor. *Am. J. Pathol.,* 97:609–22, 1979.

Kerbel, R. S., Frost, P., Liteplo, R., Carlow, D., and Elliot, B. E.: Possible epigenetic mechanisms of tumor progression: Induction of high-frequency heritable but phenotypically unstable changes in the tumorigenic and metastatic properties of tumor cell populations by 5-azacytidine treatment. *J. Cell. Physiol., Suppl.,* 3:87–97, 1984.

Lagarde, A. E., Donaghue, T. P., Dennis, J. W., and Kerbel, R. S.: Genotypic and phenotypic evolution of a murine tumor during its progression in vivo toward metastasis. *J. Natl. Cancer Inst.,* 71:183–91, 1983.

Malmgren, R. A.: Studies of circulating tumor cells in cancer patients. In Denoix, P. (ed.): *Mechanisms of Invasion in Cancer,* pp. 108–17, Springer-Verlag, New York, 1967.

Miller, F. R.: Tumor subpopulation interactions in metastasis. *Invasion Metastasis,* 3:234–42, 1983.

Miller, B. E., Miller, F. R., and Heppner, G. H.: Interactions between tumor subpopulations affecting their sensitivity to the antineoplastic agents cyclosphosphamide and methotrexate. *Cancer Res,* 41:4378–81, 1981.

Miner, K. M., Kawaguchi, T., Uba, G. W., and Nicolson, G. L.: Clonal drift of cell surface, melanogenic and experimental metastatic properties of *in vivo*-selected, brain meninges-colonizing murine B16 melanoma. *Cancer Res.,* 42:4631–38, 1982.

Neri, A., and Nicolson, G. L.: Phenotypic drift of metastatic and cell-surface properties of mammary adenocarcinoma cell clones during growth *in vitro. Int. J. Cancer,* 28:731–38, 1981.

Neri, A., Rusolahti, E., and Nicolson, G. L.: Distribution of fibronectin on clonal cell lines of a rat mammary adenocarcinoma growing *in vitro* and *in vivo* at primary and metastatic sites. *Cancer Res.,* 41:5082–95, 1981.

Neri, A., Welch, D., Kawaguchi, T., and Nicolson, G. L.: The development and biologic properties of malignant cell sublines and clones of a spontaneously metastasizing rat mammary adenocarcinoma. *J. Natl. Cancer Inst.,* 68:507–17, 1982.

Nicolson, G. L.: Transmembrane control of the receptors on normal and tumor cells. I. Cytoplasmic influence over cell-surface components. *Biochim. Biophys. Acta,* 457:57–108, 1976.

Nicolson, G. L.: Cancer metastasis: Organ colonization and the cell-surface properties of malignant cells. *Biochim. Biophys. Acta,* 695:113–76, 1982.

Nicolson, G. L.: Stability and phenotypic heterogeneity of metastatic tumor cells. In Moloy, P. J., Nicolson, G. L. (eds.): *Cellular Oncology: New Approaches in Biology, Diagnosis, and Treatment,* pp. 3–27, Praeger Press, New York, 1983.

Nicolson, G. L.: Cell-surface molecules and tumor metastasis. Regulation of metastatic diversity. *Exp. Cell Res.,* 150:3–22, 1984a.

Nicolson, G. L.: Generation of phenotypic diversity and progression in metastatic tumors. *Cancer Metastasis Rev.,* 3:25–42, 1984b.

Nicolson, G. L.: Tumor progression, oncogenes, and the evolution of metastatic phenotypic diversity. *Clin. Exp. Metastasis,* 2:85–105, 1984c.

Nicolson, G. L., and Custead, S. E.: Tumor metastasis is not due to adaptation of cells to a new organ environment. *Science,* 215:176–78, 1982.

Nicolson, G. L., Dulski, K., Basson, C., and Welch, D.: Preferential organ attachment and invasion *in vitro* by B16 melanoma cells selected for differing metastatic colonization and invasive properties. *Invasion Metastasis,* 5:144–58, 1985a.

Nicolson, G. L., Mascali, J. J., and McGuire, E. J.: Metastatic RAW117 lymphosarcoma as a model for malignant-normal cell interactions. Possible roles for cell-surface antigens in determining the quantity and location of secondary tumors. *Oncodevelop. Biol. Med.,* 4:149–59, 1982.

Nicolson, G. L., and Poste, G.: Tumor cell diversity and host responses in cancer metastasis. I. Properties of metastatic cells. *Curr. Probl. Cancer,* 7(6):1–83, 1982.

Nicolson, G. L., and Poste, G.: Tumor cell diversity and host responses in cancer metastasis. II. Host immune responses and therapy of metastases. *Curr. Probl. Cancer* 7(7):1–43, 1983a.

Nicolson, G. L., and Poste, G.: Tumor implantation and invasion at metastatic sites. *Int. Rev. Exp. Pathol.,* 25:77–181, 1983b.

Nicolson, G. L., Rotter, V., Wolfe, D., Irimura, T., Reading, C. L., LaBiche, R., and Frazier, M.: Biochemistry and molecular biology of RAW117 large cell lymphoma. *In* Liotta, L., Lopis, K. (eds.): *Biochemistry and Molecular Genetics of Cancer Metastasis,* pp. 115–27, Martinus Nijhoff/Dr. Junk, Hingham, Mass., 1985b.

Nicolson, G. L., Steck, P. A., Welch, D. R., and Lembo, T.: Heterogeneity and instability of phenotypic and metastatic properties of local tumor- and metastasis-derived clones of a mammary adenocarcinoma. In Rich, M., Hager, J., Furmanski, P. (eds.): *Understanding Breast Cancer: Clinical and Laboratory Concepts,* pp. 145–66, Marcel Dekker, New York, 1983.

North, S. M., and Nicolson, G. L.: Effect of host immune status on the spontaneous metastasis of cloned cell lines of the 13762NF rat mammary adenocarcinoma. *Br. J. Cancer,* 52:747–55, 1985.

Nowell, P. C.: The clonal evolution of tumor cell populations. *Science,* 194:23–8, 1976.

Nowell, P. C.: Tumor progression and clonal evolution: The role of genetic instability. In German, J. (ed.): *Chromosome Mutation and Neoplasia,* pp. 413–23, Alan R. Liss, Inc., New York, 1983.

Paget, S.: The distribution of secondary growth in cancer of the breast. *Lancet* 1:571–73, 1889.

Pearce, V., Pathak, S., Mellard, D., Welch, D. R., and Nicolson, G. L.: Chromosome and DNA analysis of rat 13762NF mammary adenocarcinoma cell lines and clones of different metastatic potentials. *Clin. Exp. Metastasis,* 2:271–86, 1984.

Peterson, J. A., Ceriani, R. L., Blank, E. W., and Osvaldo, L.: Comparison of rates of phenotypic variability in surface antigen expression in normal and cancerous breast epithelial cells. *Cancer Res.,* 43:4291–96, 1983.

Poste, G., and Fidler, I. J.: The pathogenesis of cancer metastasis. *Nature,* 283:139–46, 1980.

Poste, G., Doll, J., and Fidler, I. J.: Interactions among clonal subpopulations affect stability of the metastatic phenotype in polyclonal populations of B16 melanoma cells. *Proc. Natl. Acad. Sci. U.S.A.,* 78:6226–30, 1981.

Poste, G., Tzeng, J., Doll, J., Greig, R., Rieman, D., and Zeidman, I.: Evolution of tumor cell heterogeneity during progressive growth of individual lung metastases. *Proc. Natl. Acad. Sci. U.S.A.,* 79:6574–78, 1982.

Raz, A.: Clonal emergence of metastatic heterogeneity in a growing tumor. *Cancer Lett.,* 17:153–60, 1982.

Salsbury, A. J.: The significance of the circulating cancer cell. *Cancer Treat. Rev.,* 2:55–72, 1975.

Schirrmacher, V., Altevogt, P., Fogel, M., Dennis, J., Waller, C. A., Barz, D., Schwartz, R., Cheingsong-Popov, R., Springer, G., Robinson, P. J., Nebe, T., Brossmer, W., Vlodavsky, I., Paweletz, N., Zimmermann, H.-P., and Uhlenbruck, G.: Importance of cell-surface carbohydrates in cancer cell adhesion, invasion, and metastasis. *Invasion Metastasis,* 2:313–360, 1982.

Stackpole, C. W.: Generation of phenotypic diversity in the B16 mouse melanoma relative to spontaneous metastasis. *Cancer Res.,* 43:3057–65, 1983.

Steck, P. A., and Nicolson, G. L.: Cell surface glycoproteins of 13762NF mammary adenocarcinoma clones of differing metastatic potentials. *Exp. Cell Res.,* 147: 255–67, 1983.

Sugarbaker, E. V.: Patterns of metastasis in human malignancies. *Cancer Biol. Rev.,* 2:235–278, 1981.

Sugarbaker, E. V., Cohen, A. M., and Ketcham, A. S.:

Do metastases metastasize? *Ann. Surg.,* 174:161–66, 1971.

Talmadge, J. E., Starkey, J. R., Davis, W. C., and Cohen, A. L.: Introduction of metastatic heterogeneity by short-term *in-vivo* passage of a cloned transformed cell line. *J. Supramol. Struct.,* 12:227–43, 1979.

Tomasovic, S. P., Thames, H. D., Jr., and Nicolson, G. L.: Heterogeneity in hyperthermic sensitivities of rat 13762NF mammary adenocarcinoma cell clones of differing metastatic potentials. *Radiat. Res.,* 91:555–63, 1982.

Van de Velde, C. J. H., and Carr, I.: Lymphatic invasion and metastasis. *Experientia,* 33:837–840, 1977.

Wang, T.-Y. and Nicolson, G. L.: Metastatic tumor cell invasion of brain organ tissue cultured on cellulose polyacetate strips. *Clin Exp. Metastasis,* 1:327–29, 1983.

Weiss, L.: Metastasis: Differences between cancer cells in primary and secondary tumors. *Pathobiol. Ann.,* 10: 51–81, 1980.

Weiss, L.: Random and nonrandom processes in metastasis, and metastatic efficiency. *Invasion Metastasis,* 3:193–208, 1983.

Welch, D. R., and Nicolson, G. L.: Phenotypic drift and heterogeneity in response of metastatic mammary adenocarcinoma cell clones to adriamycin, 5-fluoro-2′-deoxyuridine and methotrexate treatment *in vitro. Clin. Exp. Metastasis,* 1:317–325, 1983.

Welch, D. R., Milas, L., Tomasovic, S. P., and Nicolson, G. L.: Heterogeneous response and clonal drift of sensitivities of metastatic 13762NF mammary adenocarcinoma clones to gamma radiation *in vitro. Cancer Res.,* 43:6–10, 1983.

Welch, D. R., Krizman, D., and Nicolson, G. L.: Multiple phenotypic divergence of mammary adenocarcinoma cell clones. I. *In vitro* and *in vivo* properties. *Clin. Exp. Metastasis,* 2:333–55, 1984a.

Welch, D. R., Evans, D. P., Tomasovic, S. P., Milas, L., and Nicolson, G. L.: Multiple phenotypic divergence of mammary adenocarcinoma cell clones. II. Sensitivity to radiation, hyperthermia, and FUdR. *Clin. Exp. Metastasis,* 2:357–71, 1984b.

Willis, R. A.: The spread of tumors in the human body. In *Pathology of Tumors,* 3rd ed., Butterworth, London, 1973.

Wolman, S. R.: Karyotypic progression in human tumors. *Cancer Met. Rev.,* 2:257–93, 1983.

Zeidman, I., and Buss, J. M.: Experimental studies on the spread of cancer in the lymphatic system. I. Effectiveness of the lymph node as a barrier to the passage of embolic tumor cells. *Cancer Res.,* 14:403–05, 1954.

CHAPTER 2

The Influence of Organ Microenvironment on the Development of Cancer Metastases

Isaiah J. Fidler and Janet E. Price

EDITORS' COMMENT

If we are to understand the treatment of regional metastases of head and neck cancer, we must first appreciate its origins. In this chapter, Dr. Fidler and Dr. Price lay the groundwork for this understanding. By the identification of the "seed and soil" theory proposed by Paget in 1889, these authors, like Dr. Nicolson in the last chapter, develop the scientific basis on which this hypothesis appears to be valid.

The biologic heterogeneity of the cell population of a given primary tumor makes it difficult for the clinician to treat. Add to this the influences of the host, recipient organ, and environmental factors once regional or distant metastasis has occurred, and the reader can understand the complexity of the task of the basic researcher in analyzing cancer metastases at a cellular level.

In this chapter, the authors recognize the fact that the hematogenous spread of tumor cells results in the survival of less than 0.1 percent of these cells. What then is the mechanism by which so many cells die in vivo, yet allow the few survivors to be so virulent? As we might suspect, the answers are not simple, but rather are related to a specialized metastatic subpopulation of cells, which in fact may have a unicellular or multicellular origin. Other considerations include the unexplained preferential growth of tumor cells once they become imbedded in the microvascular bed of the recipient organ. Some of the answers to these questions have been worked out in rodent models, less so in human neoplasms.

In their conclusion, the authors are careful not to translate the behavior of tumors in animals to those in humans; rather they are cautious to conclude that the "seed and soil" theory of Paget certainly is supported by well-documented basic scientific research that can aid the clinician in a better understanding of the seemingly bewildering behavior of the metastatic tumor cell.

INTRODUCTION

The concept that neoplasms are heterogeneous and contain multiple subpopulations of cells with different biologic properties no longer merits debate (Hart and Fidler, 1981; Fidler and Poste, 1982; Fidler and Hart, 1982). Nor is the concept new. In 1889, the pathologist Paget analyzed autopsies of a large number of patients with breast cancer and concluded that the nonrandom pattern of metastasis was not due to chance. Rather, some tumor cells ("seeds") traveling in the circulation with affinity for growth in the environment provided by certain organs ("soil") are responsible for the production of metastasis. Recently, this hypothesis has received considerable support (Hart, 1982). Organ-specific metastasis has been identified in many transplantable experimental tumors (Poste and Fidler, 1980; Poste, 1982; Nicholson, 1982; Nicolson and Custead, 1982), and has also been recently reported in autochthonous human tumors in patients with peritoneovenous shunts (Tarin *et al.*, 1984c).

A present-day definition of the "seed and soil" hypothesis of Paget, however, must include three important principles. First, neoplasms are not uniform entities, but consist of cells exhibiting heterogeneous metastatic capabilities. Second, the process of metastasis is not random. Third, the outcome of metastasis depends on the properties of both metastatic tumor cells and host factors, and the balance of these interactions could well vary in tumors arising in different organs and in tumors of similar histologic origin in different patients (Poste and Fidler, 1980; Fidler, 1984).

In the majority of patients, by the time of diagnosis of primary malignant neoplasms, excluding skin cancers, metastasis may well have occurred (Fidler, 1984). Therefore, despite major advancements in patient care, surgical techniques, and systemic therapies, the major cause of death from cancer remains the uncontrolled growth of metastases that are resistant to conventional therapy. The most significant obstacle to the destruction of these metastases stems from the fact that the cells ("seeds") populating both primary and secondary neoplasms are biologically heterogeneous. By the time of diagnosis, and certainly in clinically advanced lesions, malignant neoplasms contain a large variety of cell populations with different biologic characteristics. Indeed, cells obtained from individual tumors can differ with respect to cell-surface properties, antigenicity, immunogenicity, growth rate, karyotype, sensitivity to various cytotoxic drugs, and the ability to invade and produce metastases (Fidler and Hart, 1982; Heppner, 1984).

Biologic heterogeneity is not confined to cells in primary tumors, but is equally prominent among tumor cells in metastases (Fidler, 1984). Many clinical observations suggest that multiple metastases proliferating in different organs or even in the same organ of cancer patients can be biologically diverse. This could be due to the growth of different tumor cells ("seeds"), but it is not surprising that various organ environments ("soil") also influence the biologic behavior of metastases. With the discovery of neoplastic heterogeneity, a great deal of attention has been given to elucidating the various properties associated with the malignant phenotype. Less emphasis however, has been given to the various host, organ, and environmental factors that can influence the metastatic process. In this chapter, we provide a summary of our understanding of the influence of organ environment ("soil") on the process and its implications for cancer therapy.

THE FORMATION OF CANCER METASTASIS

To produce a clinically relevant metastasis, malignant tumor cells must complete a sequence of destructive interactions with host homeostatic mechanisms (which include host defense mechanisms). The pathogenesis of a metastasis begins with the invasion by malignant cells into the host stroma that surrounds the primary tumor. Once tumor cells penetrate lymphatics or blood vessels, they can detach and disseminate either as single-cells or multiple-cell emboli. While in the circulation, the tumor cells must survive mechanical traumas such as blood turbulence and evade host immune and nonimmune defenses. The few tumor cells that survive in the circulation can arrest in the capillary beds of distant organs by adhering to endothelial cells or to exposed basement membranes (Nicolson, 1982). Of those tumor cells that arrest in the capillaries, some can extravasate into the organ parenchyma where they must proliferate in order to establish new tumor foci. Newly established metastases can readily give rise to other metastases (Fidler, 1984).

Failure to complete even one step in the process of metastasis leads to the elimination of the disseminating tumor cell. The complexity of the pathogenesis of metastasis partially explains why the process is seemingly so inefficient (Weiss, 1980). Using radiolabeled mouse melanoma cells, we have observed that after entry into the circulation, fewer than 0.1 percent of tumor cells survived to produce metastases (Fidler, 1970). This observation was compatible with the "seed" hypothesis (Paget, 1889) and prompted us to question whether the few cells responsible for the development of metastases survived at random, or whether the cells represented the selective survival and growth of preexistent subpopulations of metastatic cells. Using a modified fluctuation assay of Luria and Delbruck (1943), we have shown that tumor-cell subpopulations preexisting in the same tumor exhibit heterogeneous metastatic potential (Fidler and Kripke, 1977). This finding has been confirmed in numerous laboratories using a wide range of experimental animal tumors of different origins and histologic types (Poste, 1982; Nicolson and Poste, 1982; Fidler, 1984). Moreover, by using young athymic nude mice, whose natural killer cells are not fully active, as models for metastasis of human neoplasms, it has been demonstrated recently that several human tumor lines are also heterogeneous and contain subpopulations of cells with widely differing metastatic properties (Kozlowski et al., 1984 a, b).

THE ORIGIN OF METASTASES

As stated, metastases in general do not result from the random survival of tumor cells but from the proliferation of specialized metastatic subpopulations of cells. Metastases, like primary tumors, may have a unicellular or a multicellular origin (Fidler and Hart, 1981; Talmadge et al., 1982; Poste and Greig, 1983; Poste et al., 1982). To distinguish between these possibilities, we determined whether individual metastases are clonal in origin and whether different metastases can be produced by different progenitor cells that preexist in a primary neoplasm. We examined the metastases that arose from subcutaneous tumors produced by the K-1735 mouse melanoma cells (Fidler et al., 1981), that had been X-irradiated to induce random chromosomal damage and rearrangement (Talmadge et al., 1982). We reasoned that if a metastasis were derived from a single cell, all the chromosome spreads examined within an individual metastasis would exhibit the same karyotype. In contrast, if a metastasis were produced by more than one progenitor cell, (Talmadge et al., 1982), its constituent cells were likely to exhibit different chromosomal arrangements.

The cellular compositions of 21 individual lung metastases were analyzed after cultivation of cells from each of the lesions. In 11 metastases, unique karyotypic patterns of abnormal marker chromosomes were found, suggesting that each metastasis originated from a single progenitor cell. These data allowed us to conclude that many metastases can originate from single cells and that different metastases can originate from different progenitor cells. Similar results have been obtained in experiments using B16 melanoma cell clones bearing identifiable biochemical markers. The study with the B16 cells also revealed that variant clones with diverse phenotypes are formed rapidly to generate significant cellular diversity within solitary metastases (Poste and Greig, 1983).

ROLE OF ORGAN ENVIRONMENT IN THE METASTASIS OF RODENT NEOPLASMS

Studies in experimental animal tumor systems have demonstrated that the formation and anatomic locations of metastases are determined by both host factors and tumor-cell properties (Fidler, 1984). The distribution and fate of hematogenously disseminated radiolabeled tumor cells in experimental rodent systems (Fidler, 1970, 1978; Fidler et al., 1977; Fidler and Nicolson, 1977; Poste, 1982) clearly reveal that tumor cells reach and arrest in the microvasculature of many organs. However, proliferation of tumor cells, which results in visible metastases, occurs in some but not all the organs tumor cells reach. Thus, the arrest of viable tumor cells in a particular organ does not always predict that metastasis will develop (Hart and Fidler, 1980).

In 1928, Ewing suggested that metastasis is produced as a consequence of only mechanical mechanisms such as anatomic and hemodynamic factors of the vasculature. Although circulatory anatomy may indeed influence the dissemination of many malignant cells, it cannot fully explain the patterns of distribution of numerous tumors. Why organs, such as the spleen or skeletal muscle, with highly developed vasculature should be infrequent sites of metastatic development is not understood (Zeidman and Buss, 1952; del Regato, 1977). Similarly, the propensity of certain human and animal tumors for growth in specific organs cannot be accounted for on hemodynamic grounds alone (Tarin et al., 1984c).

Experimental data in support of the alternative explanation for the nonrandom pattern of metastasis (i.e., the "seed and soil" hypothesis of Paget) were first reported by Kinsey (1960), who used the Cloudman melanoma, then by Sugarbaker et al. (1971), who used a murine fibrosarcoma system. In both studies, neonatal tissue from various organs was implanted in the thighs of syngeneic mice. Following the intraarterial or subcutaneous injection of lung-colonizing tumor cells, metastatic foci developed in the in situ lung and in the ectopically grafted lung but not in other grafted control organs. Experiments from our laboratory were carried out to determine whether metastatic tumor cells arrest specifically in some organs where metastases develop, or whether metastatic tumor cells distribute to many organs but grow in only particular sites. We also questioned whether the mechanical arrest of circulating tumor emboli can explain the unique patterns of metastasis in this tumor, or whether tumor cell and organ affinities were responsible for the growth of metastatic foci (Hart and Fidler, 1980).

The preferential growth of B16 melanoma metastases in specific organs was therefore studied. Following the intravenous injection of B16 melanoma cells into syngeneic C57BL/6 mice, tumor growths developed in the in situ lungs and in grafts of pulmonary or ovarian tissue implanted either subcutaneously or intramuscularly into the quadriceps femoris. In contrast, metastatic lesions did not develop in control grafts of similarly implanted renal tissue or at the site of surgical trauma. The formation of tumor at the transplanted organ could have been due to the arrest and growth of tumor cells immediately following intravenous injection (i.e., "initial metastases"). Alternatively, tumor cells injected intravenously could have been arrested in the lungs and developed there. Once metastases were established, tumor cells could enter the circulation, to be arrested at other organs and produce "secondary metastases."

To distinguish between these possibilities, we performed several experiments with parabiotically joined mice (Fidler and Nicolson, 1977). Two weeks after normal tumor-free mice were joined parabiotically to tumor-bearing animals, there was no evidence of any tumor growth in the "guest" animals. However, when the parabiont animals were allowed to survive for 4 weeks after separation from the tumor-bearing animals, 40 percent of the mice developed lung metastases.

To determine whether tumor growth in ectopically implanted organs was due to the organ-specific arrest of intravenously injected cells, we monitored the organ distribution of radiolabeled melanoma cells. By 10 minutes after injection of [^{125}I]IdUrd-labeled cells, no more than 0.8 percent of the total number of injected cells was lodged in the hind legs where organs (lung or kidney) were implanted. No significant difference could be detected between the number of cells lodged in limbs bearing kidney (tumor negative) or lung (tumor positive) grafts at 10 and 60 minutes and 1 day after tumor-cell injection. Likewise, no significant differences in tumor-cell lodgment were detected between transplant-bearing limbs and the opposite, nonoperated limb, which served as a control. Similarly, no significant differences in tumor cell arrest were detected among the different implanted organs or between operated and nonoperated legs.

The preceding data clearly demonstrate the organ-specific nature of a mouse melanoma and illustrate the difficulty encountered in past studies in defining tumor cell "homing." Although B16 melanoma cells do indeed produce gross metastases in the lungs and gonads (Hart and Fidler, 1980), it is not apparent that these metastases can be explained merely by the initial lodgment of tumor cells in these organs. Rather, the lung and gonads provide a receptive organ for the multiplication of a few surviving tumor cells. Thus, the use of the term "homing" in the context of tumor dissemination must refer to both the initial localization and subsequent growth of tumor cells at specific organ sites.

THE ROLE OF HOST-ORGAN ENVIRONMENT IN THE METASTASIS OF HUMAN NEOPLASMS

Patterns of metastasis formation have emerged from studies of many different human tumors whose systemic dissemination cannot be explained by blood-flow alone (Willis, 1973; Tarin, 1976). The results of more than 700 breast carcinoma cases led Paget (1889) to propose the "seed and soil" hypothesis of metastasis, pointing out the apparent predisposition of some organs (e.g., liver) to develop distant metastases, compared with others (e.g., spleen and kidneys) in which breast carcinoma metastases were much less frequent. Such findings pose the question of different susceptibilities of organs to support (or conversely to suppress) the growth of metastases. A study of the distribution of melanoma metastases in 56 patients concluded that the patterns of metastasis may be related to the embryologic derivation or functional properties of the tissues affected (de laMonte et al., 1983). That the role of organs as the "soil" is not totally passive has been suggested by studies showing that damage elicited by injury or radiation can enhance metastasis formation, a phenomenon termed "inflammatory oncotaxis" (DerHagopian et al., 1978).

Ethical considerations rule out the experimental analysis of human tumor metastasis in the ways it has been investigated in animal systems. Thus, there have been no acceptable methods for directly studying the underlying mechanisms of dissemination or identifying markers of metastatic potential of human tumor cells. The introduction of peritoneovenous shunts for palliation of malignant ascites, however, has provided an opportunity to study some of the factors affecting metastatic spread in humans.

The studies of Tarin and colleagues (1984a, b, c; Souter et al., 1983) describe the outcome of draining ascitic fluid, with the resulting vascular dissemination of viable tumor cells into the jugular veins of patients with malignant ascites. The primary concern was to show that this treatment provided real benefit to the patients and did not mediate widespread metastasis formation. The published studies included 29 patients with different primary tumors, the most common being ovarian carcinoma (12 cases), and reported good palliation with minimal complications (Souter et al., 1983; Tarin et al., 1984b). The autopsy findings from 15 patients reflect the clinical observations that the peritoneovenous shunts do not carry the risk of promoting significant metastasis, and as a valuable byproduct give insights into the dissemination of human tumor cells.

In eight patients, small metastases were found in extraabdominal organs (most commonly lungs) possibly seeded since the peritoneovenous shunts were inserted, but these tumor foci were not clinically detectable. In the other seven patients there was no evidence of tumor seedings outside the abdomen, even in cases where the peritoneovenous shunt had functioned for several months, and in one case longer than 2 years (Tarin et al., 1984a).

Malignant neoplasms do not need the intervention of peritoneovenous shunts to disseminate cells; however, the negative findings in half these patients are of great importance. The identification of cytologic markers (psammoma bodies) in the tumor of two patients confirmed the widespread distribution of cells to many organs, but tumor proliferation was seen only in few organ sites or none at all. The studies therefore provide verification of the nearly century-old "seed and soil" hypothesis of Paget. Laboratory investigation of properties of the ascites tumor cells and correlation with the metastatic behavior afford opportunities to find markers of metastatic potential and for further research into why tumor cells can grow in some organ sites and not others.

DISCUSSION

Tumor cell properties contribute significantly to organ arrest patterns. Organ-specific variant lines have been selected from parent tumor populations (Poste, 1982; Fidler, 1984), and the modification of many tumor-cell properties can lead to alterations in their dispersion patterns (Hart et al., 1980; Poste and Nicolson, 1980). Moreover, studies with the B16 melanoma in parabiotically joined mice have also demonstrated the lung-seeking nature of these cells (Fidler and Nicolson, 1977). The effect of host tissues themselves on tumor development is less well-established. Preferential growth in certain organs has been explained by the vagaries of local immune defenses (Ioachim et al., 1976; Reif, 1978; Proctor, 1976) and the fact that diffusible inhibitors of tumor development may be released by certain tissues (Houck and Hennings, 1973; Bellamy and Hinsull, 1978).

It is interesting that in an experiment in which lung and kidney tissue were placed ectopically in the same site (Hart and Fidler, 1980), there was apparently a greater reduction in tumor growth than that observed with lung tissue alone. Extracts of rat kidney have been shown to inhibit thymidine incorporation by cultured rat cells (Klein et al., 1979), but whether such a mechanism is operative in the results with the B16 melanoma study is unknown. Lung tissue, however, does not necessarily promote the growth of all metastatic tumors. The M5076 tumor, a murine reticulum cell sarcoma, injected intravenously, failed to grow in the in situ or implanted lungs. Nevertheless, this tumor did spread to and grow in visceral organs of the peritoneal cavity as well as in some implanted ovaries (Hart et al., 1981).

Clinical observations have suggested that the response of metastases in women with breast cancer is influenced by the anatomic location of the lesions. With few exceptions, the superficial metastases in lymph nodes and skin responded better than skeletal or pulmonary metastases (Canellos et al., 1974; Slack and Bross, 1975; Brambilla et al., 1976). Similar results for differential response of metastatic lesions in different organs to different cytotoxic drugs have also been reported (Donelli, 1967, 1977). Subcutaneously transplanted mouse neoplasms were sensitive to three cytotoxic agents, whereas the same tumor cells implanted intracerebrally were not (Donelli et al., 1967; Holst et al., 1971). While it is tempting to attribute the differences in the response of metastases to chemotherapy to heterogeneity in cell population, the influence of the organ environment must not be ignored.

The viability and growth of tumor cells depends on an adequate source of nutrients. The degree of tumor vascularity can control the delivery of nutrients, clearance of metabolites, and the delivery of cytotoxic drugs to a lesion. Measurements of blood flow in subcutaneous tumors of rats reveal a lack of autoregulation in response to infusions of angiotensin II. The selective increase in tumor blood flow, with no increase in normal tissues, can provide a method for enhancing chemotherapeutic drug delivery (Suzuki et al., 1981). The extent of tumor angiogenesis, a host response to a growing neoplasm, can differ among different organs and contribute to differential growth of some metastases.

Observations of human tumors in both classical pathologic studies and the more recent findings from cancer patients treated with peritoneovenous shunts show how metastasis formation is the result of an interplay between malignant cells and the target organs. The peritoneovenous shunt findings are directly comparable with those from animal tumor studies, confirming that although viable tumorigenic cells may be distributed to many organs, proliferation into metastases only occurs in a few sites, often characteristic of that particular neoplasm.

We conclude that the outcome of metastasis is dependent on both tumor cell properties and host factors. This conclusion supports the "seed and soil" hypothesis and explains the nonrandom pattern of cancer metastasis.

REFERENCES

Bellamy, D., and Hinsull, S. M.: Influence of lodgement site on the proliferation of metastases of Walker 256 carcinoma in the rat. *British J. Cancer,* 37:81–85, 1978.

Brambilla, C., Delena, M., Rossi, A., Valagussa, P., and Bonadonna, G.: Response and survival in advanced breast cancer after two noncross-resistant combinations. *Br. Med. J.,* 1:801–4, 1976.

Canellos, G. P., Devita, V. T., Gold, G. L., Chabner, B. A., Schein, P. S., and Young, R. C.: Cyclical combination chemotherapy for advanced breast carcinoma. *Br. Med. J.*, 1:218–20, 1974.

dela Monte, S. M., Moore, G. W., Hutchins, G. M.: Patterned distribution of metastases from malignant melanoma in humans. *Cancer Res.*: 3427–33, 1983.

Del Regato, J. A.: Pathways of metastatic spread of malignant tumor. *Semin. Oncol.*, 4:33–38, 1977.

DerHagopian, R. P., Sugarbaker, E. V., and Ketcham, N.: Inflammatory oncotaxis. *JAMA*, 240:374–75, 1978.

Donelli, M. G., Colombo, T., Broggini, M., and Garattini, N.: Differential distribution of antitumor agents in primary and secondary tumors. *Cancer Treat. Rep.*, 61:1319–24, 1977.

Donelli, M. G., Rosso, R., and Garattino, S.: Selective chemotherapy in relation to the site of tumor transplantation. *Int. J. Cancer*, 2:421–24, 1967.

Ewing, J.: *Neoplastic Disease*, 3rd ed., W.B. Saunders, Philadelphia, 1978.

Fidler, I. J.: Metastasis quantitative analysis of distribution and fate of tumor emboli labeled with ^{125}I-5-iodo-2′-deoxyuridine. *J. Natl. Cancer Inst.,* 45:775–82, 1970.

Fidler, I. J.: General considerations for studies of experimental cancer metastasis. *Methods Cancer Res.,* 15:399–439, 1978.

Fidler, I. J.: The evolution of biological heterogeneity in metastatic neoplasm. In Nicolson, G. L., Milas, L. (eds.): *Cancer Invasion and Metastasis: Biologic and Therapeutic Aspects*, p. 5, Raven Press, New York, 1984.

Fidler, I. J., Gersten, D. M., and Riggs, C. W.: Relationship of host immune status to tumor-cell arrest, distribution, and survival in experimental metastases. *Cancer*, 40:46–55, 1977.

Fidler, I. J., Gruys, E., Cifone, M. A., Barnes, Z., and Bucana, C.: Demonstration of multiple phenotypic diversity in a murine melanoma of recent origin. *J. Natl. Cancer Inst.*, 67:947–56, 1981.

Fidler, I. J., and Hart, I. R.: The origin of metastatic heterogeneity in tumors. *Eur. J. Cancer,* 17:487–94, 1981.

Fidler, I. J., and Hart, I. R.: Biological diversity in metastatic neoplasms: Origins and implications. *Science*, 217:998–1003, 1982

Fidler, I. J., and Kripke, M. L.: Metastasis results from preexisting variant cells within a malignant tumor. *Science*, 197:893–95, 1977.

Fidler, I. J., and Nicolson, G. L.: Fate of recirculating B16 melanoma metastatic variant cells in parabiotic syngeneic recipients. *J. Natl. Cancer Inst.,* 58:1867–72, 1977.

Fidler, I. J., and Poste, G.: The heterogeneity of metastatic properties in malignant tumor cells and regulation of the metastatic phenotype. In Owen, A., Coffey, D. S., Baylin, S. B. (eds.): *Tumor Cell Heterogeneity*, p. 127. Academic Press, New York, 1982.

Hart, I. R.: "Seed and soil" revisited: Mechanisms of site-specific metastasis. *Cancer Met. Rev.,* 1:5–17, 1982.

Hart, I. R., and Fidler, I. J.: Role of organ selectivity determination of metastatic patterns of B16 melanoma. *Cancer Res.,* 41:1281–87, 1981.

Hart, I. R., and Fidler, I. J.: The implications of tumor heterogeneity for studies on the biology and therapy of cancer metastasis. *Biochim. Biophys. Acta*, 651:37–50, 1982.

Hart, I. R., Raz, A., and Fidler, I. J.: Effect of cytoskeleton-disrupting agents on the metastatic behavior of melanoma cells. *J. Natl. Cancer Inst.*, 64: 891–900, 1980.

Hart, I. R., Talmadge, J. E., and Fidler, I. J.: Metastatic behavior of a murine reticulum cell sarcoma exhibiting organ-specific growth. *Cancer Res.,* 41:1281–87, 1981.

Heppner, G.: Tumor heterogeneity. *Cancer Res.,* 214: 2259–65, 1984.

Houck, J. C., and Hennings, H.: Chalones. Specific endogenous mitotic inhibitors. *FEBS Lett.*, 32:1–8, 1973.

Ioachim, H. L., Pearse, A., and Keller, S. E.: Role of immune mechanisms in metastatic patterns of hemopoietic tumors in rats. *Cancer Res.,* 36:2854–62, 1976.

Kinsey, D. L.: An experimental study of preferential metastasis. *Cancer*, 13:874–76, 1960.

Klein, K., Coetzee, M. L., Madhav, R., and Ove, P.: Inhibition of tritiated thymidine incorporation in cultured cells by rat kidney extract. *J. Natl. Cancer Inst.,* 62:1557–64, 1979.

Kozlowski, J. M., Hart, I. R., Fidler, I. J., and Hanna, N.: A human melanoma line heterogeneous with respect to metastatic capacity in athymic nude mice. *J. Natl. Cancer Inst.,* 72(4):913–17, 1984a.

Kozlowski, J. M., Fidler, I. J., Campbell, D., Xu, Z., Kaighn, M. D., and Hart, I. R.: Metastatic behavior of human tumor cell lines grown in the nude mouse. *Cancer Res.,* 44:3522–29, 1984b.

Luria, S. E., and Delbruck, M.: Mutations of bacteria from virus sensitivity to virus resistance. *Genetics,* 28:491–511, 1943.

Nicolson, G. L.: Organ colonization and the cell-surface properties of malignant cells. *Biochim. Biophys. Acta,* 695:113–76, 1982.

Nicolson, G. L., and Custead, S. E.: Tumor metastasis is not due to adaptation of cells to a new organ environment. *Science*, 215:176–78, 1982.

Nicolson, G. L., and Poste, G.: Tumor-cell diversity and host responses in cancer metastasis. *Curr. Probl. Cancer:* 7(6):4–83, 1982.

Paget, S.: The distribution of secondary growths in cancer of the breast. *Lancet,* 1:571–73, 1889.

Poste, G.: Experimental systems for analysis of the malignant phenotype. *Cancer Met. Rev.,* 1:141–200, 1982.

Poste, G., and Fidler, I. J.: The pathogenesis of cancer metastasis. *Nature,* 283:139–146, 1980.

Poste, G., and Greig, R.: On the genesis and regulation of cellular heterogeneity in malignant tumors. *Invasion and Metastasis,* 2:137–76, 1982.

Poste, G., and Nicolson, G. L.: Modification of the arrest of metastatic tumor cells in the microcirculation after treatment with plasma membrane vesicles from highly metastatic cells. *Proc. Natl. Acad. Sci. USA,* 77:399–403, 1980.

Poste, G., Tzeng, J., Doll, J., Greig, R., Reiman, D., and Zeidman, I.: Evolution of tumor cell heterogeneity during progressive growth of individual lung metastases. *Proc. Natl. Acad. Sci. USA,* 79:6574–79, 1982.

Proctor, J. W.: Rat sarcoma model supports both "soil and seed" and "mechanical" theories of metastatic spread. *Br. J. Cancer,* 34:651–54, 1976.

Proctor, J. W., Auclair, B. G., and Stokowski, L.: Endocrine factors and the growth and spread of B16 melanoma. *J. Natl. Cancer Inst.,* 57:1197–98, 1976.

Reif, A.: Evidence for organ specificity of defense against tumors. In H. Waters (ed.): *The Handbook of Cancer Immunology,* Vol. 1, pp. 174–240, Garland STPM Press, New York, 1978.

Slack, N. H., and Bross, J. D. J.: The influence of site of metastasis on tumor growth and response to chemotherapy. *Br. J. Cancer,* 32:78–86, 1975.

Souter, R. G., Tarin, D., and Kettlewell, M. G. W.: Peritoneovenous shunts in the management of malignant ascites. *Br. J. Surg.,* 70:478–81, 1983.

Sugarbaker, E. V., Cohen, A. M., and Ketcham, A. S.: Do metastases metastasize? *Ann. Surg.,* 174:161–66, 1971.

Suzuki, M., Hori, K., Abe, I. Saito, S., and Sato, H.: A new approach to cancer chemotherapy: Selective enhancement of tumor blood flow with angiotensin II. *J. Natl. Cancer Inst.,* 67:663–69, 1981.

Talmadge, J. E., Wolman, S. R., and Fidler, I. J.: Evidence for the clonal origin of spontaneous metastases. *Science,* 217:361–63, 1982.

Tarin, D.: Cellular interactions in neoplasia: In Weiss, L. (ed.): *Fundamental Aspects of Metastasis,* p. 151, North-Holland Publishing Co., Amsterdam, 1976.

Tarin, D., Vass, A. C. R., Kettlewell, M. G. W., and Price, J. E.: Absence of metastatic sequelae during long-term treatment of malignant ascites by peritoneovenous shunting. *Invasion Metastasis,* 4:1–12, 1984a.

Tarin, D., Price, J. E., Kettlewell, M. G. W., Souter, R. G., Vass, A. C. R., and Crossley, B.: Clinicopathological observations on metastasis in man studied in patients treated with peritoneovenous shunts. *Br. Med. J.,* 288:749–51, 1984b.

Tarin, D., Price, J. E., Kettlewell, M. G. W., Souter, R. G., Vass, A. C. R., and Crossley, B.: Mechanisms of human tumor metastasis studied in patients with peritoneovenous shunts. *Cancer Res.,* 44:3584–92, 1984c.

Weiss, L.: Cancer cell traffic from the lungs to the liver: An example of metastatic inefficiency. *Int. J. Cancer,* 25:385–92, 1980.

Willis, R. A.: *The Spread of Tumours in the Human Body,* 3rd ed., Butterworth, London, 1973.

Zeidman, I., and Buss, J. M.: Transpulmonary passage of tumor cell emboli. *Cancer Res.,* 12:731–33, 1952.

PART TWO

EVALUATION OF THE NECK SPECIMEN

CHAPTER 3

Pathological Evaluation of Neck Dissection Lymph Nodes: A Status Report

John G. Batsakis and Jesus E. Medina

EDITORS' COMMENT

In this succinct chapter, Dr. John Batsakis, the well-known head and neck pathologist, joins with Dr. Jesus Medina, a head and neck surgeon, to give us a practical update on what can and cannot be surmised from pathologic evaluation of regional lymph nodes.

In the first chapters of this book, we learned from Dr. Nicolson and Dr. Fidler of the variation in biologic character of nodal metastasis when compared not only with the primary tumor, but also with other nodal metastases in the same patient.

In this chapter, the authors establish by literature review that immunologic assessment of the lymph node matrix by histologic, histomorphometric, or immunocytochemical means has very little prognostic significance. This finding is probably related to the wide range of heterogeneity noted by Dr. Nicolson and Dr. Fidler, and is exemplified by the difficulty of identifying a uniform antigenic character of nodal carcinoma.

In their conclusion, Dr. Batsakis and Dr. Medina note that for the present we must depend on both clinical findings (location, size, fixation) and conventional pathologic evaluation (extranodal extension, number of nodes involved) in order to make a safe, rational decision regarding adjunctive treatment and prognosis in metastatic neck disease.

INTRODUCTION

Pathologic examination of cervical lymph nodes in patients with squamous cell carcinoma of the head and neck encompasses two areas: (1) *immunologic* assessment of the lymph-node matrix and characterization of the metastasis, and (2) *conventional anatomicopathologic data* such as size of nodes, number of lymph nodes involved, levels of involved lymph nodes, and gross or microscopic evidence of extranodal extension. There is no question that the extent of metastatic spread to cervical lymph nodes is an important prognostic indicator in patients with head and neck cancers. Data shown in Table 3-1 confirm this

Table 3–1. Absolute Disease-Free Survival Related to Nodal Stage for Squamous Cell Carcinoma*

SITE OF PRIMARY	NO. OF PATIENTS	SURVIVAL (%)			
		N0	*N1b*	*N2b*	*N3*
Faucial arch and tonsil	661	50	40	29	25
Base of tongue	359	41	27	25	27
Supraglottic larynx	218	56	53	57	26
Pyriform sinus	434	36	34	11	15
Nasopharynx	104	38	44	50	34

*Modified from Bataini et al. (1982).

but also suggest some anomalies. Because of these anomalies, the past decade has seen intense examination of lymph-node characteristics in order to better predict prognosis and response to therapy. This chapter evaluates the status of these studies.

LYMPHATIC METASTASIS AND LYMPH-NODE REACTION PATTERNS

Lymphatic metastasis is an important mechanism in the spread of human cancer, but less is known about lymphatic metastasis than hematogenous metastasis. Most of what is known has been derived from animal models, and it is not known how much of such information can be transferred to human lymphatic metastasis (Carr, 1983).

There are several stages of metastasis via lymphatic pathways: (1) *premetastatic invasion* by penetration of the basal lamina of the epithelium of the primary site's mucosa and extension into connective tissue spaces; (2) *approach* of the neoplastic cells and contact with lymphatic endothelium; (3) *penetration* through the endothelium; (4) *translocation* of the cells through a lymphatic; (5) *intranodal settling* in the sinusoids of a lymph node, followed by proliferation; (6) *growth and destruction* of the lymph node; and (7) *secondary metastases* to other lymph nodes, an event not necessarily predicted by destruction of the primary echelon node (Carr, 1983).

The affected lymph node may be completely replaced or may show only focal capsular invasion. The metastatic neoplasm stimulates the stroma in a variety of ways, including fibrosis, angiogenesis, or lymphoreticular reaction.

Lymph nodes react to antigenic or inflammatory stimuli in their drainage area by a B-cell response, enlargement of lymphoid follicles, and formation of germinal centers; and by a T-cell response, increase in paracortical areas due to an entry and proliferation of lymphocytes, and by sinus histiocytosis (Carr, 1983; Tsakraklides et al., 1974) (Table 3–2).

The patterns of lymphoid-cell reaction in lymph nodes draining carcinoma are of some importance in prognosis because of the implied immunologic response (Byrnes et al., 1983; Berlinger et al., 1976; Schuller et al., 1985). Several histologic patterns have been described: lymphocytic predominance, where extrafollicular parts of a lymph node are filled with lymphoid cells; follicular reaction, an intermediate or average state; and lymphocyte depletion, most often accompanied by a hyaline fibrosis. Sinus histiocytosis has also been associated with a better prognosis.

Lymph-Node Reactivity

The sharp limitations of lymph-node histomorphology, even with the addition of immunohistochemistry, are perhaps nowhere better realized that when applied to an under-

Table 3–2. Immunomorphologic Patterns in Regional Lymph Nodes*

PATTERN	DESCRIPTION OF PATTERN
Lymphocyte predominance	Increased cortical and medullary lymphocytes; cortical follicles without germinal centers; increased paracortical immunoblasts, reticular cells, possible sinus histiocytosis.
Germinal-center predominance	Increased hypertrophic germinal centers in cortex or elsewhere, enlarged medullary cords with increase mature and immature plasma cells.
Lymphocyte depletion	Decreased lymphocytes; no germinal centers, general increase in plasma cells, and often a prominent fibrosis.
Unstimulated pattern	Cortical follicules, no germinal centers, small hypocellular paracortex, prominent sinuses.

*After Tsakraklides et al. (1974).

standing of basic control mechanisms of the regional immune response in head and neck cancer. Studies of cell-mediated immunity at the systemic level have indicated that peripheral blood-derived T-cells are reduced (number and mitogen stimulation) and skin testing with recall antigens is, in most patients, depressed (Houck et al., 1983), but they do not accurately reflect immunomodulatory activity in regional lymph nodes. There also appear to be locoregional differences—e.g., an association with a good prognosis between lymphocyte predominance and uterine or breast carcinoma but not with carcinoma of the colon (Borchard and Quakulinski, 1984).

The varying significance given to sinus histiocytosis and prognosis in breast carcinoma illustrates the difficulty inherent in translating static histomorphologic observations into biologic implications. The importance of this nodal reaction was first emphasized by Black and Speer (1957) nearly three decades ago. Using enzyme histochemical and in situ immunohistochemical techniques, current opinion is that the sinus histocyte is a monocyte-derived, fixed macrophage. It functions as a first line of defense by early interception of foreign materials that enter lymph nodes—by phagocytosis and degradation and by presentation of antigens to surrounding T-lymphocytes (van den Oord et al., 1985). Whether sinus histiocytosis is an immunologic phenomenon is debatable. If it is, its effect may be regarded as only transient. Studies have also failed to disclose any relationship between sinus histocytosis and the transformation of nodal lymphocytes (Fisher et al., 1983). On balance, it is doubtful whether sinus histiocytosis has any prognostic value. The significance of other histiocytic proliferations (e.g., sarcoidal) is not clear. These reactions may be responses to necrosis or inflammatory areas in the neoplasm or they may be reactions to shed tumor antigens (Carr, 1983).

Histologic studies have attempted to relate lymph-node structure to prognosis in patients with squamous cell carcinoma of the head and neck. Berlinger et al. (1976) found that various nodal reaction patterns (Table 3-3) were associated with improved survival. These workers

Table 3-3. Lymph-Node Reactivity in Head and Neck Tumors

SOURCE	CORRELATION
Berlinger et al. (1976)*	Significant relationship between 5-year survival and "stimulated" lymph nodes (lymphocyte or germinal center predominance)
Bennett et al. (1971)*	Favorable prognosis with germinal center hyperplasia
Noone et al. (1974)*	No correlation
Gilmore et al. (1978)	No correlation
Houck et al. (1983)	No correlation and no relation to modulatory activity

*Relationships seen only in patients with cervical metastases.

found that a reactive pattern (follicular or paracortical hyperplasia) of the lymph nodes correlated with fewer metastases in the neck and hence a better clinical outlook. The relationship was seen only in patients with cervical metastases; no correlation was observed in patients with pathologically negative necks. Furthermore, many of the patients studied by Berlinger et al. (1976) had received preoperative irradiation (45%).

Of five reported series dealing with squamous cell carcinomas of the head and neck, only those of Berlinger et al. (1976) and Bennett et al. (1971) indicate a correlation between lymph-node reactivity and prognosis (Table 3-3). Noone et al. (1974) found no relationship between histologic differentiation of the primary neoplasm and lymph-node structure. A University of Michigan study by Gilmore et al. (1978), who applied the same grading scheme as Berlinger et al. (1976), determined that the pattern of lymph-node reaction is not in itself a good indicator of prognosis and does not appear to reflect the immune activity in the lymph nodes (Table 3-4). Further support for this statement comes from Houck et al. (1983), who found that immunomodulatory activity in regional lymph nodes does not correlate with the histologic pattern of nodal reactivity but does correlate with the size and histologic grade of the neoplasm.

In an elegant experimental and morphometric analysis of lymph-node response to neo-

Table 3-4. Carcinoma of the Larynx: Survival as a Function of Lymph-Node Reaction

LYMPH NODE REACTION	NO. OF PATIENTS		DEAD OF DISEASE		SURVIVAL (%)	
	*Univ. Mich.**	*Berlinger et al.*†	*Univ. Mich.**	*Berlinger et al.*†	*Univ. Mich.**	*Berlinger et al.*†
Stimulated	42	27	11	3	74	89
Unstimulated	6	13	2	6	67	54
Lymphocyte depletion	0	2	—	2	—	0
Total	48	42	13	11	70.5	71.5

*Gilmore et al., 1978.
†Berlinger et al., 1976.

plasms of difficult immunogenicity, van de Velde and associates (1978) concluded that: (1) immunogenicity is *not* relevant in evoking a morphologically evident response; (2) great caution must be exercised in the interpretation of changes in lymph-node morphology as evidence of an influence of immunologic response to tumor-cell growth; and (3) the thymus-dependent areas of lymph nodes, populated mainly by T-lymphocytes, show an early increase and subsequent decrease in time with both immunogenic and nonimmunogenic neoplasms.

From the foregoing, it can be said that to date it has not been possible to establish generally valid histologic, histomorphometric, or immunocytochemical parameters for a prognostic immunostaging in resected lymph nodes (Grundmann, 1984). Resort must be made to functional studies of the complex immune system (Trinchieri and Perussia, 1984).

Antigenic Characterization of the Carcinoma

Most monoclonal antibodies that have been raised to human epithelial tumors bind to only some of the cells in a neoplasm. A similar heterogenicity is also manifested by normal epithelia, as well as cell lines and clones of epithelial cells in culture. The variability of binding is not related to the mitotic cell cycle, but it is unclear whether differences in antigen expression reflect variations in the differentiated state of the cells or merely variations in carbohydrate structures in otherwise identical cells (Edwards, 1985).

The heterogeneous expression of antigens poses problems for diagnosis, therapy, and prognostication. It is likely that cells with different surface properties have different abilities to metastasize, but attempts to identify clones with high or low potential for metastasis have been unsuccessful, perhaps because of the rapid regeneration of cell-surface properties. The absence to date of any clear relation between antigen expression and cell proliferation is disappointing (Edwards, 1985). Whether antibodies can be produced that bind to tumor cells by avoiding antibodies to carbohydrate structures that are their antigenic determinants is unknown. If the immunocytochemical properties expressed by neoplastic cells is phenotypic as well as genotypic, it may be that heterogeneous cell populations reflect only a randomization of surface structures and not a relationship to other cell properties.

The expectations of the use of monoclonal antibodies for diagnosis certainly cannot be equated to a panjandrum, but cell-surface heterogeneity remains a problem. Even though the antibodies used do not stain all tumor cells, they can detect metastases at a higher sensitivity than by morphology alone. It remains difficult-to-impossible, however, to extract any significant prognostic index from the expression of an antigen by a neoplasm.

Table 3-5. Effects of Extracapsular Invasion on Survival*

NODAL STATUS	ABSOLUTE SURVIVAL (%)	DETERMINANT SURVIVAL (%)
Histologically negative lymph nodes	62	70
Histologically positive lymph nodes without extracapsular invasion	52	62
Extracapsular invasion	28	37

*Modified from Johnson et al. (1985).

Table 3–6. Fixed Lymph Nodes (%) in Relation to Primary and T-Stage*

SITE OF PRIMARY	NO.	T_1	T_2	T_3	T_4	TOTAL
Oral cavity	287	1.2	3.2	9.6	19.3	7.3
Oropharynx	178	11.4	10.7	18.3	33.3	16.3
Nasopharynx	31	10.5	0.0	0.0	25.0	9.7
Hypopharynx cervical esophagus	331	7.9	6.6	17.0	62.0	12.4

*Modified from Stell et al. (1984).

CONVENTIONAL PATHOLOGIC EVALUATION OF CERVICAL LYMPH NODES

Extracapsular Extension and Fixation

There is a general agreement that extracapsular spread of a metastasis to a lymph node has a substantial negative effect on survival (Johnson et al., 1985; Snyderman et al., 1985). Johnson et al. (1985) have clearly demonstrated this point (Table 3–5). It is also clear that while the probability of extracapsular extension is high with lymph nodes larger than 3 cm and highest with fixed lymph nodes, a significant number of smaller lymph nodes also show this adverse histologic feature. The number of lymph nodes involved does not have a bearing on the frequency of extranodal spread, and the degree of differentiation does not appear to influence the event (except for carcinomas of the hypopharynx). Patients whose lesions manifest extension beyond the capsule of the lymph node, however, are in high clinical stages.

The effect of fixation of a lymph node is marked when considering prognosis—i.e., a 5-year survival of 7 percent for patients with unilateral fixed lymph nodes and 0 percent for bilateral fixed lymph nodes (Stell, 1983; Stell et al., 1984). The truly fixed cervical lymph node must be distinguished from one with reduced mobility. Fixation indicates attachment to adjacent structures such as mandible, base of skull, carotid artery, clavicle, deep muscles of the triangles of the neck, and the skin of the neck.

The importance of the distinction is seen in a study of carcinomas of the oral cavity and oropharynx. The 5-year cure rate for single nodes with reduced mobility was 40 percent and 13 percent for fixed lymph nodes (Stell et al., 1984). The incidence of fixed cervical nodes differs between primary sites and increases with an increase in T-stage of the primary—e.g., 4 percent with T_1 carcinomas and 18 percent for T_4 lesions (Stell et al., 1984) (Table 3–6). Sites most likely to produce fixed nodal metastases are the oropharynx, pyriform fossa, and the lower alveolus. The highest incidence is said to be in metastases from a clinically occult primary (Stell et al., 1984). A lymph node of less than 6.0 cm is unlikely to be truly fixed.

Level of Lymph Node

The fixed lymph node and extranodal extension of a metastasis appear to be the most ominous pathologic indicators of both local recurrence and prognosis (Table 3–7). Both portend an increased tumor virulence (Cachin and Eschwege, 1975). To these we add the level of the involved lymph node. The level of the node (submandibular, upper, middle and deep cervical, and posterior triangle) is dictated

Table 3–7. Patient Survival in Relation to Cervical Lymph-Node Invasion (N = 948 Cases)*

SURVIVAL	NO METASTASIS	METASTASIS CONFINED TO NODE	METASTASIS, EXTRANODAL EXTENSION
1 yr	86% (224)	67% (273)	56% (299)
3 yr	65% (158)	33% (230)	16% (213)

*Modified from Cachin and Eschwege (1975).

Table 3-8. Nodal Size and Presence of Histologic Metastases*

NODE SIZE (CM)	HISTOLOGIC STATUS (%)		
	Negative	*Positive*	*Positive and extranodal extension*
1	67	33	14
2	38	62	26
3	19	81	49
4	12	88	71
>5	0	100	76

*Adapted from Cachin (1983).

mainly by the primary carcinoma; other factors such as T or N status are not significant predictors of node level (Stell et al., 1983). In a study of 569 patients, Stell et al. (1983) found a strong association between node level and survival: a 5-year survival for patients with level 1 (submandibular) lymph nodes of 34 percent and only 4 percent for those with positive nodes at level 4.

Other Features

As with other characteristics of metastases to cervical lymph nodes, absolute numbers and percentages of positive nodes or node size are generally not useful prognostic indicators (Schuller et al., 1980). The size of a lymph node, however, does correlate with the presence of histologic metastasis (Cachin, 1983) (Table 3-8). Fairly reliable predictions of the primary site in association with involvement of groups of lymph nodes can also be made (Table 3-9). Involvement of the posterior triangle nodes by squamous cell carcinoma or noncontiguous or multiple nodal sites are associated with a poor prognosis.

REFERENCES

Bataini, J. P., Bernier, J., Brugere, J., Jaulerry, C. H., Brunin, F., and Picco, C. H.: Approche radiotherapique des adenopathies cervicales secondaries aux cancers epidermoides du larynx et du pharynx. In Pinel, J., Leroux-Robert, J. (eds.): *Adenopathies Cervicales Malignes*, Masson Publishing Co., Paris, 1982.

Bataini, J. P., Bernier, J., Brugere, J., Jaulerry, C. H., Picco, C. H., and Brunin, F.: Natural history of neck disease in patients with squamous cell carcinoma of the oropharynx and pharyngolarynx. *Radiother. Oncol.*, 3: 245-55, 1985.

Bennett, S. H., Futrell, J. W., and Roth, J. A.: Prognostic significance of histologic host response in cancer of the larynx or hypopharynx. *Cancer*, 28:1255-65, 1971.

Berlinger, N. T., Tsakraklides, V., Pollak, K., Adams, G. L., Yang, M., and Good, R. A.: Prognostic significance of lymph-node histology in patients with squamous cell carcinoma of the larynx, pharynx, or oral cavity. *Laryngoscope*, 86:792-803, 1976.

Black, M. M., and Speer, F. D.: Sinus histiocytosis of lymph nodes in cancer. *Surg. Gynecol. Obstet.*, 105: 97-102, 1957.

Borchard, F., and Quakulinski, R.: Reaktionsformen in metastasenfreien und metastatisch befallenen Lymphknoten bei Dickdarmkarzinomen. *Verh. Dtsch. Ges. Pathol.*, 68:288-94, 1984.

Byrnes, R. K., Hunter, R. L., and Vellios, F.: Immunomorphologic changes in regional lymph nodes associated with cancer. *Arch. Pathol. Lab. Med.*, 107:217-21, 1983.

Cachin, Y.: Management of cervical nodes in head and neck cancer. In Evans, P. H. R., Robin, P. E., Fielding, J. W. L. (eds.): *Head and Neck Cancer*, Alan R. Liss, Inc., New York, 1983.

Cachin, Y., and Eschewage, F.: Combination of radiotherapy and surgery in treatment of head and neck cancers. *Cancer Treat. Rev.*, 2:177-91, 1975.

Carr, I.: Lymphatic metastasis. *Cancer Metastasis Rev.*, 2:307-17, 1983.

Edwards, P. A. W.: Heterogeneous expression of cell-surface antigens in normal epithelia and their tumours, revealed by monoclonal antibodies. *Br. J. Cancer*, 51:149-60, 1985.

Fisher, E. R., Kotwal, N., Hermann, C., and Fisher, B.: Types of tumor lymphoid response and sinus histiocy-

Table 3-9. Anatomic Groups at Presentation*

ANATOMIC SITE AT PRESENTATION	POSITIVE LYMPH-NODE GROUP (%)			
	Jugular chain	*Spinal accessory chain*	*Submandibular*	*Preauricular*
Tonsil, faucial arch	74	12	13	1
Glossoepiglottic, base of tongue	85	10	4	1
Pyriform sinus	82	18	0	0
Lateral epilarynx	82	17	1	0

*Modified from Bataini et al. (1985).

tosis: Relationship to five-year, disease-free survival in patients with breast cancer. *Arch. Pathol. Lab. Med.,* 107:222–27, 1983.

Gilmore, B. B., Repola, D. A., and Batsakis, J. G.: Carcinoma of the larynx: Lymph-node reaction patterns. *Laryngoscope*, 88:1333–38, 1978.

Grundman, E.: Die lymphogene Metastasierung. *Verh. Dtsch. Ges. Pathol.*, 68:33–46, 1984.

Houck, J. R., Panje, W. R., McCormick, K. J., and Merrick, R. H.: Immunomodulatory activity in regional lymph nodes. *Arch. Otolaryngol.,* 109:785–88, 1983.

Johnson, J. T., Myers, E. N., Bedetti, C. D., Barnes, E. L., Schrammn, V. L., and Thearle, P. G.: Cervical lymph node metastases: Incidence and implications of extracapsular carcinomas. *Arch. Otolaryngol.,* 111: 534–37, 1985.

Noone, R. B., Bonner, H., and Raymond, S.: Lymph node metastasis in oral carcinoma. *Plast. Reconstr. Surg.,* 53:158–66, 1974.

Schuller, D. E., McGuirt, W. F., McCabe, B. F., and Young, D.: The prognostic significance of metastatic cervical lymph nodes. *Laryngoscope,* 90:557–70, 1980.

Schuller, D. E., Libby, D. H., Rinehart, J. J., Milo, G. G., and Koolemans-Beynen, A.: Immunomodulation of nodal lymphocytes in head and neck cancer. *Arch. Otolaryngol.,* 111:465–68, 1985.

Synderman, N. L., Johnson, J. T., Schramm, V. L., Myers, E. N., Bedetti, C. D., and Thearle, P.: Extracapsular spread of carcinoma in cervical lymph nodes: Impact upon survival in patients with carcinoma of the supraglottic larynx. *Cancer*, 56:1597–99, 1985.

Stell, P. M.: Fixed, bilateral cervical nodes. *J. Laryngol. Otol.,* 97:851–56, 1983.

Stell, P. M., Morton, R. P., and Singh, S. D.: Cervical lymph-node metastases. The significance of the level of the lymph node. *Clin. Oncol.,* 9:101–7, 1983.

Stell, P. M., Dalby, J. E., Singh, S. D.; and Taylor, W.: The fixed cervical lymph node. *Cancer*, 53:336–41, 1984.

Trinchieri, G., and Perussia, B.: Human natural killer cells: Biologic and pathologic aspects. *Lab. Invest.,* 50:489–513, 1984.

Tsakraklides, V., Olson, P., Kersey, J. H., and Good, R. A.: Prognostic significance of the regional lymph node histology in cancer of the breast. *Cancer*, 34:1259–67, 1974.

van des Oord, J. J., de Wolf-Peaters, C., and Desmet, V. J.: The paracortical area in reactive lymph nodes demonstrating sinus histiocytosis: An enzyme and immunohistochemical study. *Virchows Arch. (Cell Pathol.)*, 48:77–85, 1985.

van de Velde, C. J. H., Cornelisse, C. J., van der Velde, E. A., van Putten, L. M., and Swaveling, A.: A morphometrical analysis of lymph-node responses to tumors of different immunogenicity. *Cancer Res.*, 38: 661–67, 1978.

CHAPTER 4

Potential Application of Flow Cytometry in the Diagnosis of Metastatic Cancer of the Head and Neck

Thomas E. Carey and Jerry L. Hudson

EDITORS' COMMENT

It is obvious from the last chapter, by Dr. Batsakis and Dr. Medina, that a more sophisticated evaluation of both the primary and metastatic tissue must be made if we are to have a lasting impact on the treatment of head and neck cancer. The logical extension of this tenet is examination of the cellular characteristics and contents of tumor in vitro; this can be accomplished by the relatively new technique of flow cytometry.

Though they are young laboratory investigators, Dr. Carey and Dr. Hudson have acquired a unique knowledge since 1980 of the use of flow cytometry in head and neck cancer. After briefly describing the components and technique of the flow cytometer, the authors identify its specific application to squamous tumor cells in vitro evaluating the DNA and chromosomal content as well as the cell-surface antigens expressed by these cancers. Using these data, they are developing monoclonal antibodies specific for membrane antigens of squamous cell carcinoma. This might be the first step in the development of a test for early detection of squamous cancer, whether primary or recurrent.

Although the clinician might not find this information immediately germane, it is obvious that basic research along the lines of flow cytometry is essential because the implications for diagnosis, staging, treatment, and prognosis are clear. All of us in clinical medicine must have an open mind and give a helping hand and a sympathetic ear to the work of basic researchers such as Dr. Carey and Dr. Hudson if we are to find the answers to the cure (and hopefully the prevention) of head and neck cancer.

Work reported in this chapter was supported in part by grants Nos. CA 28564 and CA35929 from the National Cancer Institute. Support was also received from the EPICS Division, Coulter Corporation, Hialeah, Florida. Dr. Carey is the recipient of Research Career Development Award No. CA 00621 from the National Cancer Institute.

INTRODUCTION

For the past 5 years, our laboratory has been investigating the biologic and antigenic features that characterize human squamous carcinomas (Carey, 1985). The goal of these investigations is to gain information that will be useful for more effective diagnosis and treatment of squamous cancers of the head and neck and prediction of their clinical courses. A critical feature of our approach has been the development and characterization of cell lines from primary, recurrent, and metastatic squamous carcinomas (Krause et al., 1981; Carey et al., 1983; Grossman et al., 1984). These cultured tumor lines have made it possible for us to assess the expression of cell-surface antigens that are specifically and commonly displayed by squamous cancers, and have made possible the development of monoclonal antibodies to squamous cell antigens (Carey et al., 1983; Kimmel et al., 1985). We have also used the cell lines to examine the relative DNA content and the chromosome content of cancer cells from early and recurrent or metastatic tumors, in some cases by studying multiple cell lines from the same patient (Roa et al., 1985).

Using the information gained from these in vitro studies on pure populations of malignant cells, it should now be possible to examine mixed populations from clinical specimens—particularly cervical lymph nodes—to assess whether or not tumor cells are present. In fact, recent experiments with both primary and metastatic tumor-cell lines from individual patients suggest that it may also be possible to predict the relative biologic aggressiveness of metastatic tumors (Roa et al., 1985; Kimmel and Carey, in press).

In this chapter, we will briefly describe the components and functions of the flow cytometer and show how information gained in the laboratory may soon be used with this technology to more effectively diagnose—and therefore more effectively treat—head and neck cancer metastatic to the neck.

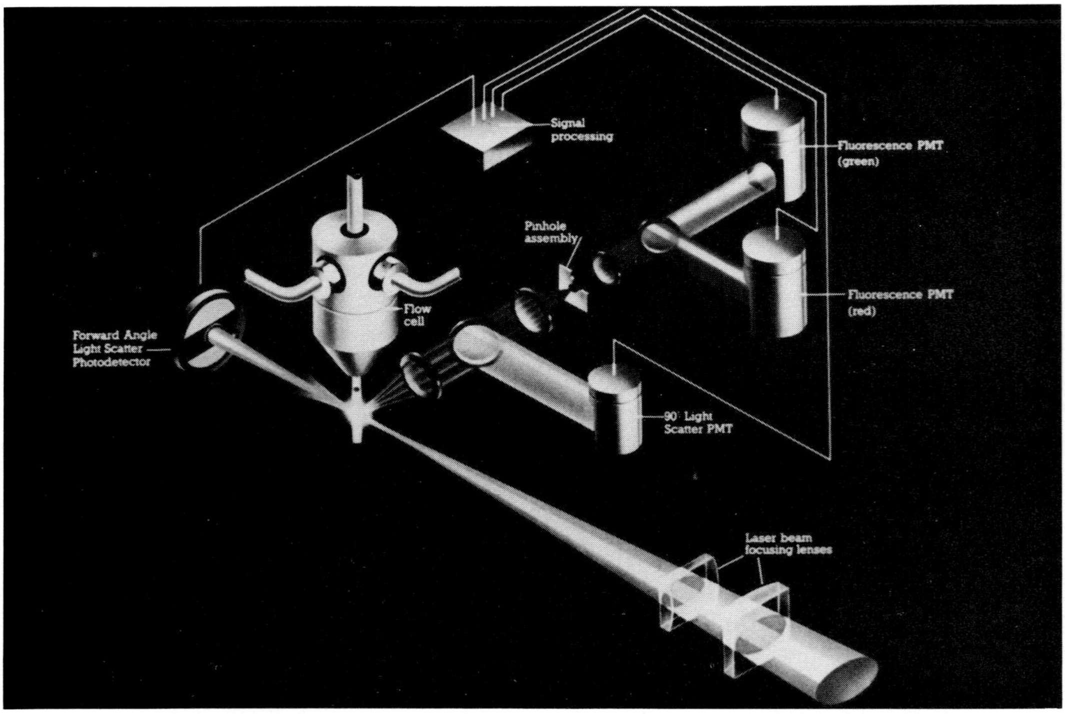

Figure 4–1. Schematic illustration of the components of a flow cytometry system. The important features include the flow cell; the laser and the light path; the optical assembly; the detectors for light signals; and the computer that stores and processes the information (PMT = photomultiplier tube). (Provided courtesy of EPICS Division of Coulter Corporation.)

THE FLOW CYTOMETER

The flow cytometer is a device that can measure and record multiple characteristics of individual cells passing one at a time through an intense beam of light (see Figures 4–1 and Figure 4–2) (for detailed reviews, see Lovett et al., 1984; Hudson et al., 1985; and Muirhead et al., 1985). This sophisticated machine can

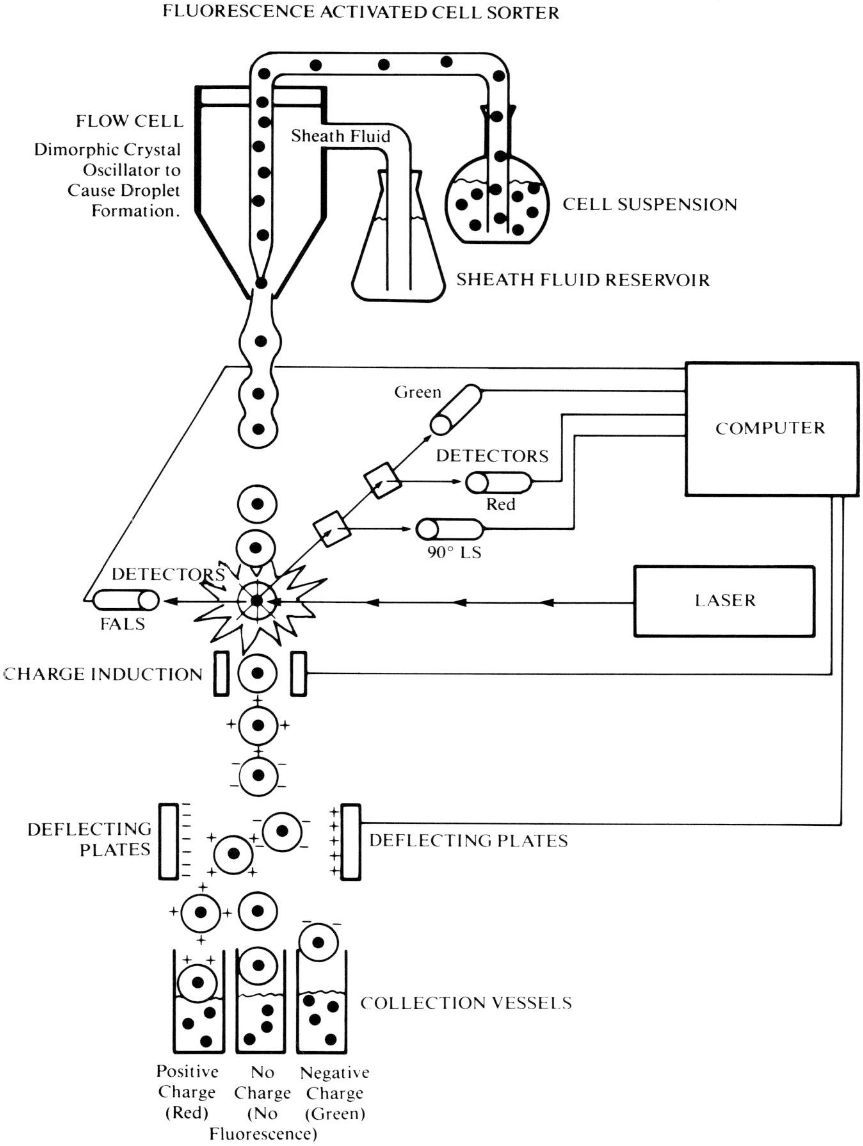

Figure 4–2. Cutaway line drawing of a flow cytometer equipped for cell sorting, showing the path of the cells as they flow through the light beam and the sorting mechanism. As individual cells pass through the light beam, they scatter and emit light in 360°. Sensors or optical detector units are arrayed both in the forward direction of the laser beam for collection of forward angle light scatter (FLS) and at 90° to the laser beam to sample the 360° light scatter. Filters and dichroic mirrors split the beam to appropriate sensors for 90°LS, red fluorescence, green fluorescence, or other wavelengths of light be emitted from specific fluorochromes in the cells. For cell sorting, the computer is programmed to induce a charge on droplets immediately following receipt of information about the light scatter or light-emitting properties of a cell. The charged droplets are then deflected by charged plates, and droplets containing cells with similar properties will be sorted together. For example, all droplets containing a cell with green fluorescence might be given a negative charge. These droplets would be deflected toward the positively charged plate while droplets with cells stained red would be given a positive charge, deflected toward the negatively charged plate. Droplets containing unstained cells would remain uncharged.

assess and store multiple data points per cell on as many as 10,000 cells each second.

Taken separately, the components of the flow cytometer are simple to comprehend. They consist of a flow cell, a light source, an optical detector system, and a computer system. The flow cell creates a fine stream of fluid that carries the cells through the interrogating light beam. The light source provides a highly focused, intense light beam that intersects the fluid stream perpendicularly. A mercury-arc lamp may be used as the light source, but lasers that can be tuned to deliver a range of wavelengths are usually used. The optical detector units consist of sensors, filters, and photomultiplier tubes designed to collect the light scattered and emitted from each cell. The photodetectors are aligned both in the laser path to collect light scattered in the forward direction, and orthogonally to the laser path to sample, at 90°, the light that is scattered and emitted in 360° by each cell. Each of the photomultiplier tubes delivers its information to the data acquisition computer, where the information is digitized and stored. In some instruments, the system operation is under computer control.

Light-Scatter Analysis

Individual cells can be interrogated by the light beam in essentially two ways. The first is by use of the inherent light-scattering properties of cells, which provides information about cell size and granularity. The second is by the use of fluorochromes, which emit light of a characteristic wavelength after excitation by the incident laser beam. Such fluorochromes can be endogenous to the cells, but they are most often dyes or fluorescent compounds used to label either surface or internal structures of the cell. Two commonly used types of fluorescent probes are fluorochrome-conjugated antibodies to cellular structures and photon-emitting dyes, which bind stoichiometrically to nucleic acids.

Cell Sorting

While much information can be gained from the analysis of light-scatter and fluorescence-emission data, many flow cytometers are also equipped for cell sorting to allow collection of separate cell populations on the basis of particular cytometric characteristics. Sorting is achieved by use of computer logic, which causes the fluid stream containing the cells to be given a positive or negative charge whenever a cell with certain preselected criteria passes the detector. The stream breaks up into individual droplets as a result of oscillation induced upstream by the nozzle, and the charged droplets containing individual cells can be deflected to the right or the left by charged plates in the sorting chamber (Figure 4–2). Using current technology, approximately 5,000 to 10,000 cells per second can be sorted by these devices (Muirhead et al., 1985).

Single-Parameter Versus Multiparameter Analysis

Multiple traits of each cell in a population are measured by the flow cytometer, and the data points for each trait of each cell are stored in a histogram. In single-parameter analysis, the intensity value of the measured parameter for each of the cells is presented in a frequency distribution. In multiple parameter analysis, two or more frequency distributions may be combined. To appreciate how flow cytometer data can be interpreted, let us consider the information conveyed by light scatter based on intrinsic cellular properties. The incident light is scattered in 360° by collision with subcellular organelles and structures. The amount of light scattered in the forward direction is proportional to cell size. This light scatter is recorded by the forward angle light scatter (FLS) detector located in the path of the laser beam.

An example of a one-parameter histogram in which frequency (i.e., number of particles) is shown as a function of FLS is shown in Figure 4–3. In this example, the mononuclear cell fraction of peripheral blood leukocytes was analyzed. When this population is studied by the single parameter of FLS, a relatively homogeneous size distribution is obtained, even though the sample contains both monocytes and lymphocytes. In a second example, shown in Figure 4–4, peripheral whole-blood leuko-

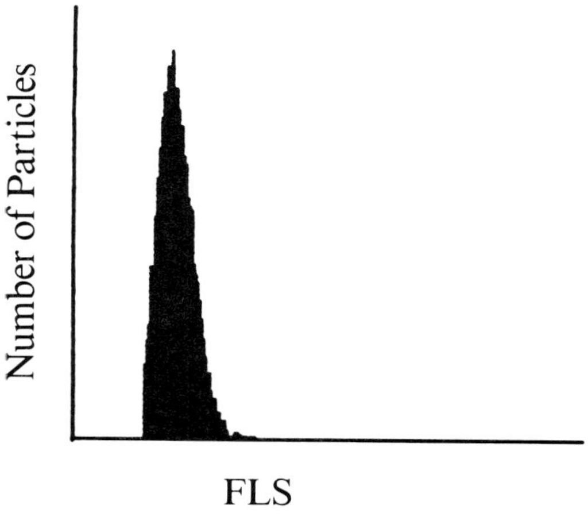

Figure 4-3. Flow cytometry histogram showing particle number as a function of forward light scatter. Forward light scatter (FLS) is used as a measure of cell size. This figure shows the results obtained when a sample of mononuclear leukocytes (lymphocytes and monocytes) from human peripheral blood was assessed for FLS.

cytes—a mixed population of cells including lymphocytes, monocytes, and granulocytes—was used. By taking advantage of a second intrinsic light-scattering parameter, this population can be resolved into three subgroups.

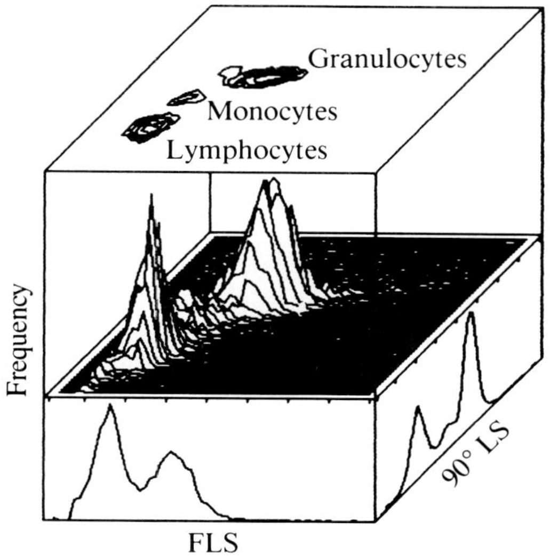

Figure 4-4. Three-dimensional representation of flow cytometric data from a sample of human peripheral blood leukocytes. Frequency (particle number) on the vertical axis is shown as a function of forward light scatter (FLS) (cell size) on the horizontal axis, and as a function of 90° LS, which is a measure of cell granularity, on the depth axis. Note that three separate populations can be discriminated in the mixed cell sample by using two-parameter analysis: cell size (FLS) and granularity (90° LS).

In this three-dimensional figure, frequency on the vertical axis is shown as a function of FLS (cell size) on the horizontal axis and as a function of 90° light scatter (90°LS), which is a measure of cell granularity, on the depth axis. Although either parameter alone can partially resolve the complex population, three populations can be distinguished when both parameters are used, as shown in the center of the figure. This can also be readily appreciated from a contour analysis or two-dimensional representation of the FLS versus the 90° LS as shown at the top of Figure 4–4 and in Figure 4–5.

In Figure 4–5, three areas of contour lines representing clustered data points can be seen. Near the origin are the small, low-granularity lymphocytes. Next along the 90°LS axis are the small size but intermediate granularity monocytes. Farthest down the 90°LS axis, and also down the FLS axis, are the highly granular, large granulocytes.

Using contour analysis it is possible to set electronic gates, as shown in Figure 4–5, to examine specific cell populations, discriminated by one set of parameters, for the expression of a different characteristic. In the example shown, leukocytes are discriminated into three populations by their FLS and 90°LS properties. By setting electronic gates or bit maps around each population, one can direct the flow cytometer to report the expression of a different parameter such as cell-surface fluorescence for each population. In the example shown in the figure, three samples of the same blood specimen were stained with fluoresceinated antibodies against three cell-surface antigens were used.

From histograms showing frequency as a function of fluorescence, it is clear that the population enclosed within the bit map includes cells that express the T4 thymic lymphocyte marker and cells that express the B1 marker of B-lymphocytes, but not the monocyte marker MO2. If the electronic gates were placed around the monocyte population, a different pattern of fluoroescence would be observed. The MO2 staining would be strong on many cells in the population, but few or no cells would express fluorescence with the T4 or B1 antibodies. Later in this chapter we will

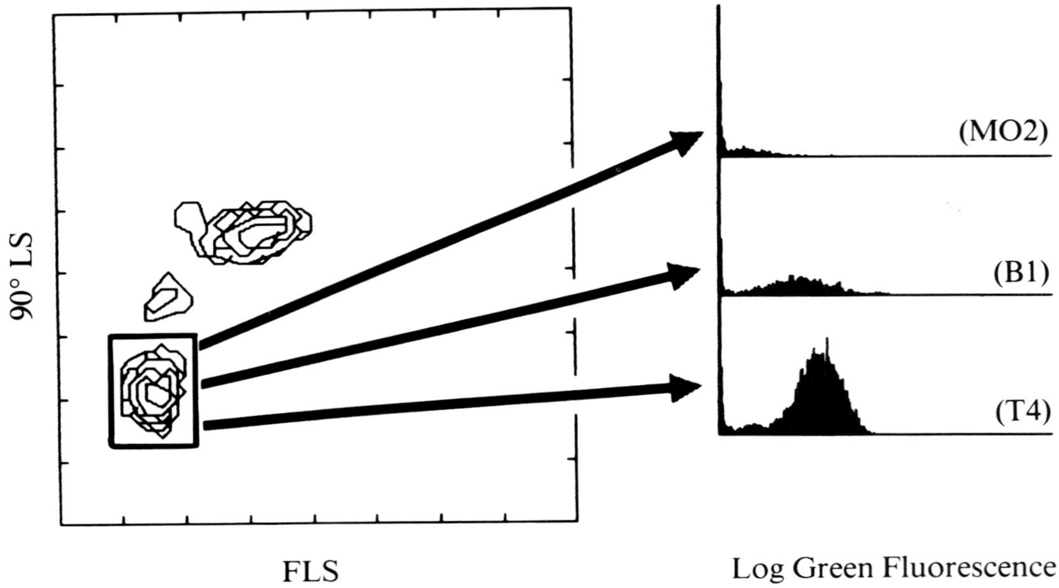

Figure 4–5. Contour maps. In the panel on the left, 90 ° light scatter (90° LS) on the y-axis is shown as a function of forward light scatter on the x-axis. Electronic gates have been placed around the contour or bit map of the lymphocyte population as discriminated by the two-parameter analysis (see Figure 4–4). A third parameter, fluorescent antibody binding, is shown on the right side of the figure. Frequency is plotted as a function of fluorescence intensity (log green fluorescence). Monoclonal antibodies to the T_4 T-lymphocyte antigen, the B-1 B-lymphocyte antigen, and the MO2 monocyte antigen were used.

suggest how this kind of multiparameter analysis can be applied to the detection of occult metastatic disease in the neck.

Flow Cytometric DNA Analysis

The analysis of cellular DNA content is an important application of flow cytometry (Vindelov et al., 1983a; Lovett et al., 1984; Muirhead et al., 1985; Hudson et al., 1985). This method can be used to detect cells with abnormal DNA content (Vindelov et al., 1983b; Moberger et al., 1984) to carry out cell-cycle analysis (Lovett et al., 1984), and even to distinguish the differences in DNA content of cells from men and women based on the greater DNA content of the x-chromosome (Vindelov et al., 1983c).

A variety of dyes have been used to stain DNA. The intercalating compounds ethidium bromide and propidium iodide are perhaps the most widely used. Although these compounds bind stoichiometrically to the DNA, they also combine with double-stranded RNA. Therefore, nuclei are usually prepared from whole cells by detergent lysis of the cell membrane in the presence of RNase before staining (Vindelov et al., 1983b). In some cases, it is useful to stain the DNA of live cells. For this purpose, the DNA-specific Hoechst stains 33258 and 33342 can be used (Muirhead et al., 1985). Vital DNA staining is useful for sorting viable cells and for dual-parameter analysis when both DNA content and membrane antigen staining are to be assessed on the same cell population.

FLOW CYTOMETRIC STUDIES OF SQUAMOUS CARCINOMA CELL LINES

Recently, we and our co-workers (Roa et al., 1985) reported the results of our studies of DNA content and chromosome number in 15 human squamous carcinoma cell lines. To determine the relative DNA content of individual tumor-cell lines, internal standards of known DNA content were used (Vindelov et al., 1983a). With these standards, it was also possible to compare the results of separate experiments over a period of several months by using the computer to adjust the histograms of separate runs so that internal standard peaks would be aligned.

The standards used in these experiments were chicken and trout nucleated red blood cells and lymphocytes from peripheral blood of normal human volunteers. Chicken red cells have approximately 20 percent of the DNA of human cells, whereas trout red cells have a DNA content equal to about 80 percent of that of human somatic cells. An example of propidium-iodide-stained nuclei from chicken and trout red cells, human lymphocytes, and one of the human squamous carcinoma lines is shown in Figure 4–6.

The histograms produced when such samples are analyzed by the flow cytometer are shown in Figure 4–7. In this figure, frequency on the y-axis is shown as a function of red fluorescence on the x-axis. Chicken red cells have the lowest DNA content, bind the least propidium iodide, and therefore have the lowest level of fluorescence; thus, the chicken cells are represented by the first large peak at the left of the histogram. The trout cells appear as the second peak, the lymphocytes as the third peak, and the squamous cancer cells, which have an abnormal DNA content with the highest fluorescent intensity, appear as the fourth peak. Only the three controls were present in the sample used for the lowest panel, whereas for the upper panels, UM-SCC-8 (top) and UM-SCC-5 (middle) were also tested.

Figure 4–8 shows the results obtained in three separate experiments with four of the squamous carcinoma lines. In each panel of the figure, the positions of the chicken red cell peak and the human lymphocyte peak were translocated by the computer to the same channel numbers, thus normalizing peak positions so that the position of the squamous cancer-cell DNA distribution could be compared. From this comparison and from a comparison of the DNA index, which is a ratio of the DNA content in the tumor cells to that of

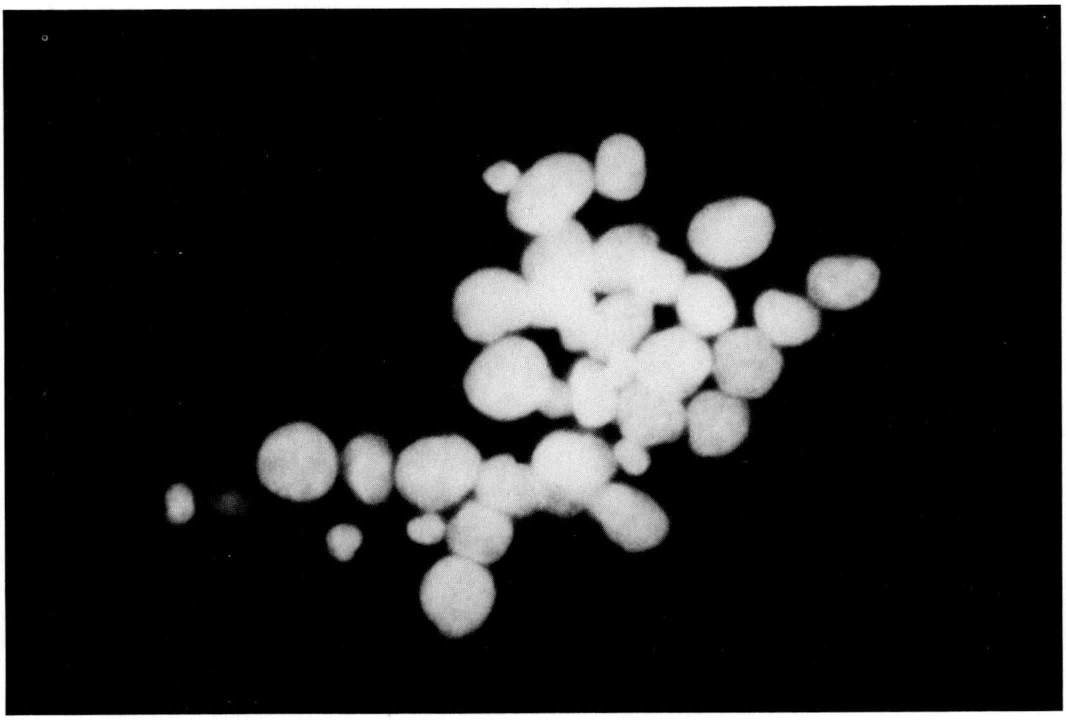

Figure 4–6. Fluorescence photomicrograph of a mixture of Propidium-iodide-stained nuclei. Nuclei prepared from chicken and trout erythrocytes, human lymphocytes, and UM-SCC-11A squamous carcinoma cells were mixed together and treated with NP-40 detergent to lyse the cell membrane and ribonuclease and digest double-stranded RNA (Vindelov et al., 1983b). The nuclei were then stained with the intercalating dye propidium iodide (PI). PI-stained nuclei emit red fluorescence on excitation with blue-green light (original magnification 100×).

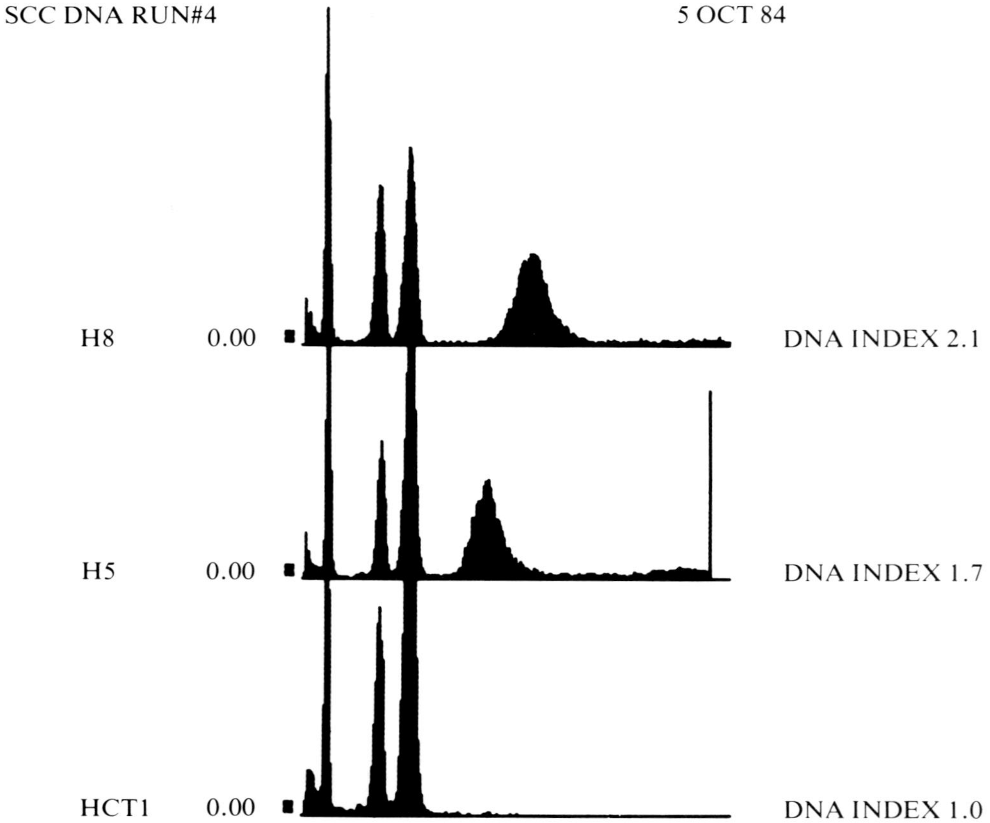

Figure 4–7. Flow cytometry histograms showing red fluorescence intensity on the x-axis and frequency on the y-axis. Propidium-iodide-stained nuclei from chicken erythrocytes, trout erythrocytes, and normal human lymphocytes serve as internal standards and have 20 percent, 80 percent, and 100 percent of the normal somatic DNA content of human cells. The standards are shown in the bottom panel. The peaks from left to right are chicken nuclei, trout nuclei, and lymphocyte nuclei. In the top panel UM-SCC-8 and in the middle panel UM-SCC-5 squamous carcinoma cells were also in the sample. In each case, the chicken red-cell peak and the human lymphocyte peak were translocated by the computer to normalize the peak positions so that individual experiments could be compared.

the normal lymphocytes, it is apparent that little variation in the DNA content of individual cell lines was observed over the 7-month period spanned by the experiments in this series. Yet wide variation in DNA content was found among the cell lines, including cell lines derived from primary and recurrent tumors from the same patient (see Figure 4–9). Since the DNA content of individual lines was stable over approximately 20 in-vitro passages, it is unlikely that the wide range of DNA content arose solely as an artifact of culture. Rather, it likely reflects an in-vivo evolution that occurs in the patients during tumor progression.

With this concept in mind, we compared the DNA content and chromosome number of each cell line. This comparison is shown in Figure 4–9. Initially, we expected that more advanced tumors would have accumulated the greatest DNA content; if so, the cell lines at the upper right end of Figure 4–9 should represent the most aggressive cancers. Instead, we found in almost every case that if more than one cell line was established from the same patient, then the first cell line established had a higher DNA content or chromosome number than the cell line established from a later recurrence or metastasis. We have noted that the cell lines from the secondary tumors that had lower DNA content than the primary tumors also exhibited more aggressive growth in vitro and in vivo in nude mice than the cell line

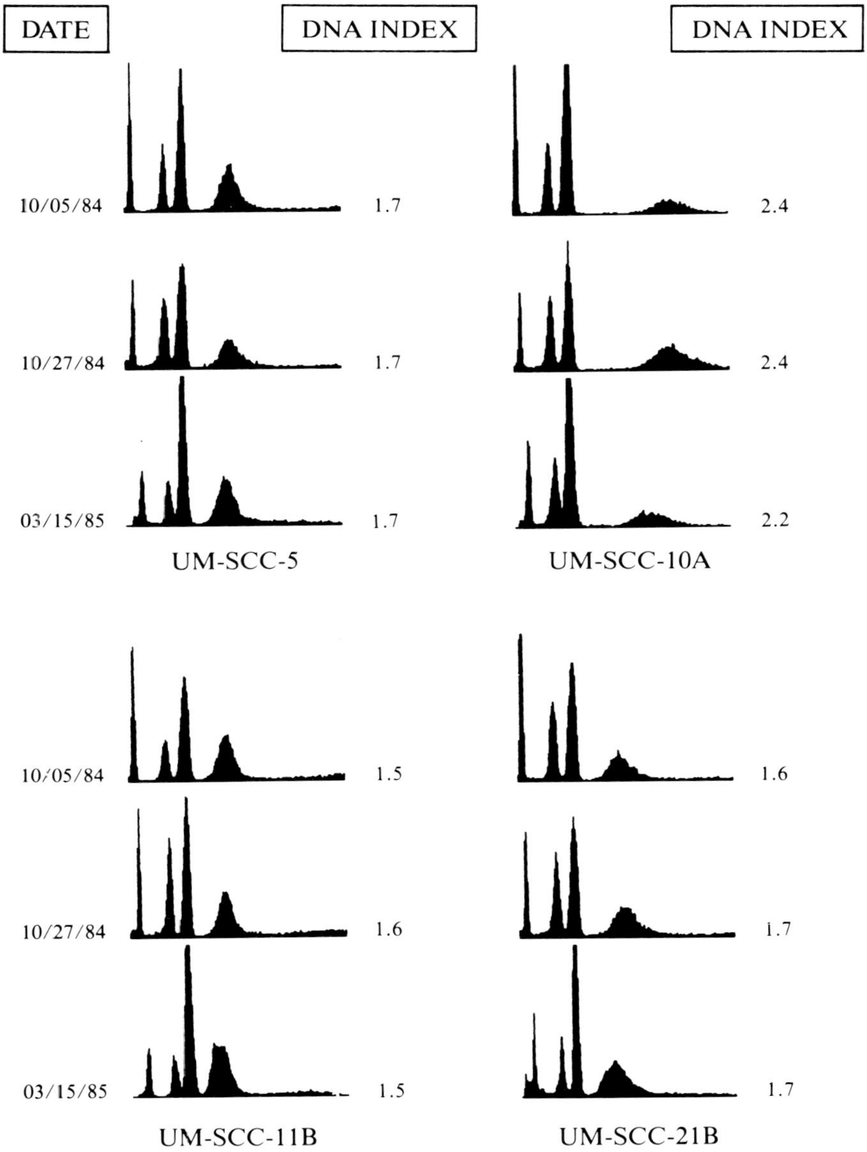

Figure 4–8. Propidium-iodide-stained DNA-fluorescence histograms showing DNA content of four different squamous carcinoma cell lines. Nuclear DNA histograms from experiments run on three separate dates are shown for each of four UM-SCC-cell lines in each panel of the figure. Note that tumor-cell DNA content showed very little change in three experiments over a 7-month interval. The stability of the DNA content is numerically represented by the DNA index values (a ratio of the tumor cell DNA to the lymphocyte DNA) shown on the right side of each histogram. (Reproduced with permission from Roa et al., 1985. Copyright 1985, American Medical Association.)

from the primary tumor from the same individual (Carey et al., manuscript in preparation).

These observations suggest that early in tumor development, perhaps even at the initial step, there is an increase in DNA content that confers abnormal growth behavior on the cells. Later in tumor progression, random loss of chromosomes may occur, reducing the DNA content toward the normal level. When such random loss decreases the requirement for total DNA synthesis without also eliminat-

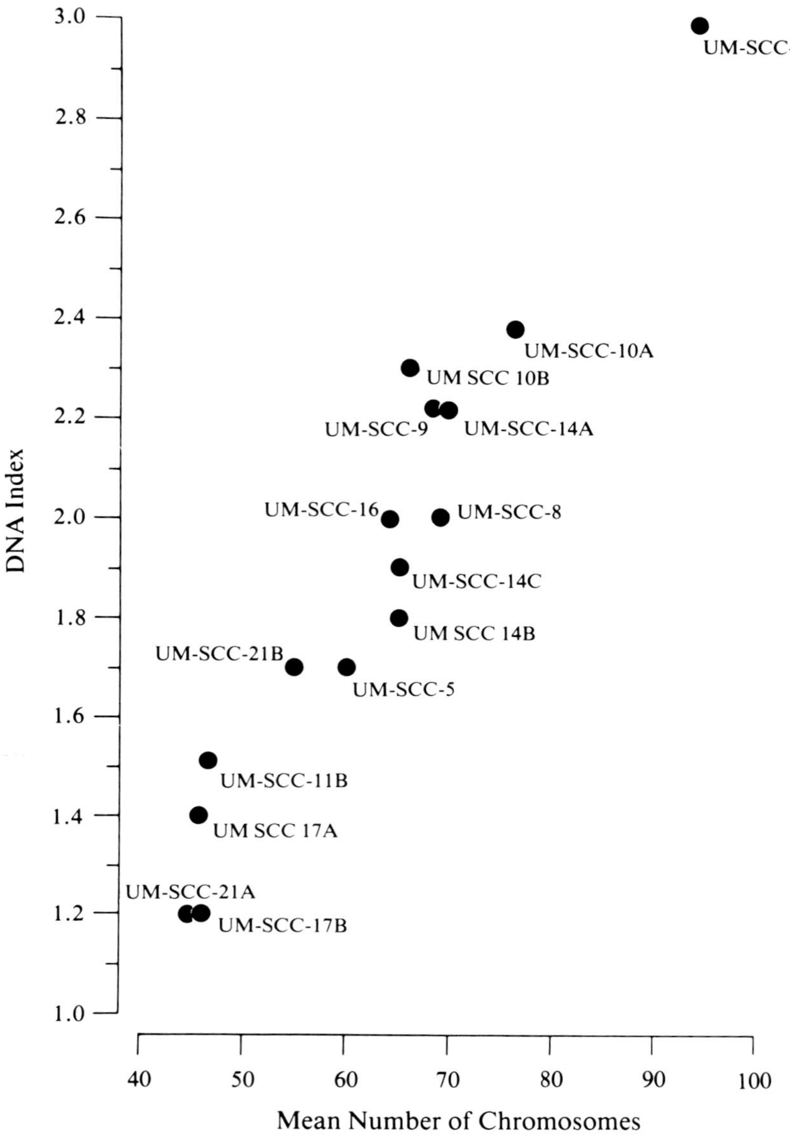

Figure 4–9. DNA index as a function of the mean number of chromosomes. DNA index determined by flow cytometry appears to be a more sensitive measure of increased DNA content than chromosome enumeration. Four cell lines with a near diploid number of chromosomes (UM-SCC-17A, 17B, 11B, and 21A) were shown by flow cytometry to have elevated DNA indices. From the data in this figure, a relationship between tumor progression and DNA content can be observed. Cell lines from early tumors (cell lines designated A) in four of five cases had higher DNA content than lines established from later recurrences or metastases in the same patients (cell lines designated B). See 10A and B, 11A and B, 14A and B, and 17A and B. Note that only 21A and 21B did not show this pattern (Reproduced with permission from Roa et al., 1985. Copyright 1985, American Medical Association.)

ing chromosomes or chromosome fragments that carry genes encoding growth factors, the emergence of cell populations with more aggressive growth characteristics is favored. In contrast, cells that accumulate or retain high DNA content must expend greater effort on DNA synthesis, and consequently may grow more slowly than cells with a decreased requirement for DNA synthesis.

Our findings indicate that most head and neck squamous cell cancers have abnormal DNA content. The flow cytometer can detect abnormal DNA content even in cancers with an apparently normal chromosome count (see

Figure 4–9), in which the net effect of chromosome translocations, duplications, and deletions results in abnormal nuclear DNA content. Together, this suggests to us that flow cytometric DNA analysis can be used diagnostically. Most likely this will be accomplished in conjunction with the use of a second marker such as a monoclonal antibody to a squamous cell-specific antigen. The initial application we envision would be the detection of subclinical lymph-node metastases among apparently uninvolved lymph nodes removed at the time of radical neck dissection. Later, this approach might be used for assessment of needle aspirates, and even to survey blood samples in the venous drainage from the site of tumor excision to monitor whether intraoperative manipulations cause tumor cells to enter the peripheral circulatory system.

MONOCLONAL ANTIBODY TO SQUAMOUS CANCER CELLS

Single-parameter analysis (i.e., DNA content measurements) to identify squamous cancer cells in cell suspensions prepared from cervical lymph nodes may not be adequate to prove the presence of metastasis, since polymorphonuclear leukocytes and granulocytes are large granular cells that may also appear to have elevated DNA content. Furthermore, a recent report by Bijman et al. (1985) using flow cytometry listed DNA indices of 1.0 for a high proportion of primary head and neck cancer specimens. Therefore, dual-parameter analysis, in which an antibody to a squamous carcinoma cell-membrane antigen and a vital DNA stain are used, should identify, among lymph-node cell populations, only those cells that have both of the cancer cell characteristics.

A main focus of our laboratory is the development of monoclonal antibodies specific for membrane antigens of squamous cell carcinoma. One of these antibodies, A9, is directed against an antigen that has been found on all the UM-SCC squamous cancer cell lines, and increases in expression on cell lines from secondary or metastatic tumors compared with lines established from early or primary tumors from the same individual (Kimmel and Carey, in press). Increased expression of this antigen is also associated with more aggressive in vitro growth behavior and the ability of cell lines to produce tumors in the nude mouse (Carey et al., unpublished observations). The antigen detected by the A9 antibody has not been found on lymphoid cells. It is resistant to trypsin and has been found on tumor cells in frozen tissue sections from 100 percent of the more than 50 head and neck cancer biopsy specimens that have been tested. These features make it likely that the A9 antibody will be useful for detecting cancer cells in cervical metastatic sites.

We are presently testing this antibody for indirect fluorescent membrane labeling of cultured squamous carcinoma cells in a mixed population of lymphocytes and tumor cells. Preliminary results show that squamous cancer cells can be detected by cell-surface fluorescence in such cell mixtures at tumor-cell densities as low as 1 in 10,000 (Baugh et al., unpublished data).

We foresee that mechanical and trypsin dissociation of cervical lymph nodes can be used to prepare dispersed cell suspensions for dual-parameter flow cytometric analysis. Dissociated intact cells will be stained wiith a DNA-specific dye and with the monoclonal antibody to assess both the DNA content and the level and intensity of A9 expression. If this method works well with lymph-node specimens, it will eventually be used to make similar preparations from primary cancer specimens to compare the DNA content and A9 antigen expression in primary and metastatic tumors to try to confirm the results predicted by in vitro cell-culture studies.

One potential problem with this approach is the dificulty that may be encountered in preparing monodispersed intact cells from squamous cancer specimens. We have great experience with the use of trypsin and ethylenediaminetetraacetic acid (EDTA) for dissociating cells in culture for flow cytometric analysis of A9 surface staining. If problems are encountered in preparing whole cells from fresh tissues and lymph nodes, however, a similar dual-parameter approach will still be possible using only nuclei because intact nuclei can be prepared routinely from both fresh and frozen head and neck cancer specimens (Lampe et al., 1984). In the latter case, markers recently described for nonhistone nuclear proteins, the expression of which is altered in cancer cells, could be used (personal communication, Dr. Kenneth Bauer, 1985).

DISCUSSION

The results of this type of flow cytometric analysis of clinical specimens should make it possible to detect subclinical metastatic disease in patients with head and neck cancer. Therefore, it may help to select those patients who should receive adjunctive therapy in the form of chemotherapy or radiation. Furthermore, information may be obtained from the intensity of cell-surface antigen expression and the relative DNA content that will have prognostic significance for patients with metastatic disease in the neck.

REFERENCES

Bijman, J. T., Wagner, D. J., van Rannes, H., Wessels, J. M. C., and van den Broek, P.: Flow cytometric evaluation of cell dispersion from human head and neck tumors. *Cytometry*, 6:334–41, 1985.

Carey, T. E.: Establishment of epidermoid carcinoma cell lines. In Wittes, R. E. (ed.): *Head and Neck Cancer*, pp. 287–314. John Wiley, London, 1985.

Carey, T. E., Kimmel, K. A., Schwartz, D. R., Richter, D. E., Baker, S. R., and Krause, C. J.: Antibodies to human squamous cell carcinoma. *Otolaryngol. Head Neck Surg.*, 91:482–91, 1983.

Grossman, H. B., Wedemeyer, G., Ren, L., and Carey, T. E.: UM-SCP-1, a new human cell line derived from a prostatic squamous cell carcinoma. *Cancer Res.*, 44:4111–17, 1984.

Hudson, J. L., Duque, R. E., and Lovett, E. J., III: Applications of flow cytometry in immunotoxicology. In Dean, J. et al.: (eds.): *Immunotoxicology and Pharmacology*, pp. 157–77, Raven Press, New York, 1985.

Kimmel, K. A., and Carey, T. E.: Altered expression in squamous cells of an orientation restricted epithelial antigen detected by monoclonal antibody A9. *Cancer Res.*, in press, 1986.

Kimmel, K. A., Carey, T. E., Judd, W. J., and McClatchey, K. D.: Monoclonal antibody (G10) to a common antigen of human squamous cell carcinoma: Binding to the H type 2 blood group determinant. *J. Natl. Cancer Inst.*, 76:9–19, 1986.

Krause, C. J., Carey, T. E., Ott, R. W., Hurbis, C., McClatchey, K. D., and Regezi, J. A.: Human squamous cell carcinoma: Establishment on a characterization of new cell lines. *Arch. Otolaryngol.*, 107:703–10, 1981.

Lampe, H., Flint, A., Wolf, G., McClatchey, K., and Hudson, J.: Flow cytometry: DNA analysis of squamous cell carcinoma of the upper aerodigestive tract. *Proc. Int. Conf. Head Neck Cancer*, Abst. #65, p. 46, 1984.

Lovett, E. J., III, Schnitzer, B., Keren, D. F., Flint, A., Hudson, J. L., and McClatchey, K. D.: Application of flow cytometry to diagnostic pathology. *Lab. Invest.*, 40:115–40, 1984.

Moberger, B., Auer, G., Forsslund, G., and Moberger, G.: The prognostic significance of DNA measurements in endometrial carcinoma. *Cytometry*, 5:430–36, 1984.

Muirhead, K. A., Horan, P. D., and Poste, G.: Flow cytometry: Present and future. *Biotechnology*, 3:337–56, 1985.

Roa, R. A., Carey, T. E., Passamani, P. P., Greenwood, J. H., Hsu, S., Ridings, E. O., Schwartz, D. R., Wolf, G. T., and Hudson, J. L.: DNA content of human squamous cell carcinoma cell lines: Analysis by flow cytometry and chromosome enumeration. *Arch. Otolaryngol.*, 111:565–75, 1985.

Vindelov, L. L., Christensen, I. J., and Nissen, N. L.: Standardization of high-resolution flow cytometric DNA analysis by the simultaneous use of chicken and trout red blood cells as internal reference standards. *Cytometry*, 3:328–31, 1983a.

Vindelov, L. L., Christensen, I. J., Jensen, G., and Nissen, N. L.: Limits of detection of nuclear DNA abnormalities by flow cytometric DNA analysis: Results obtained by a set of methods for sample-storage, staining, and internal standardization. *Cytometry*, 3:332–39, 1983b.

Vindelov, L. L., Christensen, I. J., and Nissen, N. L.: A detergent-trypsin method for the preparation of nuclei for flow cytometric DNA analysis. *Cytometry*, 3:323–27, 1983c.

CHAPTER 5

Prognostic Factors in Neck Node Metastasis

Gordon B. Snow, Alfons J. M. Balm, J. W. Arendse, A. B. M. F. Karim, H. Bartelink, I. van der Waal, and R. M. Tiwari

EDITORS' COMMENT

By following the observation of the French head and neck surgeon, Y. Cachin, Dr. Gordon Snow develops the tenet that extracapsular extension of tumor outside the lymph node results in a profound change in the prognosis of the patient with regional metastasis from head and neck cancer. Head and neck surgeons have long recognized the importance of nodal metastases, but it has been appreciated only recently that the microscopic extension beyond the capsule of the lymph node has significant bearing on the prognosis and hence the definitive treatment of the patient. The reporting of Dr. Snow in this chapter and Dr. Myers and Dr. Johnson in the next chapter has demonstrated the value of meticulous evaluation of the pathologic specimen, as noted by Dr. Batsakis in Chapter 3.

In Chapter 5, Dr. Snow identifies the importance of nodal disease as observed by both the American Joint Committee on End Results Reporting (AJC) in the United States and the International Union Against Cancer (UICC) worldwide. He then clearly outlines the importance of extranodal extension of disease by the analysis of two comparable series of patients who underwent radical neck dissection: one with 405 patients treated between 1950 and 1975 and another with 331 patients treated between 1973 and 1983. By identifying the actuarial data on the patients who failed at regional and distant sites, Dr. Snow demonstrates dramatically the profound effect extracapsular extension has on survival.

Taking this information one step further, Dr. Snow identifies the value of the neck dissection as both a therapeutic and diagnostic procedure. The impact of the pathologic evaluation of extracapsular extension should dictate more aggressive regional therapy in the form of adjunctive radiotherapy. Dr. Snow also shows that when more than three lymph nodes have extracapsular extension, there is a more than 50 percent chance of distant metastases within 24 months. Cautiously, but appropriately, he suggests that this is the patient in whom adjunctive chemotherapy might be indicated. The use of chemotherapy in this and other high-risk patients is reviewed and evaluated by Dr. Hong and Dr. Dimery in Chapters 15 and 16.

INTRODUCTION

It is generally recognized that the status of the cervical lymph nodes is the single most important prognostic factor in squamous cell carcinoma of the head and neck (Farr et al., 1972; Spiro et al., 1974; Kalnins et al., 1977; Cachin et al., 1979). Although nodal metastases, at presentation or developing subsequently, severely affect the prognosis—cure rates decrease roughly by half (Spiro et al., 1974)—the presence of nodal metastases does not imply a hopeless prognosis. Pointon et al. (1976), for instance, reviewed a series of patients with primary mouth and lip cancer undergoing radical neck dissection at some stage in the disease, and the 5-year survival figures varied from 35 to 53 percent depending on the site of the primary tumor. Similarly, in a large series of patients with squamous cell carcinoma of the head and neck we have reported an actuarial 5-year survival of 40 percent for patients undergoing radical neck dissection (Snow et al., 1982).

Clinical assessment of the status of neck nodes is still based on palpation. Fine-needle aspiration cytology (Zajicek, 1974) is an effective technique for establishing a tentative histologic diagnosis in patients presenting with a neck mass without an obvious primary tumor in the head and neck. This method is of little use, however, in the initial workup of the patient presenting with a primary squamous cell carcinoma of the upper air and food passages. Friedman et al. (1984) have shown that computed tomographic (CT) scanning can be of value in selected cases in detecting occult metastases in the neck. It is questionable, however, whether the cost justifies the results (Cantrell, 1984).

The palpability of a lymph node depends on its location, consistency, size, and type of neck. In an average-sized neck, the lower limit of palpability is approximately 0.5 cm in a superficial area, such as the submental and submandibular area, and 1 cm in a deeper area (Sako et al., 1964). Therefore, nodes containing small deposits of carcinoma may not be clinically palpable. On the contrary, not all enlarged nodes contain metastasic deposits. Moreover, large interobserver variations have been reported. It is not surprising, therefore, that the overall error in assessing the presence or absence of cervical lymph node metastasis is reported to be in the range of 20 to 30 percent (Sako et al., 1964; Spiro et al., 1974; Ali et al., 1985).

Controversies exist about the prognostic significance of various clinical parameters of cervical lymph node metastases in squamous cell carcinoma of the head and neck. This is well reflected by the fact that the AJC, (1982) and the UICC (1978) use different clinical classifications for neck lymph-node involvement. These two systems are summarized in Table 5–1. Among other factors, the AJC attaches importance to the size and number of involved homolateral nodes, whereas the UICC puts particular emphasis on the question of mobility versus fixation. Both the AJC and the UICC classifications attach importance to the point of homolateral versus contra- or bilat-

Table 5–1. Nodal Classification

AJC		UICC	
Designation	*Nodal status*	*Designation*	*Nodal status*
N0	No clinically positive node	N0	No evidence of involvement of regional nodes
N1	Single homolateral node 3 cm or less in diameter	N1	Palpable mobile homolateral nodes
N2a	Single homolateral node more than 3 cm but not more than 6 cm in diameter	N2	Palpable mobile contralateral or bilateral nodes
N2b	Multiple homolateral nodes, none more than 6 cm in diameter	N3	Fixed regional nodes
N3a	Massive homolateral node(s), one more than 6 cm in diameter		
N3b	Bilateral palpable nodes		
N3c	Contralateral palpable node(s)		

eral neck-node involvement, but not in the same way. The level of involvement of cervical lymph nodes is not incorporated in these two systems, although the UICC distinguishes four levels and recommends that these should always be recorded. Similarly, the AJC recommends that the regional nodes involved be indicated on diagrams of the neck.

Retrospective clinicopathologic analyses of large series of patients who underwent a radical neck dissection have demonstrated that histologic parameters of neck-node metastases are of much more prognostic significance than clinical parameters (Noone et al., 1974; Spiro et al., 1974; Pointon et al., 1976; Kalnins et al., 1977; Micheau et al., 1978; Cachin et al., 1979; Johnson et al., 1981; Snow et al., 1982). In this chapter, histologic prognostic factors in neck-node metastases are reviewed. Their impact on management will be discussed.

HISTOLOGIC PROGNOSTIC FACTORS

Extranodal spread—also called extracapsular spread or capsular rupture—and the number of positive nodes are the two histologic factors that are of most prognostic significance (Bennett et al., 1971; Noone et al., 1974; Shah et al., 1976; Sessions, 1976; Kalnins et al., 1977; Zoller et al., 1978; Cachin et al., 1979; Johnson et al., 1981; Snow et al., 1982).

Incidence

The incidence of extranodal spread as reported in two large series of patients from Europe (Micheau et al., 1978; Snow et al., 1982) is strikingly similar: 55 percent and 53.8 percent, respectively. Kalnins et al. (1977) from Roswell Park Memorial Institute reported a much lower incidence—23 percent—in a series of 213 patients with histologically positive neck-dissection specimens. In a more recent study from the United States by Johnson et al. (1981), however, an incidence of 70 percent extranodal spread is reported. Such differences in reported incidence may be due to the degree of conscientiousness with which pathologists examine the specimens for the presence (Figure 5-1) or absence (Figure 5-2) of extranodal spread. Also, the histology may be difficult to evaluate (Figure 5-3). It is important that pathologists agree on what is to be considered still contained within the capsule of the node

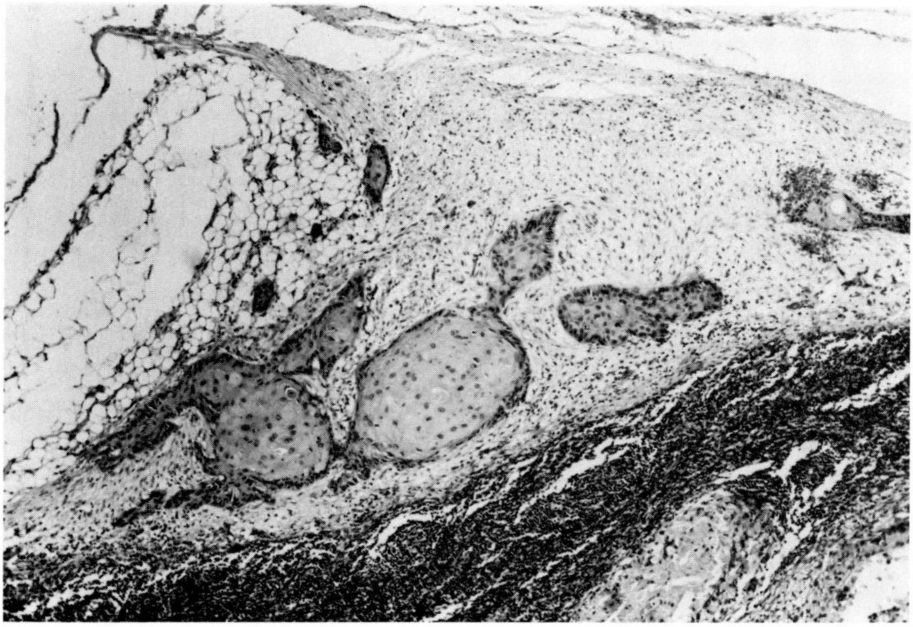

Figure 5-1. Lymph-node metastasis with extracapsular spread of tumor cells into the pericapsular fat (H&E stain; original magnification × 13).

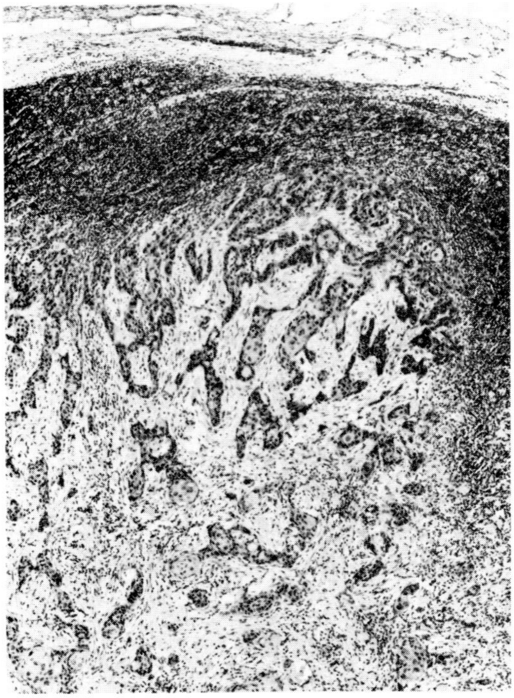

Figure 5–2. Lymph-node metastasis. The tumor cells are located well within the capsule (H&E stain; original magnification × 52).

and what should be regarded as extranodal spread.

In general, it has been thought that extranodal spread was limited to large nodes with clinical fixation. However, Cachin et al. (1979), Johnson et al. (1981), and Snow et al. (1982) have demonstrated that extranodal spread occurs from a substantial percentage of small nodes as well (Table 5–2). This appears to be in agreement with the demonstration by Toker (1963) that primary arrest of tumor emboli within the nodal capsule or juxtacapsular tissues, rather than in the subcapsular sinus, may lead to extranodal spread at a comparatively early phase in the progress of the disease.

Prognostic Value

The prognostic value of extranodal spread and the number of histologic positive nodes will be discussed on the basis of retrospective clinicopathologic analysis of two series of patients who underwent radical neck dissection: 405 patients (484 neck dissections) treated at

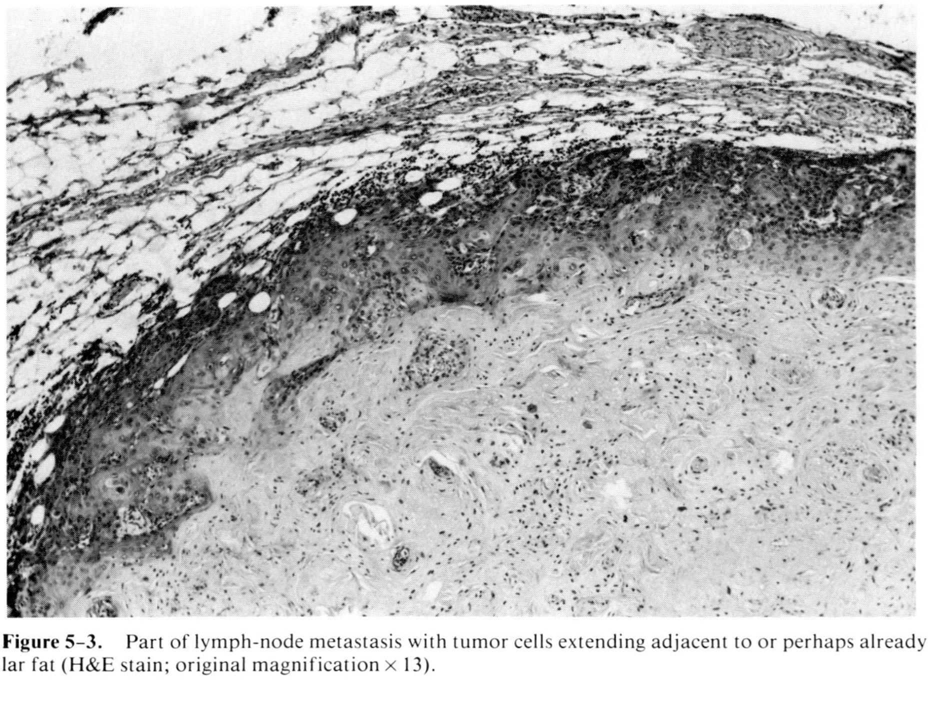

Figure 5–3. Part of lymph-node metastasis with tumor cells extending adjacent to or perhaps already into the pericapsular fat (H&E stain; original magnification × 13).

Table 5-2. Correlation of Clinical and Histologic Node Status in 253 Patients After Radical Neck Dissection

CLINICAL SIZE (CM)	HISTOLOGICAL EXTRANODAL SPREAD (%)
0—1	22.8
1—2	44.3
2—3	53.3
>3	73.7
	($p < 0.0001$)

the Netherlands Cancer Institute from 1960 to 1975 and 331 patients (383 neck dissections) treated between 1973 and 1983 at the Free University Hospital, both in Amsterdam, Netherlands. In the analysis of the earlier series, recurrence in the neck after radical neck dissection was selected as the end point of analysis, as such recurrence in the neck invariably carries a very poor, if not fatal, prognosis (Pearlman, 1979). In the analysis of the later series, interest focused on treatment failure at distant sites. In the first series, only two patients were lost to follow-up; in the second series, only one patient. At the time of analysis, all patients in the earlier series had at least a 5-year follow-up, and those in the later series, at least 2 years.

Failure in the Neck. For the whole series, recurrence in the neck occurred in 69 patients (17.3%); for the 327 patients who had histologically positive nodes, the recurrence rate in the neck was 21.1 percent. In Figure 5-4, the actuarial recurrence-free curve for neck disease is recorded. It is evident from this curve that nearly all recurrences in the neck manifested themselves within 2 years from the day of radical neck dissection. Recurrence in the

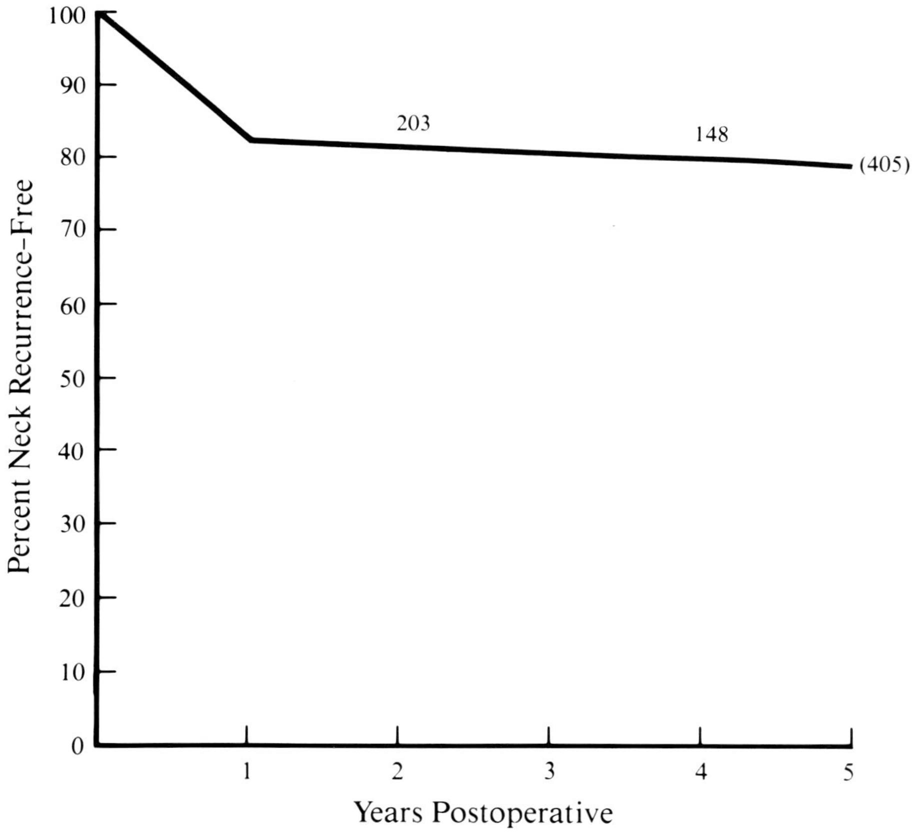

Figure 5-4. Actuarial curve delineating proportion of patients free of neck recurrence after radical neck dissection in 405 patients. (Courtesy of Balm et al., 1982, with permission of Blackwell Scientific Publications.)

neck after a standard radical neck dissection almost invariably proved fatal.

The actuarial curves delineating proportions of patients free of neck-disease recurrence after radial neck dissection are depicted according to the number of histologically positive nodes and the presence or absence of extranodal spread (Figure 5–5). When both extranodal spread and more than one positive node are present, the incidence of neck recurrence rises to 45 percent. Extranodal spread is obviously the most important single prognostic factor (p 10^{-7}).

Failure at Distant Sites. Of the total of 330 patients, 78 developed distant metastases, or a 23.5 percent incidence. The lungs were the most frequent site of metastases, accounting for 44.3 percent, followed by the skeletal system with 23.7 percent. The actuarial percentage distant metastases-free curve for the total group of patients (Figure 5–6) shows that more than 80 percent of distant metastases manifested within 2 years after radical neck dissection. Figure 5–6 also shows that patients who were found to have histologically positive nodes (N+) had a significantly greater likelihood of subsequent distant metastases than those who had histologically negative neck specimens (N0).

The incidence of distant metastases has been further analyzed for the group of patients with histologically positive nodes according to the pathologic extent of nodal metastases. In Figure 5–7, the actuarial curves delineate proportions of patients free of distant metastases according to the number of histologically positive nodes and the presence or absence of extranodal spread. Figure 5–7 shows that the patients who were found pathologically to have four or more positive nodes

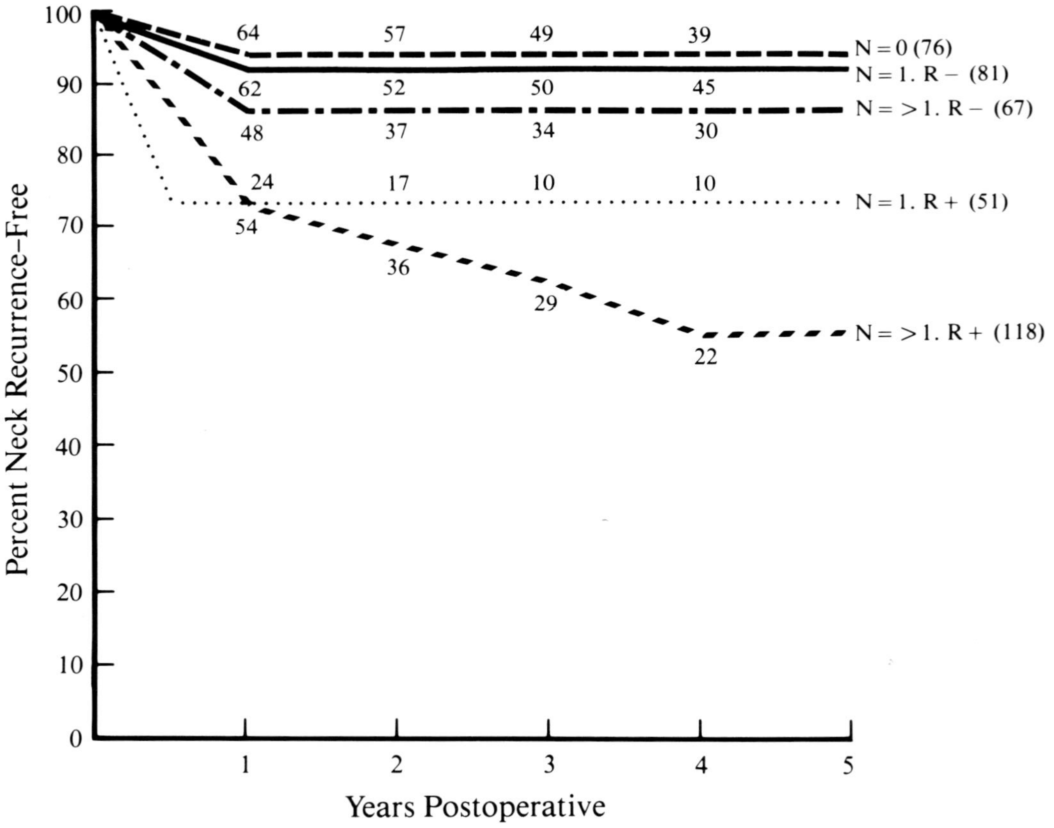

Figure 5–5. Actuarial curves delineating proportion of patients free of neck recurrence after radical neck dissection, according to the number of histologically positive nodes (n = 0, n = 1, and n > 1) and the presence (R +) or absence (R −) of extranodal spread (p = 0.00010). (Courtesy of Balm et al., 1982, with permission of Blackwell Scientific Publications).

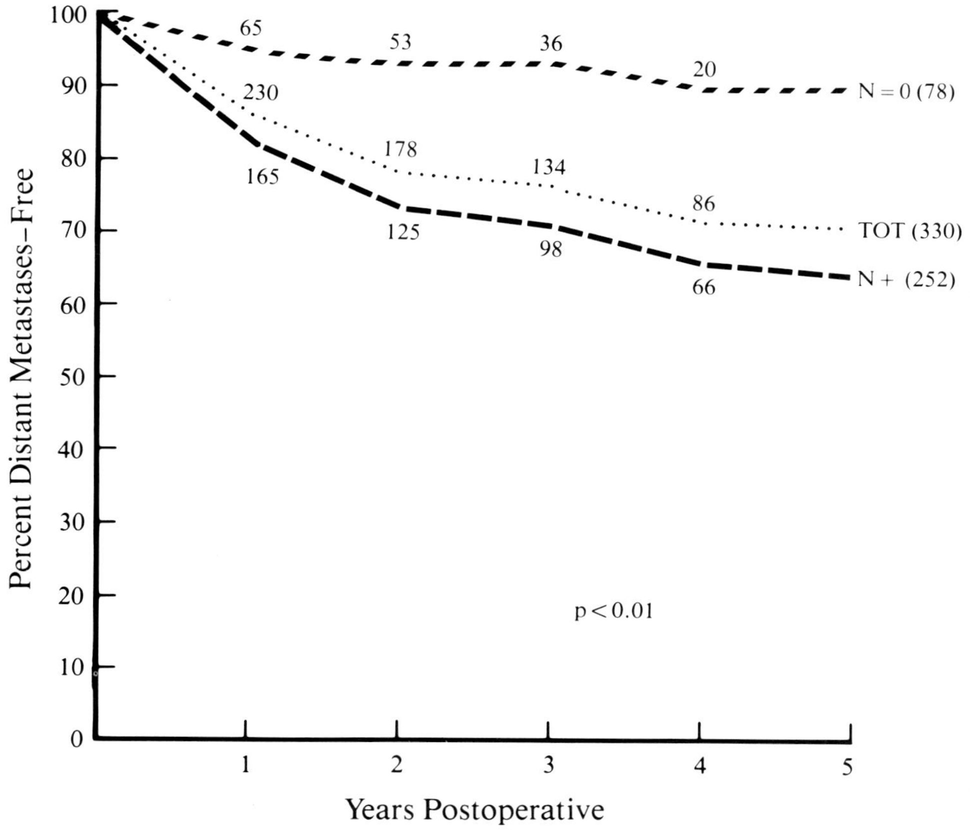

Figure 5–6. Comparison of the incidence of distant metastases between 78 patients with histologically negative and 252 patients with histologically positive neck specimens.

and extranodal spread had a greater than 60 percent likelihood of developing distant metastases. This is statistically significant when compared with the group of patients with one histologically positive node with extranodal spread ($p<0.01$), but not when compared with some of the other groups. The group of patients with three histologically positive nodes and extranodal spread is too small and has inadequate follow-up to permit definite conclusions.

IMPACT ON MANAGEMENT

At the Locoregional Level

Radical neck dissection is considered an effective method of controlling metastatic cancer in the neck. However, reported recurrence rates in the neck following radical neck dissection alone vary from 14 percent to 36 percent (Beahrs et al., 1962; Strong et al., 1966; Jesse et al., 1977; DeSanto et al., 1982). Therefore, the concept of combining surgery and irradiation to the neck has been widely applied since the 1960s. Opinions, however, are divided as to the indications and sequence of such combined treatment.

The various aspects of combined radiation therapy and surgery in the treatment of head and neck cancer have been extensively reviewed by Cachin et al. (1975). Postoperative radiation therapy has the advantage that the histopathologic information on the resection specimen can be used to select the patients most likely to benefit from combined treatment—that is, those patients with a significant probability of local regional failure after surgery alone. This study, like those of Kalnins et al. (1977), Micheau et al. (1978), Cachin et al. (1979), and Johnson et al. (1981), has shown that when extranodal spread (or

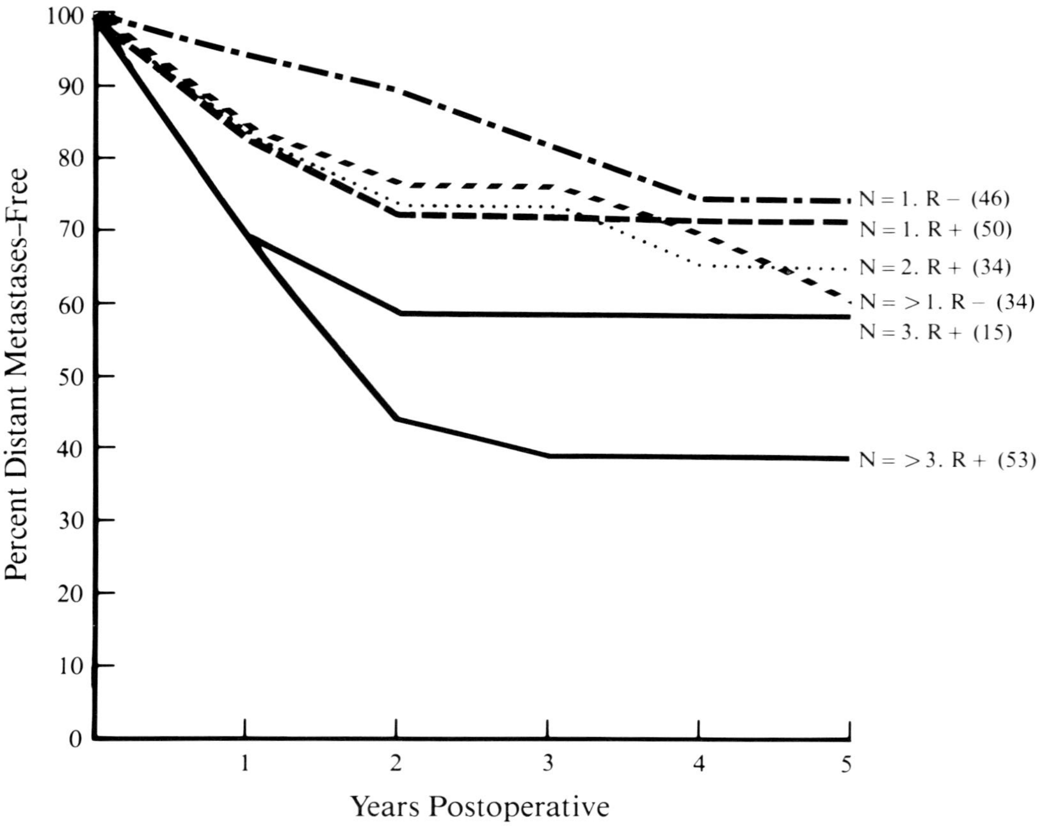

Figure 5–7. Actuarial curves delineating proportion of patients free of distant metastases after radical neck dissection, according to the number of histologically positive nodes (n = 1, n = 2, n = 3, and n > 3) and the presence (R +) or absence (R −) of extranodal spread.

multiple histologic positive nodes) is present in the neck specimen, there is a high risk of recurrence in the neck.

From the late 1960s, postoperative irradiation as an adjuvant to radical neck dissection became the routine in our institutions when extranodal spread was reported by the pathologist. Our experiences with postoperative radiotherapy in the earlier series (1960–1975) at the Netherlands Cancer Institute have been reported by Bartelink et al. (1983). In patients having extranodal spread, a lower recurrence rate in the neck was observed after surgery followed by radiotherapy than after surgery alone. The difference, however, was not statistically significant. Nevertheless, it should be emphasized that the dosages of radiotherapy given during the major part of the period concerned were often below the dose limit now considered minimal (Marcus et al., 1979).

In the series of patients treated from 1973 to 1983 at the Free University Hospital, all 106 with extranodal spread who had postoperative radiotherapy were treated with 4 MeV photons, with daily fractions of 180–200 cGy to a total dose ranging from 6000 to 7000 cGy in 7 weeks. When the neck dissection had been carried out as part of a composite resection together with that for the primary tumor, radiation therapy was directed to the primary site as well as to both sides of the neck. During this period, only 33 patients with extranodal spread had no postoperative radiotherapy. As in the earlier study, a lower recurrence rate in the neck was observed in the combined treatment group than in the group of patients who had a radical neck dissection only.

Because of the small number of patients in the surgery-only group, the difference was again not statistically significant. When the combined treatment groups and the surgery-only groups from both periods are taken together, however, the difference in recurrence rate in the neck becomes statistically significant in favor of the combined treatment group (Figure 5–8). Similarly, in retrospective studies, Jesse et al. (1977), Vikram et al. (1980), Arriagada et al. (1983), Mantravadi et al. (1983), and Goffinet et al. (1984) have shown that postoperative radiotherapy diminishes the number of recurrences in the neck.

At the Systemic Level

Failure to eradicate the disease above the clavicles is regarded as the major cause of death in patients who have local or regional advanced squamous cancer of the head and neck. But with a treatment consisting of surgery followed by radiation therapy in patients at high risk for local or regional recurrence, as just outlined, a changing pattern of failure is occurring (Vikram, 1984). Many studies report a decrease of local and regional failure rates from this type of combined therapy (Arriagada et al., 1983; Bartelink et al., 1983; Goffinet et al., 1984), but observe that this is not reflected in a proportionate increase of 5-year survival rates. As fewer patients die from uncontrolled disease above the clavicles, more are exposed to the risk of disseminated disease below the clavicles (and to the appearance of second malignant neoplasms).

It has been demonstrated that the rate of distant metastases correlates more with the appearance of cervical-node metastases than with the T-stage (Berger et al., 1971; Merino et al., 1977). This study has attempted to identify histologic prognostic indicators in neck-node metastases for distant metastases. It was found that the incidence of distant metastases was high in those patients who had more than

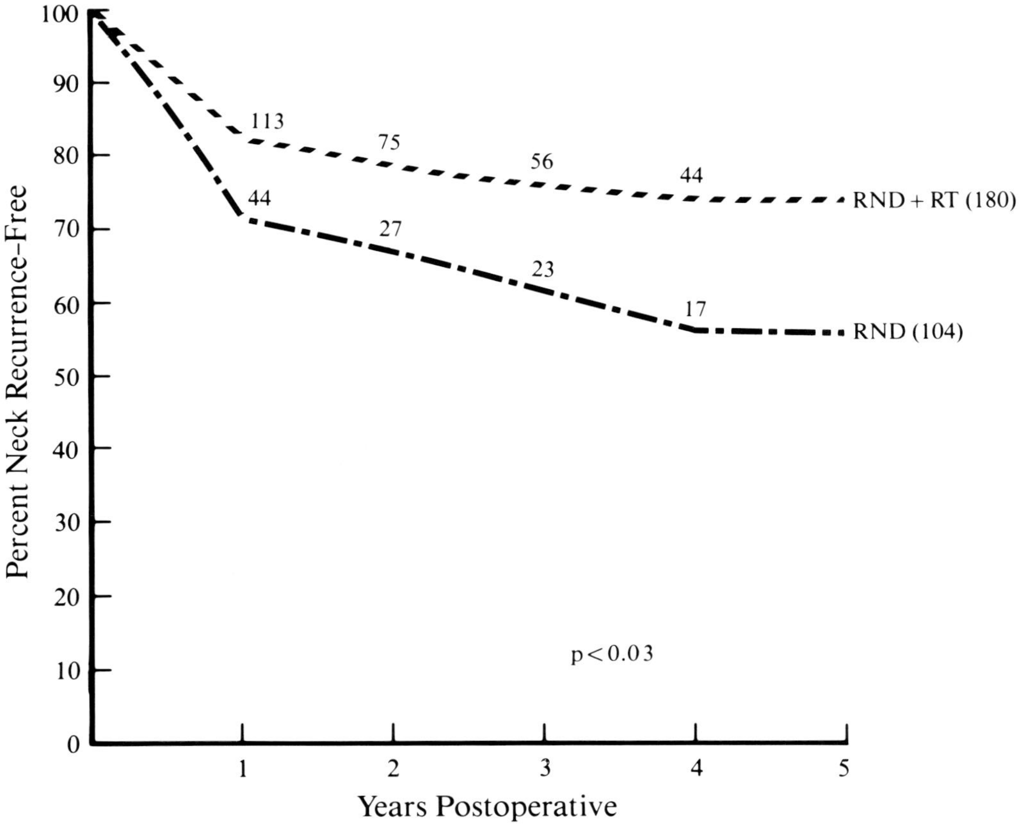

Figure 5–8. Actuarial recurrence-free percentages for neck disease in 284 patients with extranodal spread. RND = radical neck dissection; RT = postoperative radiotherapy.

three histologically positive nodes and extranodal spread. More than half these patients can be expected to develop distant metastases within the next 2 years. Likewise, Vikram et al. (1984) have shown that the pathologic extent of nodal metastases at neck dissection is the most sensitive prognostic indicator for distant metastases. These authors attach particular importance to the level of nodal involvement in the neck, and observed a significantly higher incidence of distant metastases in those patients who had pathologically demonstrated metastases at multiple levels in the neck than in those who had metastases at a single level. It should be realized, however, that the number of patients followed for longer periods of time is small in both studies. Further data, therefore, are needed to reach definite conclusions about the most sensitive indicators in neck-node metastases for distant metastases.

It is tempting to consider adjuvant chemotherapy following surgery and radiotherapy in those patients who are at the highest risk of failure at distant sites. Adjuvant chemotherapy, however, is still in the investigational stage. It is of paramount importance, therefore, that adjuvant chemotherapy studies are well designed and carried out in a prospective, randomized way to ensure meaningful data. One of the major problems with such studies will be that probably only a relatively small proportion of the population of patients with head and neck cancer will be able to complete chemotherapy programs after surgery and radiotherapy because of their age, general condition, and quality of life.

DISCUSSION

The prognosis of patients with head and neck cancer for whom either elective or therapeutic treatment of the neck is indicated is much better formulated on the basis of accurate histologic determination of lymph node metastasis than on clinical examination. This emphasizes the value of neck dissection as a staging procedure. Histologic extranodal spread is the most important prognostic factor regarding recurrence in the neck after neck dissection, followed by the number of histologically positive nodes. When these unfavorable prognostic factors are reported by the pathologist to be present in the neck specimen, postoperative radiotherapy is indicated. This treatment policy of combined surgery followed by irradiation in patients at high risk for regional failure has been shown to decrease the recurrence rate in the neck.

As fewer patients die from uncontrolled disease above the clavicles, however, more are exposed to the risk of disseminated disease below the clavicles. This study shows that the pathologic extent of nodal metastases at neck dissection is the most sensitive prognostic indicator for distant metastases. Further studies are needed to more accurately define the group of patients with the highest risk of failure at distant sites. Prospective randomized adjuvant chemotherapy studies should then be designed for this group of patients.

REFERENCES

Ali, S., Tiwari, R. M., and Snow, G. B.: False positive and false negative neck nodes. *Head Neck Surg.*, 8:78–82, 1985.

American Joint Committee for Cancer Staging. *Manual for Staging of Cancer*, 1982.

Arriagada, R., Eschwege, F., Cachin, Y., and Richard, J. M.: The value of combining radiotherapy with surgery in the treatment of hypopharyngeal and laryngeal cancers. *Cancer*, 51:1819–25, 1983.

Bartelink, H., Breur, K., Hart, G., Annyas, B., van Slooten, E. A., and Snow, G. B.: The value of postoperative radiotherapy as an adjuvant to radical neck dissection. *Cancer*, 52:1008–13, 1983.

Beahrs, O. H., and Barber, K. W.: The value of radical neck dissection of structures of the neck in the management of carcinomas of the lip, mouth and larynx. *Arch. Surg.*, 85:49–56, 1962.

Bennett, S. H., Futrell, J. W., Roth, J. A., et al.: Prognostic significance of histologic host response in cancer of the larynx and hypopharynx. *Cancer*, 28:1255–65, 1971.

Berger, D. S., and Fletcher, G. H.: Distant metastasis following local control of squamous cell carcinoma of the nasopharynx, tonsillar fossa, and base of tongue. *Radiology*, 100:141–43, 1971.

Cachin, Y., and Eschwege, F.: Combination of radiotherapy and surgery in treatment of head and neck cancers. *Cancer Treat. Rev.*, 2:177–91, 1975.

Cachin, Y., Sancho-Garnier, H., Micheau, Ch., and Marandas, P.: Nodal metastasis from carcinoma of the oropharynx. *Otolaryngol. Clin. North Am.*, 12:145–54, 1979.

Cantrell, R. W.: Computed tomography for cervical adenopathy. *Arch. Otolaryngol.*, 110:441–42, 1984.

DeSanto, L. W., Holt, J. J., Beahrs, O. H., and O'Fallon, W. M.: Neck dissection: Is it worthwhile? *Laryngoscope,* 92:502–09, 1982.

Farr, H. W., and Arthur, K.: Epidermoid cancer of the mouth and pharynx, 1960–1964. *J. Laryngol. Otol.,* 86:243–53, 1972.

Friedman, M., Shelton, V. K., Mafee, M., Bellity, P., Grybauska, V., and Skolnik, E. M.: Metastatic neck disease. *Arch. Otolaryngol.*, 110:443–47, 1984.

Goffinet, D. R., Fee, W. E., and Goode, R. L.: Combined surgery and postoperative irradiation in the treatment of cervical lymph nodes. *Arch. Otolaryngol.,* 110:736–38, 1984.

Jesse, R. H., and Fletcher, G. H.: Treatment of the neck in patients with squamous cell carcinoma of the head and neck. *Cancer*, 39:868–72, 1977.

Johnson, J. T., Barnes, E. L., Myers, E. N., Schramm, V. L., Borochovitz, D., and Sigler, B. A.: The extracapsular spread of tumors in cervical node metastasis. *Arch. Otoloaryngol.*, 107:725–29, 1981.

Kalnins, I. K., Leonard, A. G., Sako, K., Razack, M. S., and Shedd, D. P.: Correlation between prognosis and degree of lymph node involvement in carcinoma of the oral cavity. *Am. J. Surg.,* 134:450–54, 1977.

Mantravadi, R. V. P., Skolnik, E. M., Haas, R. E., and Applebaum, E. L.: Patterns of cancer recurrence in the postoperatively irradiated neck. *Arch. Otolaryngol.,* 109:753–56, 1983.

Marcus, R. B., Jr., Million, R. R., and Cassissi, N. J.: Postoperative irradiation for squamous cell carcinomas of the head and neck: Analysis of time-dose factors related to control above the clavicles. *Int. J. Radiat. Oncol. Biol. Phys.*, 5:1943–49, 1979.

Merino, O. R., Lindberg, R. D., and Fletcher, G. H.: An analysis of distant metastases from squamous cell carcinoma of the upper respiratory and digestive tracts. *Cancer*, 40:145–51, 1977.

Micheau, C., Sancho, H., and Gerard-Merchant, R.: Prognostic des adenopathies cervicales metastatiques en fonction des facteurs anatomo-pathologiques. *Nuovo. Arch. Ital. Otol.* VI, 1:5–14, 1978.

Noone, R. B., Bonner, H., Raymond, S., Brown, A. S., Graham, W. P., and Lehr, H. B.: Lymph-node metastases in oral carcinoma: A correlation of histopathology with survival. *Plast. Reconstr. Surg.*, 53:158–66, 1974.

Pearlman, N. W.: Treatment outcome in recurrent head and neck cancer. *Arch. Surg.,* 114:39–42, 1979.

Pointon, R. C. S., and Jelly, G. O.: Block dissection of the neck for squamous cell carcinoma of the mouth and lip. *Proc. R. Soc. Med.,* 69:414–16, 1976.

Sako, K., Pradier, R. N., Marchetta, F. C., and Pickren, J. W.: Fallibility of palpation in the diagnosis of metastases to cervical nodes. *Surg. Gynecol. Obst.,* 118:989–90, 1964.

Sessions, D. G.: Surgical pathology of cancer of the larynx and hypopharynx. *Laryngoscope*, 86:814–39, 1976.

Shah, J. P., Cendon, R. A., Farr, H. W., Strong, E. W.: Carcinoma of the oral cavity (factors affecting treatment failure at the primary site and neck). *Am. J. Surg.,* 132:504–7, 1976.

Snow, G. B., Annyas, A. A., van Slooten, E. A., Bartelink, H., and Hart, A. A. M.: Prognostic factors of neck node metastasis. *Clin. Otolaryngol.,* 7:185–92, 1982.

Spiro, R. H., Alfonso, A. E., Farr, H. W., and Strong, E. W.: Cervical node metastasis from epidermoid carcinoma of the oral cavity and oropharynx. A critical assessment of current staging. *Am. J. Surg.,* 128:562–67, 1974.

Strong, E. W., Henschke, U. K., Nickson, J. J., Frazell, E. L., Tollefsen, R., and Hilaris, B. S.: Preoperative x-ray therapy as an adjunct to radical neck dissection. *Cancer*, 19:1509–16, 1966.

Toker, C.: Some observations on the deposition of metastatic carcinoma within cervical lymph nodes. *Cancer*, 16:364–74, 1963.

Union Internationale Contre de Cancer: *TNM Classification of Malignant Tumors.* UICC, Geneva, 1978.

Vikram, B.: Changing patterns of failure in advanced head and neck cancer. *Arch. Otolaryngol.*, 110:564–65, 1984.

Vikram, B., Strong, E. W., Shah, J. P., and Spiro, R.: Elective postoperative radiation therapy in stages III and IV epidermoid carcinoma of the head and neck. *Am. J. Surg.,* 140:580–84, 1980.

Vikram, B., Strong, E. W., Shah, J. P., and Spiro, R.: Failure at distant sites following multimodality treatment for advanced head and neck cancer. *Head Neck Surg.,* 6:730–33, 1984.

Zajicek, J.: Cytology of Supradiaphragmatic Organs. In *Monographs in Clinical Cytology*, Vol. 4, *Aspiration Biopsy Cytology*, Part 1, 90–124. S. Karger, Basel, 1974.

Zoller, M., Goodman, M. L., and Cummings, C. W.: Guidelines for prognosis in head and neck cancer with nodal metastasis. *Laryngoscope*, 88:135–40, 1978.

CHAPTER 6

The Significance of Extracapsular Extension of Squamous Cancer in Lymph Nodes

Eugene N. Myers and Jonas T. Johnson

EDITORS' COMMENT

In this chapter, which is a U.S. companion to Dr. Snow's European experience, Dr. Myers and Dr. Johnson confirm the retrospective work of Snow and Balm as well as their own important study reported in 1980 in Tucson, Arizona, and published in 1981. This chapter is a logical extension of their original work that adds an additional 2-year period of retrospective review, for a total of 548 neck dissections in 510 patients over a 4-year period. As well as reaffirming their original conclusion that extracapsular spread (ECS) could occur in any size of lymph node and appeared to be the single most important prognostic indicator of survival, the authors have determined with the new data that there is a decrease in the mean disease-free interval.

Other important data gleaned from this chapter include the fact that neither tumor differentiation nor the number of involved lymph nodes has as much prognostic significance as the presence or absence of ECS. In fact, survival was similar between an pathologically negative and pathologically positive neck specimen as long as ECS was not present. Myers and Johnson found ECS present at all sites in the head and neck, though somewhat less prevalent in the larynx. One of the most impressive statistics was that the identification of ECS in stage III and IV disease resulted in a two- to fourfold increase in distant metastases and decrease in long-term survival of the patients.

In this important study, the authors conclude that ECS is a more sensitive prognostic indicator than the TNM classification, but we must remember that we are comparing a pathologic classification with a clinical classification, so we would expect it to be more sensitive. Dr. Myers and Dr. Johnson, like Dr. Snow in the previous chapter, identify the need to select the high-risk patient with ECS, and attempt to incorporate adjunctive chemotherapy into the treatment regimen. They suggest a maintenance program of drug therapy. We look forward to their results.

INTRODUCTION

Spread of metastatic squamous cell carcinoma through the capsule of cervical lymph nodes is associated with a poor prognosis. It had been assumed that this route of soft tissue invasion was limited to large fixed cervical lymph nodes until Snow et al. (1982) undertook a retrospective evaluation of 326 patients who underwent radical neck dissection for squamous cell carcinoma. They found ECS in 23 percent of nodes less than 1 cm in diameter. Of lymph nodes 2 to 3 cm in diameter, 53 percent demonstrated ECS, and 74 percent of lymph nodes greater than 3 cm in diameter had ECS. Johnson et al. (1981), in a retrospective review of 177 radical neck dissections, demonstrated that ECS occurred in 65 percent of the lymph nodes less than 3 cm in diameter.

Patients who had ECS had a statistically reduced survivorship in our initial series (Johnson et al., 1981). We retrospectively examined additional records to bring the total to 548 neck dissections done in 510 patients and once again found a statistically significant reduction in survivorship in patients with ECS. Tumor differentiation and the number of involved lymph nodes did not appear to be of prognostic significance. The survivorship of patients who had no evidence of metastasis in the lymph nodes was similar to the survivorship of patients who had metastasis confined to the lymph nodes.

METHODS

All patients treated by us for squamous carcinoma of the head and neck who received a radical neck dissection in the period 1978 through 1982 were identified. The histologic specimens were then reviewed without knowledge of any patient's eventual outcome. All specimens were classified according to the following schema: negative neck, no histologic evidence of cervical metastasis; no ECS, cervical metastasis confined to the lymph nodes; or ECS, cervical metastasis with involvement of the extralymphatic soft tissue. Patients' charts were then reviewed with respect to site and stage of disease, treatment, and eventual outcome.

All patients underwent radical neck dissection. During the period studied, modified or conservation neck dissection was not employed, except that in some patients with clinically disease-free necks the spinal accessory nerve was preserved.

Many patients received radiation therapy, some of them having previously undergone full-course radiotherapy with curative intent. Recurrent disease was subsequently treated surgically. Alternatively, patients who had not received prior radiation therapy were commonly referred for postoperative radiation therapy based on the best judgment of the physicians treating the patient. In some instances, radical neck dissection was not undertaken until recurrent disease developed. For instance, a small group of patients with T_1 squamous carcinoma of the floor of the mouth subsequently developed cervical metastases. These patients were then treated by radical neck dissection.

Patients who developed recurrent disease were studied to determine the site of first recurrence and the length of the disease-free interval between radical neck surgery and the diagnosis of recurrence. Survival statistics were

Table 6–1. Patient Population According to Primary Site and Stage of Disease

SITE	STAGE I	STAGE II	STAGE III	STAGE IV
Tongue	1	4	6	17
Tonsil	0	4	31	20
Floor of mouth	7	7	7	16
Base of tongue	0	0	4	15
Epiglottis	3	24	37	39
Glottis	0	4	12	9
Hypopharynx	0	3	14	22
Miscellaneous	0	5	12	19
Unknown primary	0	0	3	4
Total	11	51	126	161

Table 6–2. Histologic Findings in Radical Neck Specimens

NODE STATUS	NUMBER	%
Negative nodes	129	37
No extracapsular extension	85	24
Extracapsular spread	118	34
Could not be reviewed	17	5

prepared for patients with a follow-up of 2 years or more.

RESULTS

A total of 371 radical neck dissections were done on 349 patients between January 1978 and December 1982. Twenty-two patients had undergone bilateral radical neck dissection. The sites and stages of disease in the patients studied are shown in Table 6–1. The histologic findings in the radical neck dissection specimens are characterized in Table 6–2. Patients undergoing bilateral neck dissections were classified according to the most involved area.

The histologic status of the neck nodes was correlated with the site of the primary tumor in patients with stage III (Table 6–3) and stage IV (Table 6–4) carcinoma. ECS was noted with primary tumors arising in every head and neck site. The distribution of cases of stage I and stage II carcinoma was similar by site; however, the smaller number of patients made the data evaluation less valuable. Patients with glottic tumors demonstrated ECS less commonly compared with patients whose primary tumors occurred at other sites. ECS was observed in more patients with stage IV carcinoma than in patients with stage III carcinoma (Tables 6–3 and 6–4).

Follow-up data were obtained on all patients for 2 years or longer after completion of treatment. Table 6–5 shows disease-free survival in patients with stage III carcinoma. The incidence of recurrent carcinoma was similar in patients in whom nodes were histologically free of disease and in patients with carcinoma limited to within the lymph node capsule. The histologic finding of ECS was associated with a 50 percent reduction in survival. This observation is similar to the survival results in patients with stage IV carcinoma (Table 6–6).

The site of the first recurrence of disease was evaluated in all patients. Patients who were free of recurrent disease at their last follow-up, who died of intercurrent disease, or who were lost to follow-up are not considered. Recurrence was categorized as either local, regional (in the cervical area), or distant metastases. When patients developed recurrent carcinoma in more than one site simultaneously, the site closest to the primary tumor was indicated as the site of recurrent disease. In this way, each patient was counted only once. Similarly, when patients with local disease subsequently developed distant metastases, they were counted as having local disease. Patients indicated as having distant metastases had distant metastases as their only site of recurrent disease.

Fourteen percent (10 of 71) of patients with stage III carcinoma and no evidence of ECS (either no cervical metastases or cervical metastases limited to the lymph node) developed local or regional disease. Four percent of pa-

Table 6–3. Histologic Status of Neck Nodes in Stage III Patients

SITE	NEGATIVE NODES	NO ECS	+ ECS	UNKNOWN
Tongue	2	1	3	—
Tonsil	11	8	10	2
Floor of mouth	4	1	2	—
Base of tongue	1	1	2	—
Epiglottis	15	11	11	—
Glottis	5	6	1	—
Hypopharynx	5	4	3	2
Miscellaneous	4	3	4	1
Unknown primary	2	1	0	—
Total	49	36	36	5

Key: Negative nodes = no histologic evidence of cervical metastasis; No ECS = cervical metastases limited to lymph node; + ECS = cervical metastasis has spread beyond lymph-node capsule to soft tissue of neck; Unknown = histologic findings of extracapsular extent could not be ascertained.

Table 6–4. Histologic Status of Neck Nodes in Stage IV Patients

SITE	NEGATIVE NODES	NO ECS	+ ECS	UNKNOWN
Tongue	7	3	6	1
Tonsil	6	1	11	2
Floor of mouth	4	4	6	2
Base of tongue	4	4	6	1
Epiglottis	11	12	14	2
Glottis	6	1	2	—
Hypopharynx	3	8	11	—
Miscellaneous	6	3	9	1
Unknown primary	3	0	1	—
Total	50	36	66	9

Key: Negative nodes = no histologic evidence of cervical metastasis; No ECS = cervical metastases limited to lymph node; + ECS = cervical metastasis has spread beyond lymph-node capsule to soft tissue of neck; Unknown = histologic findings of extracapsular extent could not be ascertained.

tients (3 of 71) developed distant metastases in spite of local or regional control. By contrast, 42 percent of evaluable patients with stage III disease and evidence of ECS (14 of 33) developed local or regional recurrence. Eighteen percent (6 of 33) developed distant metastases with no evidence of local or regional recurrence.

Stage IV patients were similarly evaluated. Twenty-one percent of patients with no ECS (15 of 72) developed local or regional recurrence, whereas 14 percent (10 of 72) developed distant metastases in spite of local or regional tumor control. By contrast, 45 percent with ECS (24 of 53) developed local or regional recurrence and 19 percent (10 of 53) developed distant metastases in spite of local or regional control.

Patients indicated as having regionally recurrent disease had either recurrence in the ipsilateral (treated) or contralateral cervical nodes. An important subgroup of patients developed contralateral cervical metastases. In this series, the patients who presented with negative nodes did not develop contralateral cervical metastasis (Table 6–7). Table 6–8 indicates the therapy delivered to patients who subsequently developed cervical metastasis as their only evidence of recurrent disease. Two-thirds of the patients who developed cervical metastases as their sole site of recurrence had been treated with postoperative radiation therapy.

The disease-free interval of those patients with recurrent carcinoma is displayed in Table 6–9 according to stage and histologic findings in the radical neck dissection. Patients with ECS had a reduced disease-free interval compared with other patients, but the difference was not statistically significant.

Radiation therapy was frequently used in combination with surgery (Table 6–10). One subgroup of patients had received prior radiation therapy; most of these patients underwent surgery for recurrent disease or a new primary. A limited number, however, had been entered into a planned program of preoperative irradiation therapy and surgery. Patients with ECS were routinely treated with postoperative radiation therapy whenever possible. Other patients were referred for radiation therapy depending on the judgment of the attending surgeon.

We sought to ascertain the outcome of pa-

Table 6–5. Two-Year Disease-Free Survival According to Histologic Finding in Neck of Stage III Patients

NODAL STATUS	NO. OF PATIENTS	DIED OF DISEASE	NO EVIDENCE OF DISEASE	DIED OF SECOND PRIMARY	DIED OF OTHER CAUSES OR LOST TO FOLLOW-UP
Negative nodes	49	5 (13%)	34 (87%)	2	8
No ECS	36	8 (25%)	24 (75%)	1	3
+ ECS	36	20 (61%)	13 (39%)	1	2

Table 6–6. Two-Year Disease-Free Survival According to Histologic Finding in Neck of Stage IV Patients

NODAL STATUS	NO. OF PATIENTS	DIED OF DISEASE	NO EVIDENCE OF DISEASE	DIED OF SECOND PRIMARY	DIED OF OTHER CAUSES OR LOST TO FOLLOW-UP
Negative nodes	50	12 (29%)	30 (71%)	2	6
No ECS	36	10 (33%)	20 (67%)	2	4
+ECS	66	34 (64%)	19 (36%)	2	11

tients who underwent a cohesive treatment program involving surgery plus planned postoperative radiation therapy. Patients with pathologic indications of surgical margins involved with tumor were excluded. The only patients evaluated were those with stage III or stage IV disease who received a minimal dose of 5000 cGy in 5 weeks of external beam radiation therapy to the primary site and lymphatic distribution in the cervical nodes instituted within 6 weeks of surgery. Patients lost to follow-up or those who died of intercurrent disease were not eligible. One hundred and five patients were identified.

Survival following surgery and postoperative radiation therapy was improved to a statistically significant extent ($p<0.03$) in the group of patients with no ECS (32/44, or 73%) compared with patients with ECS (30/61 or 49%). Evaluation of these data according to cervical histology and stage demonstrated that the increased survival was observed in patients with stage III (80% vs. 48%) or stage IV (67% vs. 50%) disease. The difference was statistically significant in patients with stage III disease ($p<0.05$), but not in patients with stage IV disease ($p>0.05$). By contrast, the tumor stage (American Joint Committee) did not show a statistically significant difference in survival for either stage III (62%) or stage IV (57%) disease ($p>0.05$). The pattern of recurrent disease noted in the population of patients treated with surgery and postoperative radiation therapy was similar to the pattern of current disease noted in the entire group (Table 6–11).

Table 6–7. Site of Cervical Recurrence According to Original Stage and Cervical Node Histology in Patients With Recurrence in Neck Only

NODAL STATUS	RECURRENCE SITE		
	No. of patients	*Contralateral*	*Ipsilateral*
Stage III			
Negative nodes	2	0	2
No ECS	5	2	3
+ECS	11	4	7
Stage IV			
Negative nodes	2	0	2
No ECS	5	2	3
+ECS	14	4	10

DISCUSSION

We reported our original observations on a group of 161 patients who had undergone neck dissection for squamous cell carcinoma of the head and neck (Johnson et al., 1981). Our second series contains 349 previously unreported cases (Johnson et al., 1985). All patients received a minimum 2-year follow-up. In our first series, we observed that ECS was commonly encountered even in patients with involvement of small lymph nodes. We found that 65 percent of the patients with N1 lymph nodes had ECS, and that 75 percent of the nodes greater than 3 cm in diameter had ECS. The incidence of ECS in the combined group of patients is 60 percent.

Such a finding is very important, since patients with ECS have a significant reduction in survival compared with patients with similar stage disease in whom no cervical metastases are found or in whom cervical metastases to the lymph nodes. Patients with metastasis to the lymph nodes with no ECS have survival similar to patients with no cervical metastasis.

An equally dramatic finding is that the mean disease-free interval between radical neck dissection and the development of recur-

Table 6-8. Therapy for Patients with Cervical Recurrence

SITE	NODAL STATUS	PRIOR XRT	POST-OP XRT	NO XRT
Contralateral	Negative nodes	0	0	0
(30.7%)	No ECS	2	2	0
	+ECS	0	7	1
Ipsilateral	Negative nodes	1	0	3
(69.2%)	No ECS	1	4	1
	+ECS	1	13	3

rent disease is less than 18 months (Table 6-9). The mean disease-free interval in patients with ECS was, in fact, 6 months (Johnson et al., 1985). This indicates that patients with ECS experience not only an actual increased incidence of recurrence, but also a markedly reduced disease-free interval.

Our observations corroborate earlier reports that ECS is an indicator of poor prognosis (Johnson et al., 1981; Snow et al., 1982; Zoller et al., 1978). The evaluation of the end results of treatment according to the tumor staging system (American Joint Committee) did not show a statistically significant difference in survival between stage III and stage IV patients. These data suggest that the histologic findings in the cervical lymphatics—more specifically, the presence or absence of ECS—is a more sensitive indicator of prognosis than the TNM staging system as it is currently employed.

The poor prognosis in patients with ECS has led to an effort to improve the treatment results by the inclusion of postoperative irradiation therapy. Snow et al. (1982) noted that the addition of radiation therapy after radical neck dissection improved the results in patients whose specimens showed ECS. Zoller et al. (1978) also demonstrated that radiation therapy seemed to improve the control rate in these patients.

We have combined surgery and radiation in all patients with ECS who could tolerate both. In this study, 49 percent of patients with ECS treated with combined surgery and radiation therapy were alive without evidence of disease at 2 years. Therapeutic alternatives should be offered to this high-risk group.

The observation that the disease-free interval is reduced in patients with ECS also has treatment implications. Early efforts have been undertaken in our department to study the effects of a maintenance chemotherapy program in this group of patients.

Table 6-9. Disease-Free Interval in Patients with Recurrent Cancer According to Stage and Histologic Status of Cervical Lymph Nodes

NODAL STATUS	NO. OF PATIENTS	AVERAGE INTERVAL (MONTHS)	RANGE
Stage III			
Negative nodes	5	14	5-24
No ECS	8	17	5-36
+ ECS	20	10	4-35
Stage IV			
Negative nodes	12	8	1-14
No ECS	10	17	3-36
+ ECS	34	6	1-35

Table 6-10. Treatment Received According to Histologic Status of Cervical Nodes

NODAL STATUS	NO. OF PATIENTS	PRIOR RADIATION (%)	POST-OP RADIATION (%)
Negative nodes	133	34 (25.5)	38 (28.5)
No ECS	83	5 (6)	59 (71)
+ECS	116	11 (9)	94 (81)

Table 6-11. Site of First Recurrence According to Stage and Cervical Histology for Patients Who Underwent Surgery Plus Post-Op Radiation

STAGE	RECURRENCE SITE		
	Local	*Regional*	*Distant*
No ECS			
Stage III	1	2	1
Stage IV	2	3	3
+ECS			
Stage III	1	9	3
Stage IV	5	8	5

REFERENCES

Johnson, J. T., Barnes, E. L., Myers, E. N., Schramm, V. L., Jr., Borochovitz, D., and Sigler, B. A.: The extracapsular spread of tumors in cervical-node metastasis. *Arch. Otolaryngol.*, 107:725–29, 1981.

Johnson, J. T., Myers, E. N., Bedetti, C. D., Barnes, E. L., Schramm, V. L., Jr., and Thearle, P. B.: Cervical lymph-node metastases: Incidence and implications of extracapsular carcinoma. *Arch. Otolaryngol.* (in press).

Snow, G. B., Annyas, A. A., Van Slooten, E. A., Bartelink, H., and Hart, A. A.: Prognostic factors of neck node metastasis. *Clin. Otolaryngol.*, 7:185–92, 1982.

Zoller, M., Goodman, M. L., and Cummings, C. W.: Guidelines for prognosis in head and neck cancer with nodal metastasis. *Laryngoscope*, 88:135–40, 1978.

PART THREE

RADIOTHERAPEUTIC CONSIDERATIONS

CHAPTER 7

Basic Principles of Radiobiology in Head and Neck Oncology

Lester J. Peters

EDITORS' COMMENT

Although it is not essential to know the exact details of all modes of therapy of the head and neck cancer patient, it behooves clinicians to have a basic understanding and appreciation of the fundamental principles of the treatment modalities other than their own. In this chapter, Dr. Peters offers us an unusually lucid and well-documented treatise on the principles of radiobiology for the nonradiotherapist.

Beginning with the different mechanisms of cell death related to radiation at the molecular, cell membrane, and parenchymal levels, the author identifies the loss of tissue function as being dependent on both time and the rate of cell turnover. A description of the dose-response curve and the importance of the "shoulder" of the survival curve is stressed by Dr. Peters, in addition to its use in fractionated doses of radiation therapy. The effect of radiation quality, linear energy transfer (LET), and its identification with conventional radiation (x-ray, gamma-ray, electrons with low LET) and radiation with a high LET such as neutrons and heavy nuclei is discussed. Other basic concepts, including the effects of oxygenation, cell age, and mitotic activity, are outlined in an understandable format. Fractionation of radiation receives attention from the author in noting both the rationale and the two types (accelerated and hyperfractionation) of fractionation and their effect on the cell kinetics of a given tumor.

As noted by Dr. Fidler and Dr. Nicolson in earlier chapters, Dr. Peters also identifies tumor heterogeneity as a problem in predicting tumor-control probability. Other factors influencing dose-response curves include the dose specifications and the definition of tumor control as noted by different authors. The author notes pitfalls in attempting to predict tumor regression and regrowth as well as interpretation of biopsy results in the postirradiation period.

Concepts known to all head and neck surgeons, such as the rationale of planned radiation and surgery, sterilization of the N0 neck with 5000 cGy in 5 weeks, and the appropriate application of preoperative versus postoperative radiation therapy are covered satisfactorily. There are also some very practical points for the surgeon to remember when operating in an irradiated field, including the fact that "late radiation injury results from a progressive depletion of functional cells in slowly proliferating tissues." This translates into "unexplained" tissue necrosis when submitting radiated tissue to surgical trauma. Dr.

Peters rightly recommends the introduction of new, well-vascularized tissue into such a field.

In noting the causes of failure of tumor control, the author identifies the commonly held, though rather simplistic, concept of tumor radiosensitivity, and puts it into a logical perspective within the context of other equally important factors, including the proportion of tumor-stem cells, tumor-cell mitosis, and oxygenation. He reviews other mechanisms of failure, including tumor volume, hypoxia, tumor regeneration, underdosage, second primaries, and altered host factors (i.e., malnutrition and altered immunologic status). One exciting new area still in its infancy, noted by Dr. Peters is the concept of determining cellular radiosensitivity of a given tumor obtained from a biopsy specimen. This would enable the radiotherapist to tailor the quality, quantity, and variety of radiation to a specific tumor.

Finally, the chapter notes an area well known to the head and neck surgeon—radiation complications in normal tissue, which classically present themselves long after the fear of tumor has past. In an honest and practical approach, Dr. Peters relates these problems to the volume and dose of radiation, the quality of radiation (high vs. low LET), the concommitant use of chemotherapy, surgical trauma, and the general nutritional status of the patient. By noting the concept of normal tissue tolerance and the appropriate therapeutic ratio, Dr. Peters rounds out a most concise and pointed discussion of a highly technical topic without sacrificing its obvious clinical application.

INTRODUCTION

A working knowledge of the biologic principles underlying radiotherapy for head and neck tumors is desirable for all the disciplines involved in the management of patients with these cancers. This chapter provides an overview of radiation biology oriented toward surgeons involved in the management of patients with cancer of the head and neck.

CELLULAR EFFECTS OF IONIZING RADIATION

Cell Death

Cellular radiation biology has its origins in the development of techniques to assay clonogenic cell survival (i.e., the ability of single cells to grow into visible clones analogous to those formed by bacteria plated on an appropriate culture medium). The ability to form a clone is dependent on the reproductive integrity of the cell; thus, from the point of view of radiation biology, cell death is defined as loss of reproductive integrity or a clonogenic capacity (Puck and Marcus, 1956). Although morphologic disruption of a cell is clearly incompatible with reproductive survival, the converse is not true: a cell may appear intact morphologically, yet have lost its reproductive capability by virtue of injury to its genetic apparatus, the injury not being manifested until the cell attempts mitotic division. This is not necessarily the first division after radiation exposure, and pedigree studies have shown that mitotic death may occur after several apparently successful cell divisions have been accomplished. The essence of clonogenic survival, however, is the ability to reproduce indefinitely, and if none of the progeny of an irradiated cell retains this capability, that cell is effectively sterilized. In general, the higher the dose received, the fewer the divisions that will be accomplished before a lethally irradiated cell undergoes lysis (Elkind and Whitmore, 1967).

Less frequently, cell death following radiation injury is not linked to cell division, and is therefore called "interphase death." Unlike mitotic death, interphase death occurs soon after radiation exposure, presumably because of damage to the plasma membrane; histologically, it creates the impression of extreme sensitivity of the cell type to ionizing radiation. Classical interphase death with rapid cell lysis is manifested by certain types of lymphocytes (Anderson and Warner, 1976). In the head and neck region, the serous cells of the salivary glands, but not the mucous cells, also undergo interphase death after modest doses of radiation (Figure 7–1), which accounts for the acute changes in salivary flow and composition that occur during radiotherapy (Mossman, 1983). The reason for this selective sensitivity of serous cells has not been elucidated. Irradiation can also enhance apoptosis (Searle et al., 1982), a natural phenomenon by which defunct or injured tissue cells collapse into electron-dense bodies with preservation of organelles; these are subsequently phagocytosed by adjacent parenchymal cells. Indeed, in some tumors this appears to be the predominant mode of cell deletion after irradiation (Kerr and Searle, 1980).

Loss of Tissue Function

Unlike reproductive integrity, the vegetative functions of most mammalian cells are not detectably altered by doses of radiation in the range used clinically. Thus, loss of function of an organ following irradiation is not due to loss of an increment of function of individual cells but rather to a depletion of the total number of functional cells in the tissue. Depending on the kinetic and organizational status of a particular tissue, its functional response to radiation may vary widely. In general, tissues that are rapidly turning over and have definable stem-cell, maturation, and functional-cell compartments, manifest radiation injury soon after exposure, with a rate of onset that is not greatly dose-dependent. Examples of such tissues include most epithelia and the bone marrow. Depending on the extent of stem-cell depletion, these tissues may recover essentially all of their function following irradiation.

On the other hand, tissues characterized by low cell turnover rates and populations of functional parenchymal cells that retain the ability to revert to a reproductive function in the event of tissue loss manifest more delayed radiation injury. At the time of onset, such injury is dependent on radiation dose and tends to increase in severity with time because of an "avalanche" phenomenon (i.e., the drawing into the division cycle of cells harboring latent reproductive injury). Examples of such tissues with reference to radiotherapy in the head and neck region include bone and neuroglial and endocrine tissues.

DOSE-RESPONSE CURVES FOR REPRODUCTIVE SURVIVAL

Single Doses

The deposition of radiant energy is random and discrete. Thus, cell killing by radiation is approximately an exponential function of dose. For this reason, it has become customary to plot radiation survival curves on semilogarithmic coordinates, in which the surviving fraction of clonogenic cells is plotted on a logarithmic scale as a function of dose on a linear scale. Exponential survival is represented there by a straight line, the slope of which may be defined in terms of the mean lethal dose of radiation, D_0. This is the dose that would be sufficient to kill all the cells in the population if the dose were targeted to the critical site of each cell individually. Since dose deposition is in fact random, however, the mean lethal dose kills on average only 63 percent of the cells in a population; in other words, each dose of D_0 reduces survival to 37 percent of its former level.

For most mammalian cells exposed to x-rays or gamma-rays, however, the shape of the cell survival curve over the range of the first few hundred cGy is not exponential but curves downward on semilogarithmic coordinates (Figure 7–2). This means that over this dose range, the efficiency of cell killing progressively increases to a limit corresponding with the terminal exponential slope. The curved portion of the survival curve is known as the "shoulder," and is the region of greatest interest for clinical radiobiology because it corresponds to the dose range of conventional dose fractionation.

Various biophysical theories have been proposed to account for the shoulder on the dose-survival curve, including accumulation of sublethal radiation injury, interaction of molecular lesions, and saturation of cellular repair mechanisms. Along with these theories, different mathematical models of survival have been developed. In recent years, the trend has been toward use of the "linear-quadratic" survival-curve equation $S = e^{-(\alpha D + \beta D^2)}$ because it gives a satisfactory

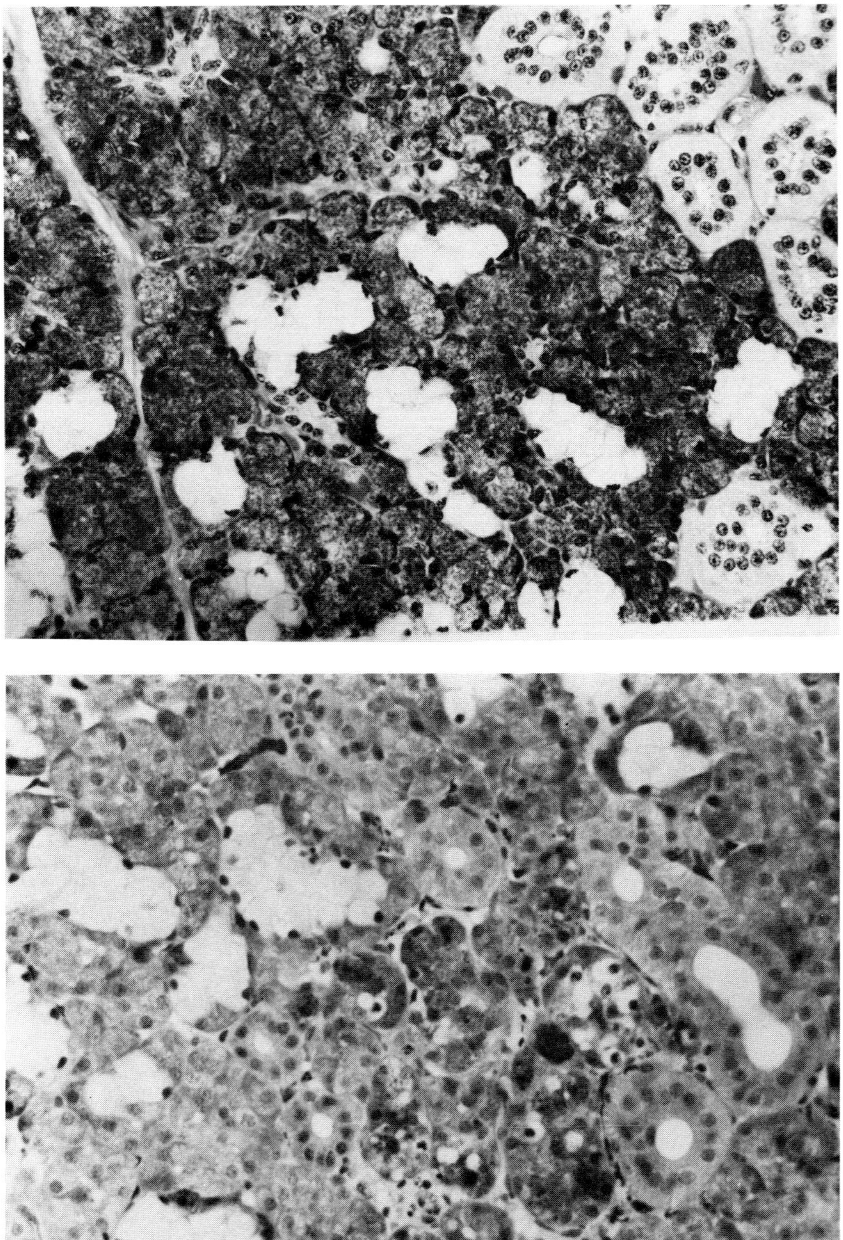

A

B

Figure 7-1. (*A*) Rhesus monkey submandibular salivary gland. Unirradiated specimen. The circular structures on the right side are ducts. Serous acini are composed of cells filled with dark granules. Mucous acini are composed of cells with unstained cytoplasm. (*B*) Specimen treated with six fractions of 1.7 Gy and biopsied 12 hours after the last fraction. A focus of necrotic serous acini is infiltrated with inflammatory cells. Mucous acini are unaffected.

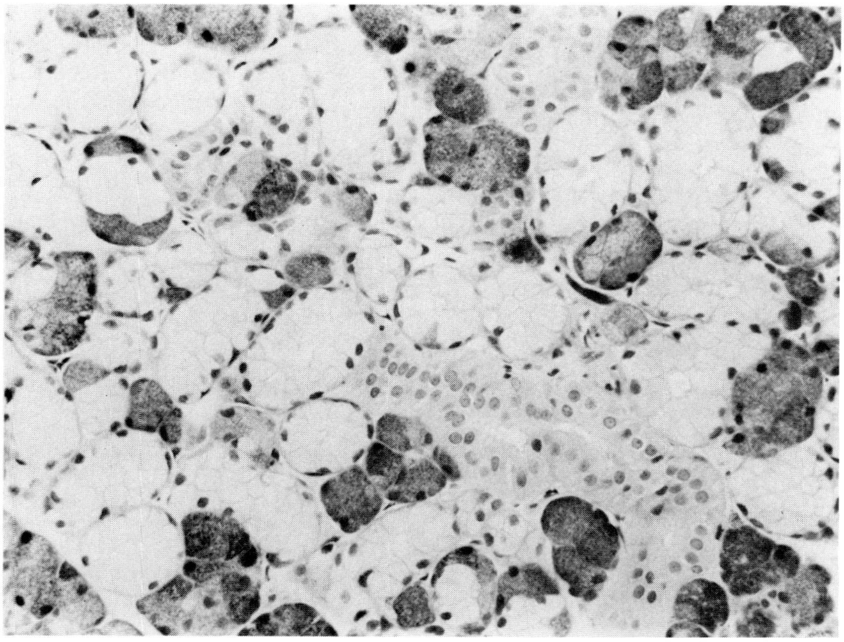

Figure 7-1 (cont.). (*C*) Specimen treated with six fractions of 1.7 Gy and biopsied 20 weeks later. Compared with (*A*), numbers of serous acini are reduced, whereas mucous acini are increased. H&E, ×250. (Photographs courtesy of L. C. Stephens, D.V.M., Ph.D., Department of Veterinary Medicine and Surgery, UTMDAH.)

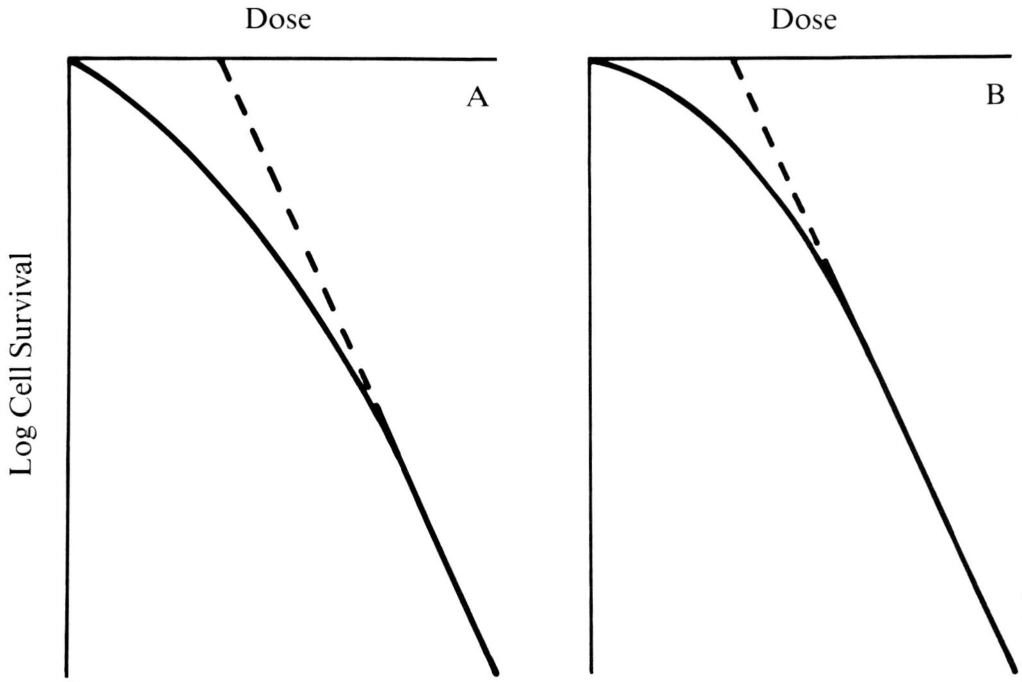

Figure 7-2. Radiation cell survival curves. Typical examples of mammalian cell-survival curves, showing an initial shoulder followed by an exponential region on semilogarithmic coordinates. While the width of the shoulder is the same as these two curves, the shape of the shoulder is markedly different. In terms of the "linear quadratic model, curve A would have a much higher α/β ratio than curve B. Differences of this type have a profound effect on the response of cell populations to fractionated irradiation with small dose increments. (Reprinted with permission from Peters, 1985a, in press.)

description of experimental data and is the simplest of the equations to manipulate mathematically. In the equation, S is the surviving fraction of cells exposed to a dose D, while α and β are constants representing cell killing by single-hit and two-hit mechanisms, respectively. The ratio of these two constants describes the shape of the shoulder region of the survival curve. Thus, a high α/β ratio typifies a curve with a steep initial slope and little curvature in the shoulder region, whereas a low α/β ratio characterizes a curve with shallow initial slope and a greater degree of curvature in the shoulder region (Figure 7–2).

The absolute values of α and β define the size of the shoulder on the radiation survival curve. This varies according to cell type and position in the division cycle. In addition, for the same cell type the size of the shoulder is affected by whether the cells are irradiated in a disaggregated state or in contact with each other, the latter leading to a wide shoulder on the survival curve (Sutherland and Durand, 1976).

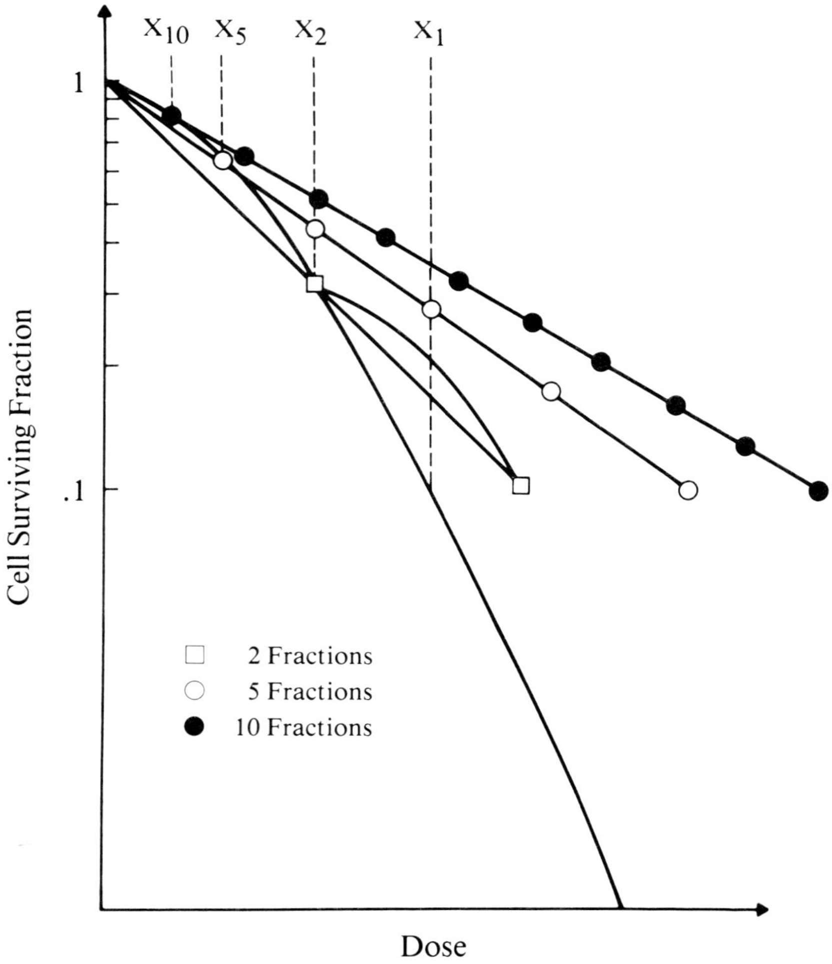

Figure 7–3. Example of single-dose and fractionated-dose cell-survival curves. The single-dose curve is characterized by a shoulder that is repeated in fractionated exposures. The figure shows that a cell-surviving fraction of 0.1 may be produced by a single dose of $\times_1$, 2 doses of $\times_2$, 5 doses of $\times_5$, or 10 doses of $\times_{10}$. Note that because the single-dose survival curve is almost straight between 0 and $\times_{10}$, any further reduction in size of dose per fraction would not significantly increase the total dose required to produce the same surviving fraction. (From Peters L. J., and Ang, K. K., Unconventional fractionation schemes in radiotherapy. In DeVita, V., Hellmas, S., and Rosenberg, S. A. *Important Advances in Oncology*. J.B. Lippincott, Philadelphia, 1986.)

Fractionated Doses

When the radiation dose is fractionated—i.e., individual doses are separated in time by several hours—the shoulder on the survival curve reconstitutes itself. This means that after an adequate period of recovery, cells surviving the first dose of radiation respond to subsequent doses as if they had never been previously irradiated. Thus, regardless of the shape of the single-dose survival curve, equal doses of radiation may be considered to produce equal decrements in cell survival, so that the resulting plot of net cell survival versus total fractionated dose can be represented by a simple exponential function (Figure 7-3). The effective slope of this fractionated irradiation survival curve allowing for full recovery between dose fractions becomes progressively shallower as the dose per fraction decreases. Eventually, however, the dose per fraction reaches a size below which no detectable bending of the dose survival curve occurs and where all cell killing can be attributed to single-hit (α-type) cell killing. Below this size of dose per fraction, there is no further increase in surviving fraction with further dose fractionation. This limit of resolvable effect of dose fractionation is designated by D_f, and for various tissues D_f lies in the range of 0 to 200 cGy (Table 7-1) (Tucker and Thames, 1983). The lower the α/β ratio, the lower will be the value of D_f; conversely, the higher the α/β ratio, the higher will be the value of D_f (Figure 7-3). This has important implications for the rationale for hyperfractionation (see page 84).

Table 7-1. Experimental Estimates of D_f for Various Normal Tissues

TISSUE	D_f* (cGy)
Bone marrow	45–134
Gut endothelium	40–198
Skin	47–162
Kidney	2–20
Lung	6–32
Spinal cord	13–74

*D_f represents the range of dose per fraction below which there is no further sparing of tissue reactions by increased dose fractionation. Note that D_f is consistently lower for late-reacting normal tissues. Modified from Tucker and Thames (1983).

Repair Mechanisms

The presence of a shoulder on the radiation dose-survival curve that is reconstituted with dose fractionation implies that cells can recover from nonlethal radiation injury between dose fractions. This phenomenon was first described by Elkind and Sutton (1959) and was called "repair of sublethal injury." Because of continued debate about the biophysical explanation of the shoulder region of the survival curve, the term "repair of sublethal injury" is giving way to the simple designation "Elkind recovery." By definition, Elkind recovery requires at least two doses of radiation for its detection, because it is manifested by the return of the shoulder on the single-dose survival curve.

An operationally different type of intracellular repair mechanism is called "potentially lethal-damage repair." This refers to the increase in proportion of cells surviving a given dose of irradiation that can be achieved by modification of the postirradiation environment (Little, 1971). In generally, the holding of cells in an environment not conducive to cell division for several hours before assaying their clonogenic survival results in an increase in the surviving fraction (Figure 7-4). This can be conceptually explained in terms of successful completion of repair of DNA lesions that would have been lethal had DNA replication been attempted prior to their repair.

Although Elkind recovery and potentially lethal-damage repair are operationally different, the consensus of radiobiologists is that they probably involve the same enzymatic pathways.

Effect of Dose Rate

The preceding sections describing cell survival after single fractionated doses of irradiation refer to acute exposures—i.e., dose rates on the order of several Gy per minute. These dose rates apply to most external beam megavoltage radiation sources. At dose rates below about 100 cGy/min, however, the efficiency of cell killing decreases (Hall, 1972). This can be attributed to Elkind recovery occurring during radiation exposure analogous to that observed

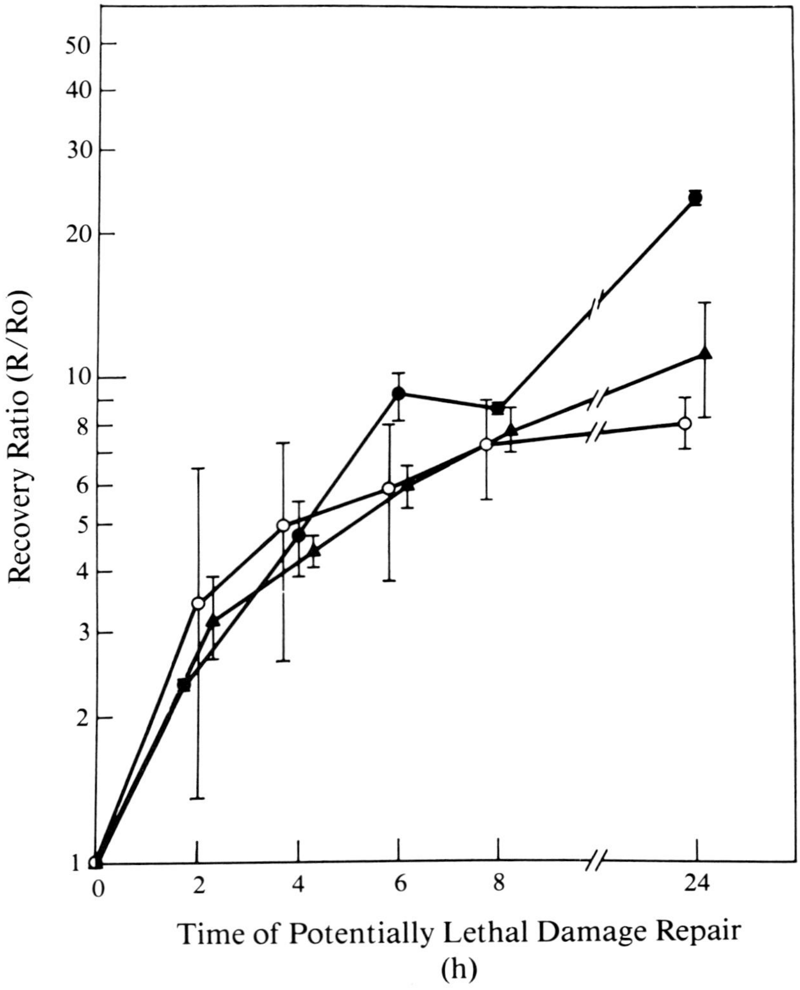

Figure 7–4. Increase in survival of human tumor cells, irradiated in density-inhibited cultures, as a function of time between irradiation and plating for assay of clonogenic survival. Two melanoma cell lines (o and ▲) and one osteosarcoma cell line (•) were exposed to 700 cGy at time 0. All show significant repair of potentially lethal damage. (From Weischselbaum et al., 1982. Used with permission.)

between acute dose fractions. Low dose-rate continuous irradiation can therefore be conceived of as a large number of very small dose fractions and, as with dose fractionation, the limit of effect of reduced dose rate is reached when essentially all cell killing results from single-hit (α-type) inactivation (Figure 7–3). This occurs at different dose rates for different cell types, but as a clinical rule of thumb one can take 1 cGy/min as the lower limit of dose rate associated with significant changes in cell-killing efficiency. Thus, in clinical radiotherapy, dose rate rarely has to be considered in calculating total doses because dose rates associated with external beam therapy are above the critical range, whereas those associated with interstitial techniques are below it.

Effect of Radiation Quality

The biological effect of a given absorbed dose of radiation can vary markedly according to the quality of the radiation. The relative biologic effect (RBE) of a given beam in relation to a reference standard is calculated as the dose of the reference standard divided by the dose of the beam in question that will produce the same biologic effect. In relation to ^{60}Co gamma-rays, kilovoltage x-rays are somewhat more effective—Gy for Gy—by a factor of 10 percent to 15 percent. Recent data suggest that protons and high-energy electrons spread by a scanning electron pencil beam, but not by a scattering foil, are also more biologically effective by about the same factor.

All of these beams of x-rays, gamma-rays, electrons, and protons are characterized as having low linear-energy transfer (LET)—i.e., the density of ionization produced by such beams is sparse. On the other hand, irradiation with particles, such as fast neutrons or heavy nuclei, produces tracks of dense ionization, and the beams are said to have high LET (Figure 7–5). High-LET beams are much more damaging—Gy for Gy—to biologic material

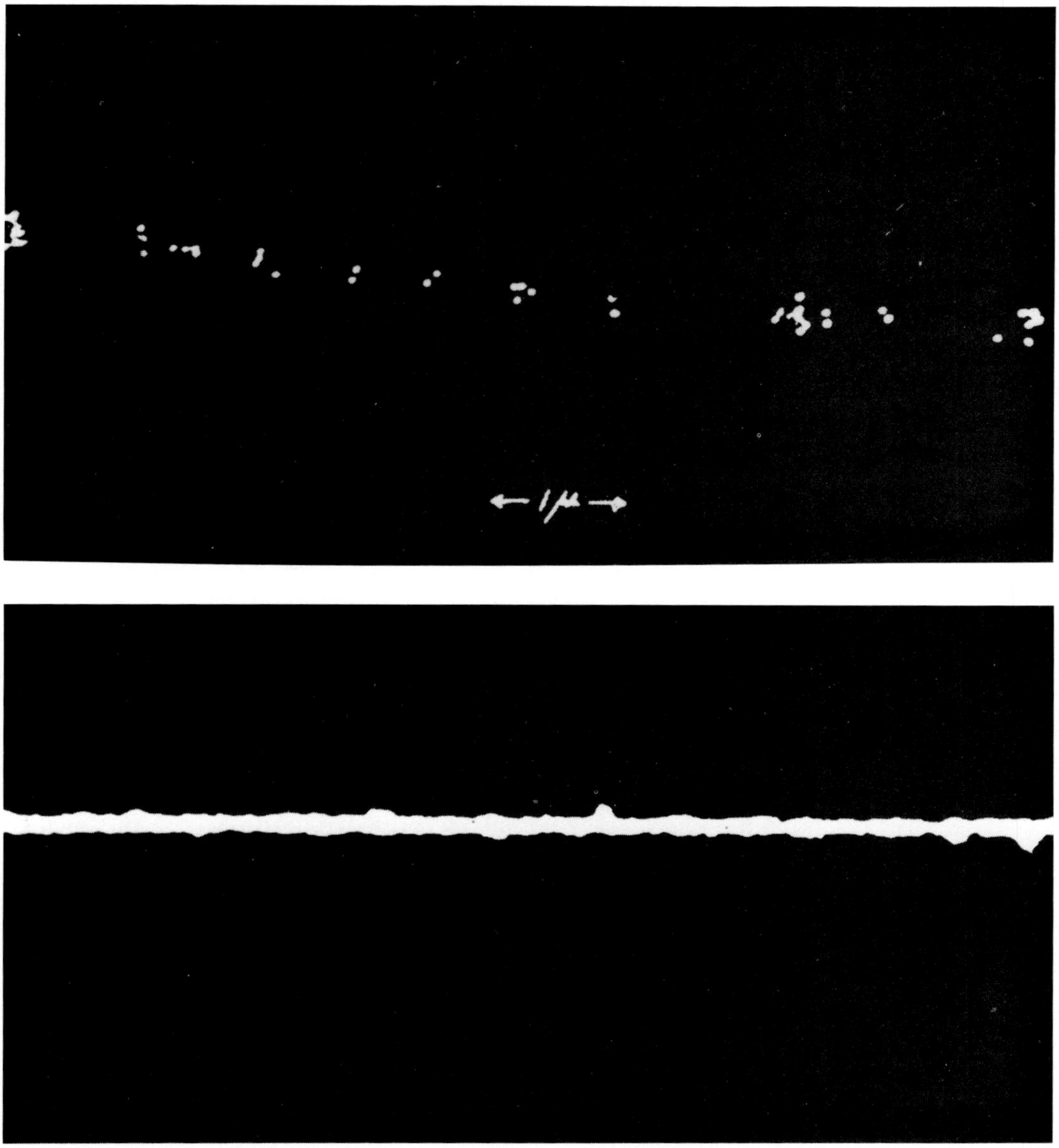

Figure 7–5. (*A*) Cloud chamber track of a fast electron illustrates that ionization occurs in clusters. Successive clusters are separated by approximately 1μm. (*B*) Cloud chamber track of a proton ejected by a neutron; note the high, confluent density of ion pairs. (Reprinted with permission from Bacq, Z. M., and Alexander, P., *Fundamentals of Radiobiology*, Copyright 1961, Pergamon Press.)

than low-LET beams. No constant factor is applicable for stating these differences in biologic effect, however, because the shape of the survival curves of cells irradiated with high-LET radiations is different from that following low-LET radiation.

The most notable differences are that the shoulder of the radiation survival curve is markedly reduced or abolished and the terminal slope is steeper. Furthermore, cells show little or no ability to repair intracellular radiation injury between doses of high-LET radiation. For these reasons, variations in dose fractionation and dose rate with high-LET radiation have much less effect, and the RBE of high-LET beams in relation to conventionally fractionated low-LET radiation is determined largely by the fractionation response of the tissue in question to the low-LET beam (Withers et al., 1982). In other words, those tissues most spared by dose fractionation with low-LET radiation will have the highest RBE for high-LET radiation. High- and low-LET radiations also differ in that cell killing by high-LET beams is less influenced by oxygen or cell-age distribution (see next section).

Effect of Oxygen

Since the early 1950s (Read, 1952), it has been appreciated that the presence of molecular oxygen at the time of irradiation determined cellular radiosensitivity. Oxygen appears to fix labile radiation injury that would otherwise be repaired within milliseconds of irradiation. Thus, although the same number of radiochemical lesions are produced by irradiation in the presence or absence of oxygen, many more are repaired if oxygen is absent. The range of oxygen tensions over which the maximum change in radiosensitivity occurs is 0 to 20 mmHg. Within this range, there is considerable variability among cell types in the effect of oxygen tension on cell survival. Oxygen is usually considered to be dose-modifying—i.e., the dose required to produce a certain level of cell survival is greater by a constant factor in the absence of oxygen than in well-oxygenated conditions. This factor is known as the oxygen enhancement ratio (OER), and for most mammalian cells it is 2.5 to 3. Some evidence, however, shows that the OER may be somewhat lower for small doses per fraction or low dose-rate irradiation because of the preponderance of cell killing by single-hit mechanisms (Hall, 1972).

Effect of Cell Age

Experiments with synchronized cell populations have demonstrated significant variations in the radiosensitivity of the same cell type as it traverses the division cycle. In virtually all cell lines, the late G_2 and mitotic phases are the most sensitive, the next most sensitive phases being late G_1 and early S phase. Many cell lines show a peak of resistance in late S phase, whereas those with a long G_1 phase tend to show a peak of resistance in early G_1 (Figure 7–6). In spite of these differences, however, cell killing by radiation is not phase specific, by contrast with certain chemotherapeutic agents: cells in all phases of the division cycle are susceptible to radiation killing. The potential clinical importance of cell age-related differences in radiosensitivity was pointed out by Sinclair (1969). He showed that with V-79 cells, the survival of the most resistant, late S-phase cells receiving 200 cGy in oxygen, was higher than that of the most sensitive, G_2M-phase cells in hypoxia.

RATIONALE FOR DOSE FRACTIONATION: THE FOUR R'S

Early in the history of radiation therapy it became apparent that better results were obtained when the total dose was fractionated into many small increments rather than being delivered as a single dose or in a few large increments. The rationale for dose fractionation is based on the 4 R's.

Repair of Intracellular Radiation Injury

As indicated, when doses of low-LET radiation are fractionated, the shoulder of the survival curve reconstitutes itself between dose fractions. This results in a sparing effect of dose fractionation, with cells having the lowest ratio α/β in the survival-curve equation

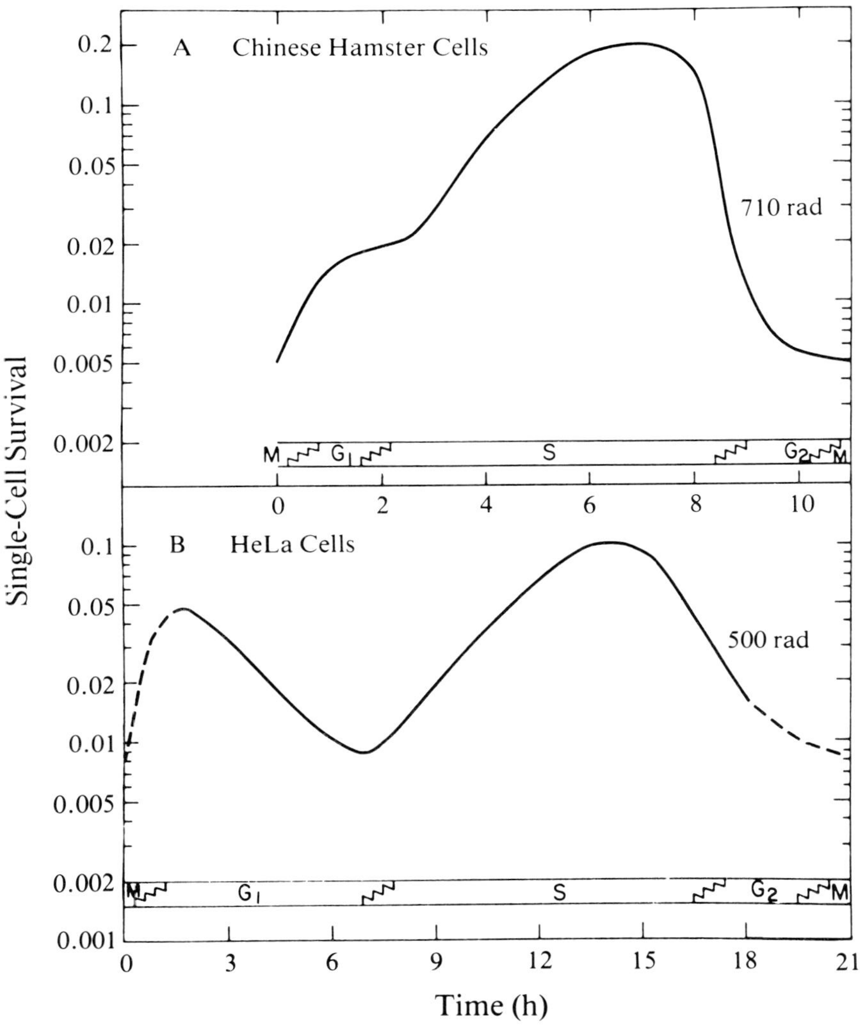

Figure 7–6. Forms of age response for cells with short G_1 (*A*), represented by hamster cells, and cells with long G_1, represented by HeLa cells (*B*). The time scales have been adjusted so that the S period has a comparable length on the figure for both cell lines. (Reprinted with permission from Sinclair, 1969.)

$S = e^{-(\alpha D + \beta D^2)}$ being spared most by dose fractionation. In practice, cells of late-reacting, normal tissues tend to belong to this class, so that dose fractionation increases the tolerance of the tissues that normally limit the total dose that can be given clinically. The rationale for predicting a therapeutic advantage with dose fractionation based on repair mechanisms is that acutely reacting tissues in general have higher α/β ratios than late-reacting, normal tissues and are therefore less spared by dose fractionation (Thames et al., 1982).

By kinetic analogy, most tumors are more akin to acutely reacting normal tissues than late-reacting ones, so that a therapeutic advantage of fractionation might be expected for tumor control compared with late, normal-tissue injury. While the analogy between acutely reacting normal tissues and tumors is obviously a gross oversimplification, a recent analysis of human tumor cell-survival data (Williams et al., 1985) supports the contention that most have rather high α/β ratios.

Another possible advantage of dose fractionation is that repair of potentially lethal radiation damage (PLDR) may be less effective after small dose fractions because tumors showing a large capacity for PLDR would not be spared as much as they would be if large dose fractions were used (Weichselbaum and Little, 1982).

Reoxygenation

Molecular oxygen is undoubtedly the best known modifier of radiation response, and for most mammalian cells the OER is 2.5 to 3.0. Although the range of partial pressures of oxygen over which cellular radiosensitivity varies most markedly (0–20 mmHg) is well below the pO_2 of venous blood, Thomlinson and Gray (1955) combined histologic observations with oxygen diffusion calculations to predict that radiobiologic hypoxia would exist in human solid tumors, as it undoubtedly does in experimental animal tumors. Based on these observations, many treatment strategies aimed at overcoming the resistance of such cells have been tested. These strategies include the use of hyperbaric oxygen, mixtures of oxygen and carbon dioxide (to induce vasodilatation), chemical analogs of oxygen, metabolic approaches to inhibit oxygen consumption, selective vasoconstriction in normal tissue, and tourniquet hypoxia. A fair summary of the clinical results of these strategies is that the beneficial results have been associated with the use of large doses of radiation, whereas results with conventionally fractionated radiation have been disappointing (Henk, 1981). This suggests that the oxygen status of hypoxic cells surviving one dose of radiation improves during the interval between fractions, and that with small sizes of dose per fraction the proportion of radiobiologically hypoxic cells does not increase sufficiently to affect net cell survival significantly.

The phenomenon of improvement in oxygen status of tumor cells between dose fractions is called "reoxygenation," and has been conclusively demonstrated in a variety of animal tumors. Postulated mechanisms for reoxygenation include: (1) reduced total tumor cell population relative to the surface area of existing tumor blood vessels; (2) reduced separation of hypoxic cells from blood vessels resulting from preferential killing and lysis of well-oxygenated cells near the blood vessels; (3) increased effective oxygen diffusion radius due to decreased consumption of oxygen by lethally injured cells; (4) decreased intratumoral pressure permitting reopening of compressed blood vessels or increased blood flow rates; (5) cyclic shunting of blood flow within the tumor microvasculature and; (6) continual ameboid movement of tumor cells in relation to one another, by which a lethally injured cell near a blood vessel may be displaced by a viable, formerly hypoxic cell.

Whatever the mechanism of reoxygenation, its clinical significance is that by delivering the total radiation dose in multiple fractions, the chances of a given cell remaining in a viable but hypoxic state throughout the course of treatment are minimized. The fact that many human tumors are cured by doses of radiation that would be inconsistent with the presence of a significant number of hypoxic tumor cells, and the fact that strategies to improve tumor control based on the oxygen effect have been largely unsuccessful with conventionally fractionated treatment, leads to the conclusion that reoxygenation does indeed occur in those human tumors controlled by radiation therapy. The failure of reoxygenation is, of course, a possible cause of failure to control a given tumor, but it is only one of many (see page 88).

Redistribution

By delivering a course of radiation in multiple fractions, the chances of irradiating a given cell in a sensitive phase of the division cycle are increased, particularly with respect to cell populations that have a moderately rapid turnover rate. This applies both to acutely reacting normal tissues and to tumors. Conversely, late-reacting normal tissues with a very low turnover rate would not be sensitized to any extent by redistribution during a conventional course of therapy. This results in a net gain in the therapeutic ratio between tumor control and late normal-tissue injury.

Regeneration

Both normal tissues and tumors can respond to depopulation by regeneration—i.e., by increasing their net cell production. A tissue's capability of regenerating itself depends on the number of stem cells present at the time of radiation able to be recruited into the stem cell pool. As with redistribution, the effect of regeneration is most marked in acutely reacting normal tissues and tumors, whereas late-reacting normal tissues with a slow turnover rate usually do not manifest sufficient radiation injury during treatment to trigger a regenerative response. Regeneration is the major determinant in deciding the optimum length of a course of radiation treatment in a given clinical situation. Protraction of the total duration of radiation spares acute reactions by allowing a regenerative response to proceed concomitantly with depopulation by radiation. The same is true for split-course regimens. This must be balanced against the fact that tumor cells also regenerate to a greater extent with protraction of overall treatment time. In circumstances where the regenerative potential of the tumor exceeds that of the critical acute-reacting normal tissue, the therapeutic ratio will be adversely affected by protraction, and accelerated fractionation should be used (Thames et al., 1983).

ALTERED FRACTIONATION SCHEDULES

Radiation dose-fractionation schedules have evolved empirically over the years, with a general tendency toward protraction of treatment to prevent acute mucosal reactions from interrupting the course of radiotherapy. So-called conventional fractionation schemes vary in different parts of the world, but in the United States the term "conventional fractionation" is generally held to mean incremental doses of 180 to 200 cGy delivered 5 days per week for periods of 6 to 8 weeks. Recently, on the basis of radiobiologic considerations, attempts have been made to improve the therapeutic ratio by using multiple dose fractions per day. There are two distinct rationales for the use of more than one daily dose fraction, and this is reflected in the following terminology: *accelerated fractionation*—overall treatment time is reduced by giving two or more daily dose fractions of close to conventional size; *hyperfractionation*—the overall time is conventional or slightly protracted, but an increase in total dose is achieved by giving two or more small dose fractions on each treatment day.

The major difference from conventional treatment with accelerated fractionation is the shortening of overall treatment time, whereas with hyperfractionation it is a reduction in size of dose per fraction with a corresponding increase in total dose. The basic concept underlying accelerated fractionation is the prevention of treatment failure because of tumor-cell regeneration during treatment. Such failure is more likely when clonogenic cells are characterized by a short potential doubling time (see "Tumor Regeneration," p. 96).

By contrast, hyperfractionation has its rationale in the different ways in which acute and late radiation responses are affected by dose fractionation (Figure 7-7). Conventional fractionation schedules are limited in total dose by late normal-tissue injury. The use of smaller fractions increases the tolerance of late-reacting normal tissues and therefore allows the total dose to be increased. This increased total dose has a greater relative effect on acutely reacting tissues, and insofar as most tumors kinetically resemble acutely reacting tissues, an improvement in the therapeutic ratio for tumor control in relation to late normal-tissue injury may be anticipated.

The choice of strategy—i.e., whether to use accelerated fractionation or hyperfractionation in a given clinical circumstance—depends basically on the tumor cell kinetics: the greater the regenerative potential of the tumor, the more accelerated fractionation would be preferred. The reverse, however, is not the case: hyperfractionation would not be the preferred strategy for extremely slow-growing tumors because the rationale for hyperfractionation depends on tumors behaving kinetically like acutely responding normal tissues. On radiobiologic grounds, such indolent tumors would be best treated with high-LET radiation, since cell radiosensitivity in different phases of the division cycle varies much less with such beams, and resistance conferred by failure of redistribution between dose fractions is minimized.

The ideal application of hyperfractionation

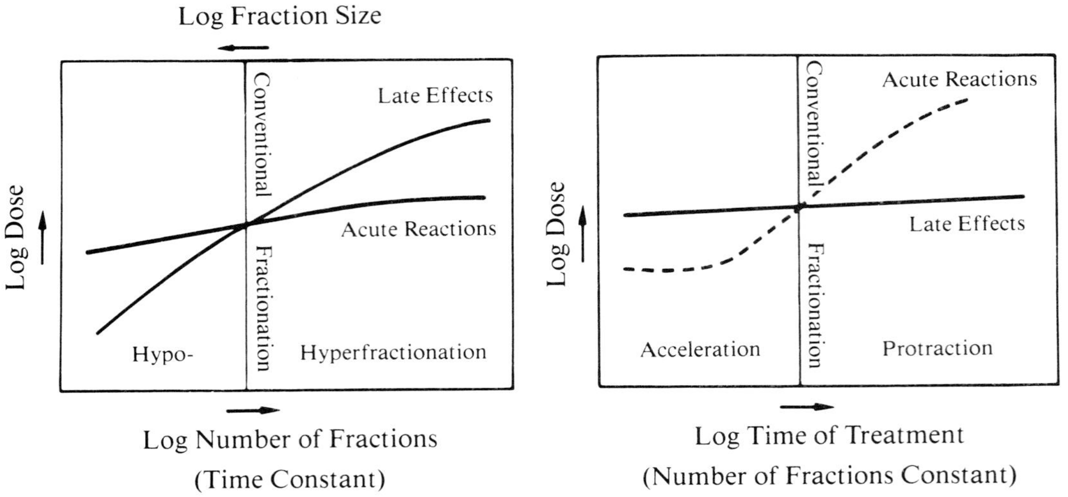

Figure 7-7. Effect of changes in time-dose relationships in fractionated radiotherapy on acute and late normal-tissue reactions. Curves represent isoeffective doses for a given level of reactions, normalized to the point designated "conventional fractionation"—i.e., 1.8 to 2.0 Gy, 5 fractions per week. The left panel shows that with overall time held constant a change in the number (and size) of dose fractions has a relatively greater effect on the isoeffective doses for late effects than for acute reactions. In particular, it should be noted that hypofractionation carries the risk of overdosage for late effects if doses are adjusted to equalize acute reactions. The right panel shows the effect of varying overall time of treatment, with the number of fractions held constant. The influence of time on the isoeffect dose for actue reactions is complex. If the treatment time is less than the turnover time of the tissues in question, registration of the radiation injury will occur after treatment is completed, and the ensuing regenerative response will not affect the isoeffect dose. When the treatment time extends into the regeneration phase, however, the isoeffect dose for a given acute reaction increases steeply, flattening off again as treatment times exceed the most active regenerative spurt. With any protraction beyond conventional treatment times, acute reactions are preferentially spared, leading to excessive late effects if doses are made isoeffective for acute reactions. Thus both hypofractionation and protraction are hazardous strategies if based on acute normal-tissue reactions. (Reprinted with permission from Peters, 1985, in press.)

is in the treatment of tumors of moderate regeneration potential growing in sites where late normal-tissue injury is a serious constraint to the dose that can be delivered using conventional fractionation—for example, when the whole larynx must be included in the high-dose volume.

TUMOR CONTROL PROBABILITY

For a tumor to be controlled, it must by definition contain no surviving clonogenic cells at the end of treatment. When the average number of surviving clonogens per tumor is known, the probability of there being zero survivors in a particular tumor is obtained from Poisson statistics ($p = e^{-n}$, where n is the average number of surviving clonogenic cells per tumor). For example, if the probability of cure is 50 percent, then $n = 0.693$. This does not, of course, mean that there is a fraction of a cell surviving in each tumor, but rather that half the tumors contain no surviving clonogens and are cured, while the other half contains one or more and will recur. For a homogeneous population of tumors, a very marked change in tumor control probability occurs over a small dose range. Figure 7-8 illustrates this change: if the TCD_{50} of a homogeneous population of tumors is 65 Gy, tumor control would increase from a little more than 5 percent at 60 Gy to a little less than 85 percent at 70 Gy.

In clinical practice, tumor-control probability curves are never so steep because of the heterogeneity of the clinical material; indeed, in some analyses, no dose-response relationship has been demonstrated. The issue of dose-response relationships for control of human tumors by radiotherapy is of great importance because it affects the philosophy of radiotherapy, both with regard to dose prescription and to accuracy of treatment planning and delivery. Clearly, if tumor control is not considered dose-dependent, these aspects of radiotherapeutic practice become less critical. Even

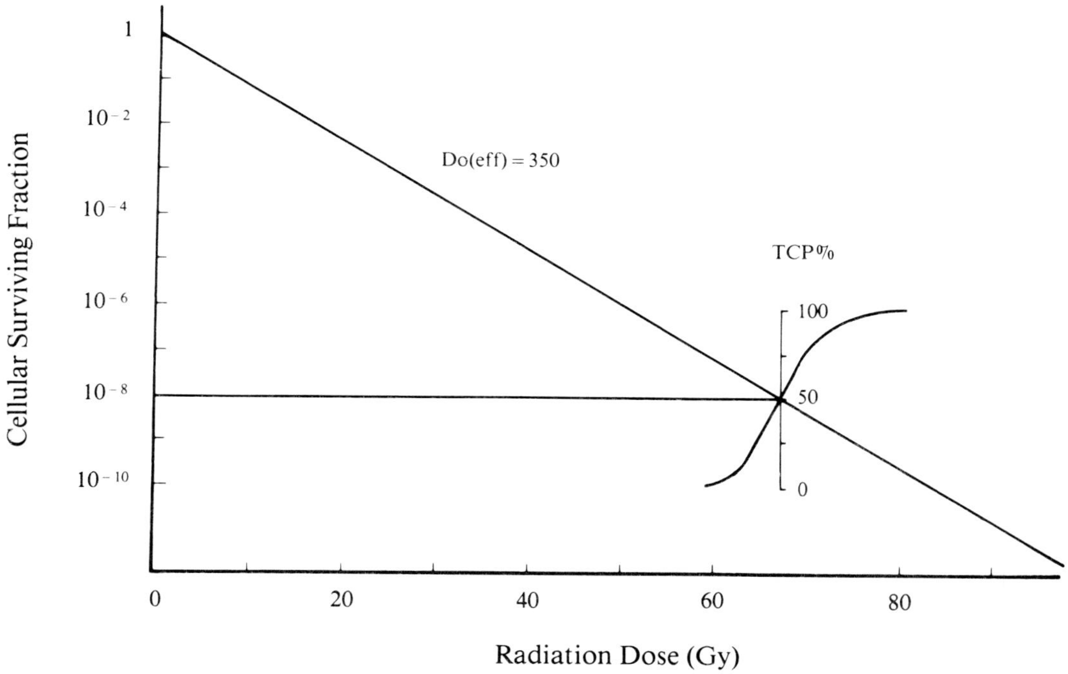

Figure 7-8. The relationship between D_0 (eff) with fractionated irradiation and the tumor control probability (TCP). In this case, the TCP was assumed to be 50 percent, with a cell survival fraction of 10^8. The effective slope of the fractionated survival curve, D_0 (eff), was set at 350 cGy, a typical value for fractional doses of 2 Gy. (Reprinted with permission from Fletcher et al., 1981.)

when no dose-response relationship can be demonstrated for various types of human cancers, it is inescapable that tumor control is dose-dependent for individual cancers, unless one postulates subpopulations of tumor cells that are absolutely resistant to ionizing radiation. This has never been demonstrated, and the only circumstance in which it could be true is when a geographic miss occurs and part of the tumor is not adequately irradiated. Thus, any analysis of clinical dose-response relationships must include a critical assessment of radiotherapeutic technique and quality control. Although it is axiomatic that tumor control is dose-dependent from a radiobiologic point of view, several factors combine to make it difficult or impossible to demonstrate steep dose-response relationships in clinical material.

Factors Influencing Dose-Response Relationships

Tumor Heterogeneity. Any variability in tumor clonogen number or other dose-limiting radiobiologic property will flatten the dose-response relationship for tumor control (Peters et al., 1982). Subsets of tumors, each with a steep dose-response function, may be separated by some distance on the dose axis, and when analysis is done of the group as a whole, the observed segment of the composite dose-response curve will be shallow or flat (Figure 7-9). Within such dose ranges, it is true that no dose-response relationship for tumor control exists for the population as a whole. It is particularly dangerous, however, to conclude that the total dose can therefore be safely reduced, since control of the most curable subsets of tumors will be most affected as the dose is reduced.

Existing Level of Tumor Control. Even with a uniform group of tumors, little change in tumor control probability with changes in dose is to be expected when the existing control level is either very high or very low. This is because of the sigmoid shape of the Poisson curve, which defines the probability of sterilizing all the clonogenic cells in a given tumor.

Assignment of Patients to Dose Groups. Virtually all clinical analyses of tumor-control

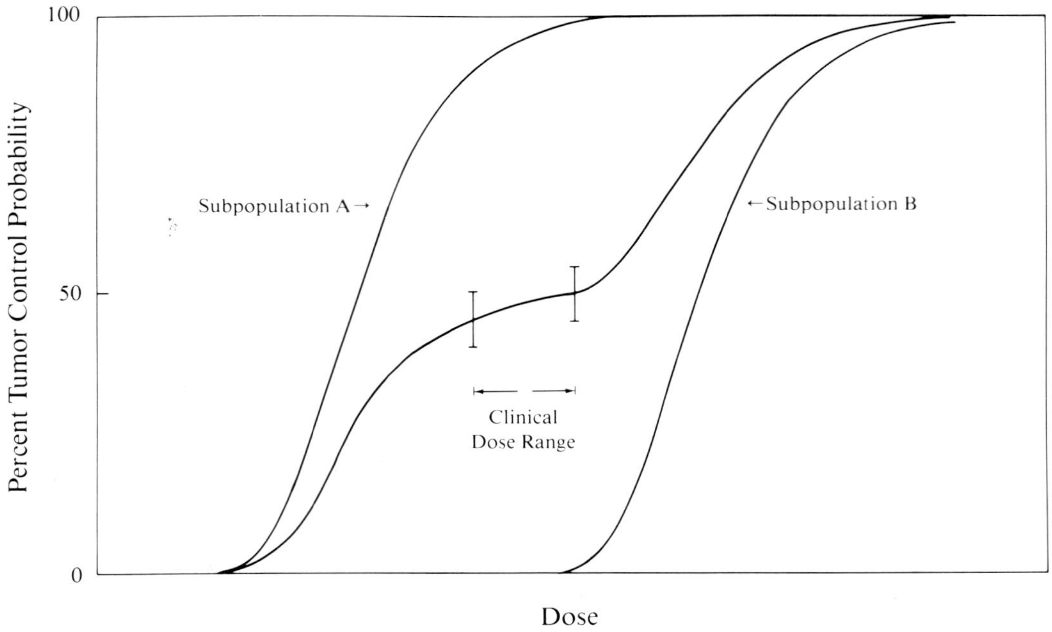

Figure 7–9. Effect of tumor heterogeneity on observed tumor control-dose response. This simple example is based on two equal subpopulations of tumor differing substantially in their radiocurability, regardless of reason. If the clinical dose-range were in the region indicated, then even with tumor control-probability rates defined accurately to within ± 5 percent, no significant dose response for tumor control could be demonstrated. (Reprinted with permission from Peters, 1985, in press.)

probability as a function of dose have been done by retrospective analysis, and the assumption has been implicitly made that patients were randomly assigned to the various dose groups. In fact, this is almost certainly not the case because of the tendency of most radiotherapists to give a slightly bigger dose to those tumors having adverse prognostic features or that have responded poorly to the initial prescribed dose of radiation. Such selection loads the high-dose groups with more unfavorable cases and inevitably acts to flatten the dose-response relationship.

Dose Specification. For an accurate analysis of dose response, one needs to know the radiation dose received at the actual site of recurrence, and not simply the prescribed tumor dose. This is rarely, if ever, available in retrospective analysis, and there is the problem of normalizing doses corresponding to different fractionation schedules. We have previously argued that less error is involved by interpolating toward the median of the range of fractionation schedules than by extrapolating to notional single doses because the isoeffect lines describing tumor control for a variety of tumors are unlikely to be parallel (Thames et al., 1980). Finally, with regard to dose specification, the range of total doses over which the analysis is made must be sufficiently wide to arrive at some reasonable definition of the slope of the curve for tumor-control probability.

Definition of Tumor Control. The definition of tumor control is of great importance when attempts are made to combine data from different series for dose-response analysis. Different conventions have been used by different authors to define tumor control: absolute tumor-control rates in patients who have survived an arbitrary period after therapy; actuarially calculated control rates; and the nonfailure rate—the number of patients who did not fail locally divided by the total number of patients treated. Each of these conventions gives different results for the same data set, with the trend being toward increases in the stated tumor-control rate from the first to the last of the three methods. Other problems with linking different series are also apparent, including different criteria for staging, tumor-dose specification, quality control, and accuracy of follow-up information. For these reasons, little, if any, reliance can be placed on analyses of different series lumped together, however elegant the statistical procedures may be.

Notwithstanding these inherent difficulties, significant dose-response relationships have been demonstrated for a variety of tumors in the head and neck region (Thames et al., 1980).

Rationale for Shrinking Fields

The concept of dose-response relationship for tumor control based on the number of clonogenic cells to be sterilized underlies the use of shrinking-field techniques in radiotherapy and combinations of irradiation and limited surgery. Since cell killing by radiation is essentially an exponential function of dose, it follows that the dose required for a given level of tumor-control probability is directly proportional to the logarithm of the number of clonogenic cells in the tumor (Figure 7–10). Thus, subclinical extensions of disease can reach the same probability of tumor control as gross palpable tumor after treatment with a lower total dose. This is true even when one assumes that the radiosensitivity of cells in small and large aggregates is identical. In fact, since the former have a higher growth fraction, one would predict them to show in-

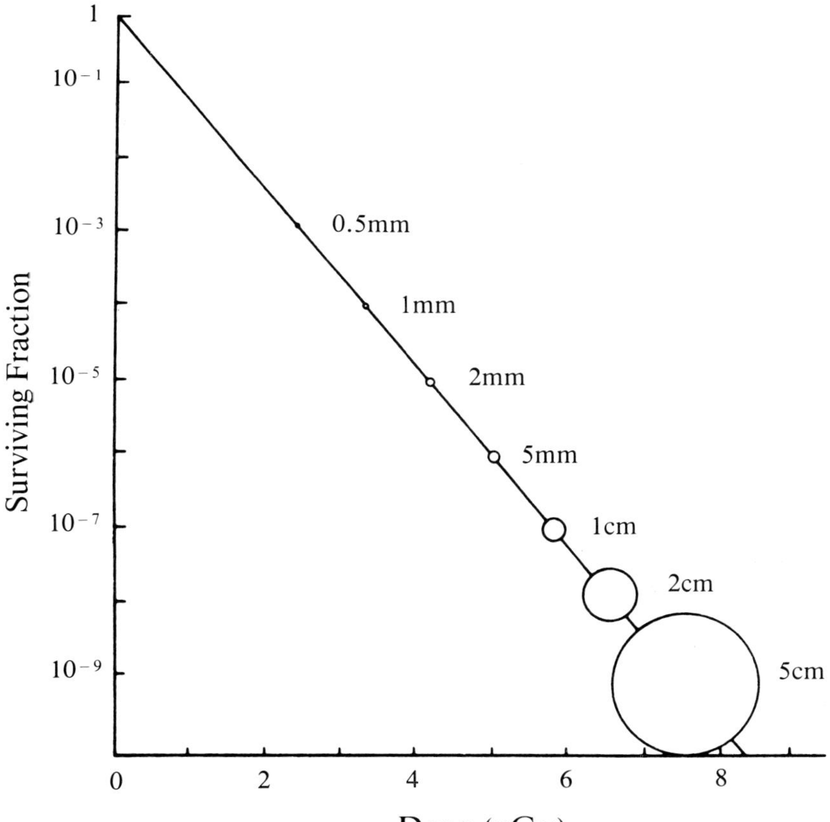

Figure 7–10. Representative fractionated survival curve for 200 cGy increments based on an "effective D_0" of approximately 350 cGy. If a dose of 65 Gy results in a given (say 80%) probability of controlling a lesion 2 cm in diameter, then the dose to produce the same level of control probability for deposits of the same tumor of different sizes can be read from the figure. For simplicity, the assumption is made that the cellular radiosensitivity and clonogenic fraction of cells in lesions of different size is constant. In practice, both would tend to be higher for smaller lesions. (Reprinted with permission from Peters et al, 1980.)

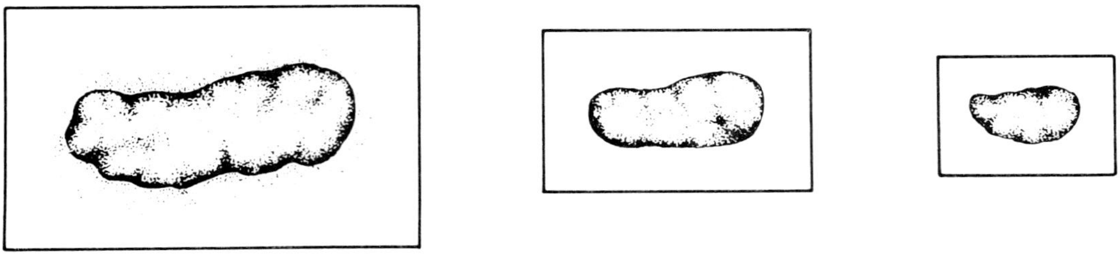

Figure 7–11. Example of shrinking field technique in treating a large cervical neck node by irradiation alone. (*A*) The whole neck receives 50 Gy (10 Gy/week), or 54 Gy (9 Gy/week), followed by (*B*) 15 to 20 Gy through a field directed to the primary or by glancing fields or electron beam. (*C*) For very large nodes to be treated by external irradiation only, an additional 5 to 10 Gy is given with electron beam or glancing fields, for a 75 to 80 Gy total dose. (Reprinted with permission from Fletcher, 1980.)

creased radiosensitivity. However, the proportion of clonogenic cells in small tumors would also more likely be higher, so these two influences would tend to cancel each other out. The ideal dose distribution to be achieved in radiotherapy is one in which the physical dose is graded to provide a homogeneous tumor-control probability throughout the treatment volume rather than a homogeneous dose distribution. This is normally achieved by the so-called shrinking field technique (Figure 7–11), or the use of body contours to provide built-in dose gradients to the site of maximum disease bulk.

TUMOR REGRESSION AND REGROWTH

The rate of regression of tumors following radiotherapy varies widely and is determined by many factors, including the turnover rate of the tumor, its cellularity in relation to stromal content and necrosis, and the efficiency of removal of dead tissue from the tumor site. In general, tumors with the most rapid cellular turnover rate will respond most rapidly to radiotherapy; those with a low cell-turnover rate will respond slowly, and these have historically been called radioresistant.

Prognostic Significance of Tumor-Regression Rates

The prognostic significance of residual tumor at the completion of a course of radiotherapy depends on the type of tumor. Most squamous cell carcinomas of the upper aerodigestive tracts have a moderately rapid turnover rate, and the presence of gross residual tumor at the end of a course of radiotherapy is associated with a lower probability of tumor control (Table 7–2) (Barkley and Fletcher, 1977). For this reason, additional boosts or limited surgical procedures are frequently carried out to remove residual disease following a planned definitive course of treatment. From a radiobiologic viewpoint, the most plausible explanation for the fact that residual tumor at the end of treatment carries a worse prognosis is that complete tumor regression is almost axiomatically associated with full reoxygenation of tumor cells during treatment. Coversely, when a tumor does not regress completely it is possible, but by no means certain, that reoxygenation may not have been complete.

Biopsies in the Postirradiation Period

Differences in the rate of regression of tumors following radiotherapy lead to difficulty in interpreting biopsy specimens taken in the postirradiation period. Because radiation killing is generally not expressed until cells attempt mitosis, it is impossible to determine on

Table 7–2. Recurrence Rates for Squamous Cell Carcinomas of the Faucial Arch, Tonsillar Fossa, and Base of Tongue (All Stages) According to Clinical Status at Completion of Radiotherapy

	RESIDUAL TUMOR	NO RESIDUAL TUMOR
Recurrence Rate*	71/117 (60.7%)	76/249 (30.5%)

*$p < 0.005$. Adapted from Barkley and Fletcher, 1977. Used by permission.

the basis of histologic examination whether apparently intact tumor cells do in fact retain clonogenic ability. For this reason, biopsies of residual tumor in the absence of any clinical evidence of regrowth should be discouraged. Such biopsies do not aid in diagnosis, and increase the risk of radionecrosis. Patients with residual disease at the end of treatment should therefore be closely followed, and biopsy confirmation of recurrence should be sought only if there are clinical signs of regrowth.

COMBINATIONS OF RADIATION THERAPY AND SURGERY

Pre- and Postoperative Irradiation

The same basic rationale underlies the boosting of gross disease with extra radiation doses or its removal with limited surgery. Frequently, the latter is to be preferred because the total dose of radiation can then be kept down to reduce the risk of normal tissue complications. The concept of elective treatment of subclinical disease with radiation doses causing little or no morbidity was pioneered by Fletcher (1973), and has recently been extensively reviewed (Fletcher, 1984). When radiation precedes surgery, a dose of about 50 Gy in 25 fractions over 5 weeks is usually adequate to sterilize subclinical disease; however, when radiation is given postoperatively, as is more usually the case in head and neck cancer, the extent of ''subclinical'' residual disease varies widely because of altered proliferation kinetics in the healing phase, and tumor cells are more likely to be radiobiologically hypoxic because of disturbance of the tissue planes. Higher doses may therefore be necessary postoperatively, depending on an assessment of the risk of residual disease after surgical dissection.

The combination of limited surgery with radiotherapy exploits the strengths of both modalities: with surgery, gross disease can usually be extirpated but microscopic residual disease cannot be excluded, whereas with radiotherapy, microscopic disease is most easily sterilized and failures are more likely at sites of gross tumefaction. Perhaps the most successful application of this complementary aspect of the two modalities in head and neck cancer has been the abandonment in all but a few cases of radical neck dissection at The University of Texas M.D. Anderson Hospital and Tumor Institute in Houston in favor of limited ''functional'' neck dissections, supplemented by radiotherapy or limited surgical procedures to remove residual disease following a basic course of radiation therapy to the neck (Jesse et al., 1978).

The sequencing of radiation and surgery is a trade-off between the radiobiologic advantages of preoperative irradiation and the practical and logistic advantages of operating first. The advantages of preoperative irradiation can be summarized as follows: radiotherapy is more effective in a surgically undisturbed bed, tumor regression resulting from radiotherapy may facilitate surgical dissection, and the risk of implantation or dissemination of viable cells at the time of surgery is greatly reduced. On the other hand, preoperative irradiation carries the following disadvantages: accurate surgical staging is precluded; margins of surgical resection are difficult to define; and delays in wound healing occur when major resections are undertaken after preoperative irradiation. For these reasons, the majority of combined procedures in the United States use radiation postoperatively. However, the option for preoperative treatment should not be overlooked, especially when a tumor is marginally resectable and a surgical cut-through is likely, or when a tumor is rapidly growing, in which case, gross recurrence may occur rapidly following surgery even before postoperative irradiation can be initiated.

The essential rationale of combined radiation and surgery is that the two modalities complement each other. It is important that the use of each modality be planned accordingly. For example, if postoperative irradiation is deemed necessary on the basis of the extent of primary disease in a patient with a node-negative neck, there is no need to dissect the neck because any subclinical disease in this region will be effectively sterilized by the postoperative radiation therapy. Conversely, for a patient in whom definitive radiation therapy for the primary tumor is planned but in whom a neck dissection is indicated on the basis of bulky nodal disease, efforts should be made to choose beam energies and port arrangements that avoid excessive doses to the neck, which would increase the risk of surgical complications.

Surgery in a Previously Irradiated Field

Attempted surgical salvage for recurrence or surgery for complications of radiation therapy call for specialized techniques and for a thorough understanding of the pathophysiology of the irradiated tissues by the surgeon. As indicated previously, acute radiation reactions are mainly due to a depletion of stem cells in rapidly cycling tissues, such as epithelia, whereas late radiation injury results from a progressive depletion of functional cells in slowly proliferating tissues. In the context of surgery months to years after previous high-dose radiation therapy, devitalization of the vasculoconnective tissues is a major deterrent to healing. Indeed, surgical trauma may precipitate an avalanche of cell death in previously irradiated, late-responding normal tissues, such that attempted conservative excision of a small area of osteoradionecrosis, for example, leads only to a larger volume of necrosis.

Neck dissections after previous irradiation call for the avoidance of trifurcate incisions because these frequently lead to flap necrosis and exposure of underlying vessels. With excellent surgical technique, neck dissections can usually be accomplished following previous radiotherapy without importation of new tissue. When major resection is necessary, however, the only really satisfactory way of ensuring wound healing following previous high-dose radiotherapy is to import new tissue with an intact blood supply and fibroblastic vitality, which is possible using myocutaneous flaps or free microvascular tissue transfer.

CAUSES OF FAILURE OF TUMOR CONTROL

It is instructive to review the causes of radiation therapy failure in order to identify those that can be minimized by optimal application of concepts and techniques readily available at present, those that are not amenable to any modification of any radiotherapeutic technique, and those that are potentially remediable by new treatment strategies based on the radiobiologic attributes of individual tumors. Cancers of the head and neck region lend themselves to accurate evaluation of causes of failure because they are generally easier to stage and to evaluate on follow-up than tumors in other sites of the body.

Histology and Intrinsic Cellular Radiosensitivity

For the first half of the century, radiosensitivity was considered to be a simple function of histology, and different histologic tumor types were classified as being radiosensitive, moderately radiosensitive, or radioresistant (Paterson, 1949). Furthermore, within the moderately radiosensitive group, differences in sensitivity were attributed to anatomic location. For example, squamous carcinoma of the mobile tongue was considered to be more sensitive than squamous carcinoma metastatic to the cervical lymph nodes. This conclusion can be traced to the fact that higher doses of radiation could be delivered to the oral tongue using interstitial techniques. Although it is undoubtedly true that tumors of certain histologic types are more radiocurable than others, this does not necessarily imply that the differences lie in inherent cellular radiosensitivity as opposed to epigenetic and environmental factors, such as the proportion of tumor-stem cells, tumor-cell kinetics, and oxygen status.

Recently, Deacon et al. (1984) collated the published data on the in vitro survival of human tumor-cell lines of diverse histologies. The authors found a broad correlation between the surviving fraction at 200 cGy and the category of tumor ranked by five levels of perceived clinical radiosensitivity (Figure 7–12). It is clear, however, that there is marked variability in cellular radiation response within each tumor category and overlap between the ranges of sensitivity reported for the most sensitive and most resistant clinical categories. These data also demonstrate the range of radiosensitivity of human tumor-cell lines

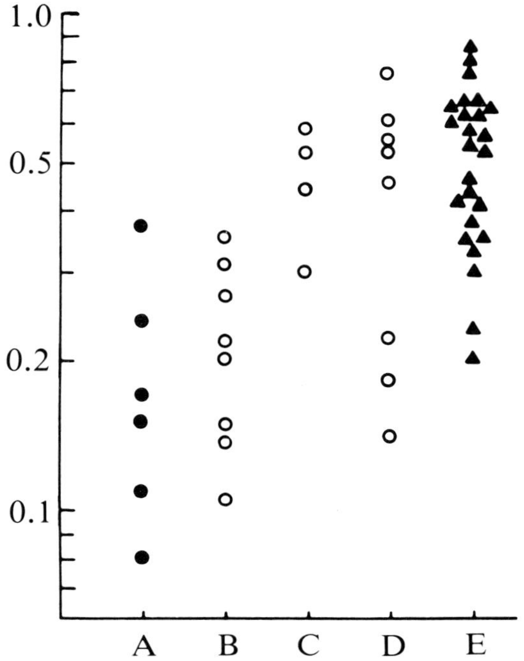

Figure 7-12. The initial slope of the cell-survival curve indicated by the surviving fraction at 2 Gy, in relation to the clinical response categories. (*A*) neuroblastoma, lymphoma, myeloma. (*B*) medulloblastoma, small-cell lung carcinoma. (*C*) breast, bladder, cervic carcinoma. (*D*) pancreas, colorectal, squamous lung carcinoma. (*E*) melanoma, osteosarcoma, glioblastoma, renal carcinoma). (Reprinted with permission from Deacon et al., 1984.)

to small doses of radiation, which would be greatly magnified in a fractionated course of treatment. For example, if the surviving fraction after 200 cGy was 50 percent in one tumor compared with 60 percent in the second, and the dose required to produce a certain cell kill in the first tumor was 70 Gy in 35 fractions, then the dose required to produce the same cell kill in the second tumor would be 95 Gy.

The data referred to in Figure 7-12 were obtained with standard in vitro cell survival techniques, which do not measure the extent of repair of potentially lethal damage (PLDR). When this has been measured, some correlation has also been observed between the clinically perceived radioresistance of different tumor histologies and the extent of PLDR seen in cell lines derived from the same histology (Weichselbaum et al., 1982).

In summary, available data demonstrate that significant differences in cellular radiosensitivity exist within human tumors, not ones necessarily related to histology, and support the concept of predicting radiocurability in individual patients by direct or indirect assays of cellular radiosensitivity from biopsy specimens (Peters et al., 1985).

Volume of Cancer

Tumor volume is one of the most fundamental determinants of radiocurability (Figure 7-10). This principle is illustrated in Table 7-3 with regard to control of cervical-node metastases from squamous carcinoma of the laryngopharynx. These data show not only a decreasing probability of control with increasing size of lymph node within each dose range, but also a dose-dependence for control within each size range.

Tumor Cell Hypoxia

For many years, hypoxic cells have been considered the single most significant cause of treatment failure, and most new radiotherapy strategies have been based on overcoming their radioresistance. Although the presence of such cells is indisputable in solid tumors, the question of how frequently they determine treatment failure with optimal fractionation

Table 7-3. Control Rates* as a Function of the Size of the Node(s) and Radiation Dose in the Squamous Cell Carcinomas of the Laryngopharynx

SIZE OF NODE (CM)	DOSE (GY)			
	≤65 Gy	*>65 Gy*	*≤70 Gy*	*>70 Gy*
<3	15/26 (58%)	86/95 (91%)		
3.5			3/9 (33%)	11/13 (85%)
>5			1/9 (11%)	11/15 (73%)

*Determinate group. From Bataini, et al., 1982. Used by permission.

techniques is still the subject of controversy (see "Reoxygenation," page 86).

Tumor Regeneration

Most human tumors have a relatively slow growth rate (Charbit et al., 1971), and tumor-cell regeneration during a conventional course of fractionated treatment lasting 6 to 8 weeks has generally been discounted as a cause of failure. However, the critical parameter is not the volume doubling time but the potential doubling time of the clonogenic tumor-stem cell population. The most direct evidence implicating tumor-cell regeneration as a cause of failure in head and neck cancer comes from the data of Parsons et al. (1980). These authors showed that when the same total dose in the same number of fractions was given either continuously or as split-course, better results were obtained in all stages with the continuous treatment. This implies that regeneration occurring during the 2-week gap in the split-course regimen contributed to failure. The rapid rate of proliferation of tumor cells surviving unsuccessful radiotherapy is attested to by the fact that the great majority of failures in head and neck cancer are manifest within 2 years of treatment, regardless of tumor growth rate prior to treatment. Furthermore, delay between surgery and the initiation of postoperative radiotherapy has been shown to have a major deleterious influence on the success of combined treatment (Table 7-4).

In certain circumstances, even the continuous administration of 10 Gy/week may not be sufficient to counter tumor regeneration. For example, it is not uncommon for neck-node metastasis to increase in size during treatment, and occasionally patients who had no palpable disease at the initiation of postoperative irradiation can develop overt disease during treatment (Figure 7-13). In these circumstances, accelerated fractionation in the form of a concomitant boost is indicated (Knee et al., 1985).

Failure of Redistribution

Since cellular radiosensitivity is very significantly related to cell age in the division cycle, it follows that tumors having a large non-growth fraction of clonogenic cells are relatively resistant to fractionated treatment because of nonprogression of cells from the more resistant phases of the division cycle.

A long tumor-cell turnover time also correlates with a slow volume regression after commencement of radiotherapy, and it is possible that failure of redistribution could account for the fact that tumors that do not clear completely during a course of treatment are less likely to be cured (Barkley and Fletcher, 1977). However, other factors, such as failure of reoxygenation, cannot be excluded. Since variation in radiosensitivity with cell age is much less with high-LET radiation, Withers and Peters (1979) predicted that the RBE of tumors that redistributed poorly would be high, providing a "kinetic gain factor" for neutron therapy. Limited clinical confirmation for this prediction has been provided by studies on lung metastases with widely varying growth rates (Batterman et al., 1981a), and kinetic analysis of tumors to select those with a low turnover rate for fast neutron therapy trials would appear to be rational and justified.

Table 7-4. Recurrences in the Head and Neck of Patients Electively Irradiated Postoperatively for Stages III and IV Epidermoid Carcinoma of the Head and Neck

NODAL STATUS AT SURGERY	RADIOTHERAPY ≤ 6WK POSTOPERATIVELY		RADIOTHERAPY > 6WK POSTOPERATIVELY*	
	No.	*%*	*No.*	*%*
Negative	0/5	0	0/3	0
Positive at one level	0/18	0	3/11	27
Positive at multiple levels	2/25	8	12/32	37
Total	2/48	4	15/46	32.5

*In the patients with a delay of more than 6 weeks there was no palpable disease at the time of the initiation of irradiation. From Vikram et al., 1980. Used by permission.

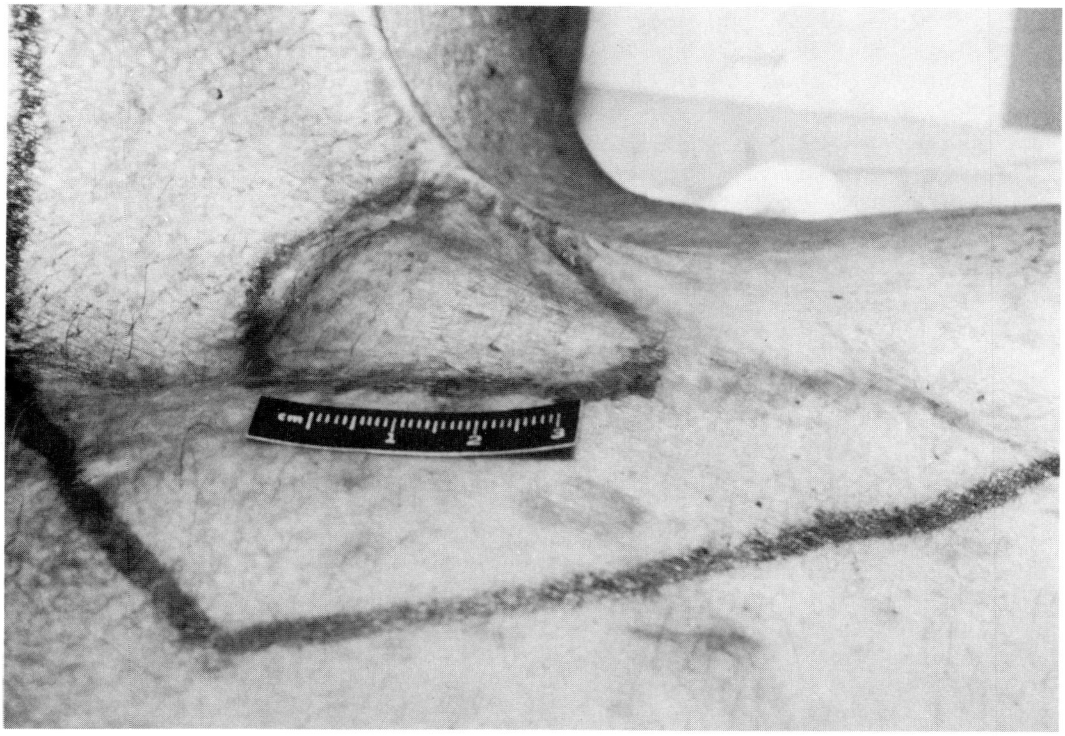

Figure 7–13. Patient was referred in June 1979 for postoperative irradiation after extensive surgery for a squamous cell carcinoma of the ear. At the start of irradiation, there was no palpable disease in the entire area. Approximately one week after the start of irradiation at 10 Gy/week, a suspicious area was palpated in the supraclavicular area; by the second week it was definite. Through a small field within the large field, 5 × 200 cGy was added in one week. The second treatment was given as a concomitant boost 3 hours after the first. At the completion of treatment, there was moist desquamation of the skin in the field-within-the field area. The total dose to the nodule was 66 Gy in 5 weeks. Although the patient subsequently relapsed at 3 years outside of the treated area, his neck remained free of disease. (Reprinted with permission from *Int. J. Radiat. Oncol. Biol. Phys.*, Vol. 9, Fletcher, G. H.: Keynote address: The scientific basis of the present and future practice of clinical radiotherapy. Copyright 1983, Pergamon Press, Ltd.)

Fraction Size

As indicated earlier, the proportionality between acute and late normal-tissue reactions varies as a function of size of dose per fraction, with large dose fractions being associated with an increase in severity of late reactions (Figure 7–7). Insofar as most tumors can be considered kinetically to resemble acutely reacting normal tissues more closely than late-reacting ones, it can be argued that the use of small dose fractions would increase the therapeutic ratio between tumor control and late normal-tissue injury. This is the rationale for hyperfractionation (see page 84). Using the same argument, one would predict that the use of larger fractions would be associated with poorer therapeutic ratios. This prediction is supported by the analysis of results by Cox (1985) showing that hypofractionated regimens with the same NSD were associated with poorer local disease control than conventional fractionation schemes. Conflicting results, however, have been reported by Henk and James (1978), who observed no difference in disease control in a randomized study comparing 30 or 10 fractions for definitive treatment of head and neck cancer.

Sigmoid Dose-Response Curves

Because tumor control probability is determined by Poisson statistics, there is always a finite probability that treatment will be unsuccessful on purely statistical grounds. As tumor-control probability increases, the likelihood that the few failures seen are due to such "probabilistic radioresistance" also increases, and the therapeutic ratio may be adversely affected by increasing the dose of radiation beyond the dose that produces tumor-control probabilities of 90 percent or better—e.g., in the treatment of early-stage glottic cancer.

Inadvertent Underdosage

The surest cause of radiotherapy failure is the geographic miss or inadvertent underdosage, and this factor must always be excluded first in any analysis of causes of treatment failure.

Second Primary Tumors

Apparent failure of radiotherapy can result from the development of a second primary cancer within or adjacent to the previous irradiated area. This is particularly relevant in the head and neck region, since multiple primary cancers are common. In some circumstances, it is difficult to distinguish between a marginal recurrence due to inadequate radiation portals and a genuine second primary cancer. In general, however, a long time to "recurrence" after apparently successful treatment points toward the development of a new primary lesion because approximately 90 percent of all true recurrences manifest themselves within 2 years of irradiation.

Host Factors

The prognosis of debilitated and malnourished patients is undoubtedly worse than that of patients in good physical condition, and the analysis of Griffin et al. (1984) showed that performance status was the single most significant factor determining tumor-control probability for radiation therapy of head and neck cancer.

Another host factor affecting radiation response is anemia, although the data for head and neck cancer (Taskinen, 1969) are less compelling than those for cancer of the uterine cervix (Bush et al., 1978). The influence of immunological parameters on treatment outcome has been studied by a number of authors (Deegan et al., 1977; Mason et al., 1977; Otkowski and Wilkins, 1975; Stefani et al., 1976; Wanebo et al., 1975), but no convincing correlation has emerged between immunologic reactivity and the response of head and neck tumors to treatment that includes radiation therapy. An interesting recent observation, however, is that the probability of metastatic disease correlates with pretreatment natural kill (NK) cell activity (Schantz et al., 1985).

Whatever the role of host factors in treatment outcome may be from the biologic viewpoint, it is undoubtedly true that debilitated patients tolerate treatment poorly by all modalities, and every effort should be made to correct nutritional deficiencies before and during cancer therapy.

CAUSES OF NORMAL TISSUE COMPLICATIONS

Simple Overdosage

The probability of any deleterious normal tissue reaction is, like the probability of tumor control, a sigmoid function of effective radiation dose. Because normal tissues are less heterogeneous than tumors, however, the dose-response curves for normal-tissue injury are frequently steeper than those for tumor control (Battermann et al., 1981b). Dose ranges associated with normal-tissue complications of conventional radiation therapy have been defined by clinical experience over the years and tend to be highly reproducible, although a few patients do manifest a greater susceptibility to radiation injury than the norm (Vaeth, 1972). In addition to the definition of dose-response relationships, clinical experience with conventional fractionation schedules has also led to a sense of proportionality between acute and late radiation effects—i.e., for any given level of acute reactions occurring during treatment, a certain level of late normal-tissue injury can be predicted, provided treatment is given in the same manner.

When changes are made in fractionation

schedules or beam quality, however, or when concomitant chemotherapy is given, this proportionality no longer applies, and the potential for severe late reactions is increased.

Volume Effect

The vulnerability of normal tissues to radiation injury varies according to the volume of tissue irradiated. The volume effect can be nonspecifically related to the ability of all normal tissues to recover functionally following irradiation injury, or can be related specifically to the functional reverse of vital organs. This latter aspect of the volume effect is best illustrated with reference to an organ such as the liver, for which functional tolerance to partial irradiation is very much greater than that for whole-organ exposure because functional compensation can be provided by the unirradiated part of the liver. The nonspecific volume effect is less well understood, but it may be related to codependence of adjacent tissue elements for functional integrity.

Size of Dose Per Fraction

Changes in size of dose per fraction have an important bearing on the relative severity of acute and late normal-tissue reactions (Figure 7–7). Thus, increase in the size of dose per fraction causes a relatively greater increase in late normal-tissue injury than in acute reactions, and it will lead to severe late normal-tissue complications if doses are matched according to acute reactions. It is important to note that all commonly used isoeffect formulations (NSD, TDF, and CRE) overestimate isoeffective doses for late and normal tissue injury when large doses per fraction are used.

Protraction of Treatment

Since acutely reacting normal tissues regenerate during a course of treatment, protraction of a course of radiotherapy results in relative sparing of acute reactions relative to late normal-tissue injury (Figure 7–7). Indeed, it is possible with prolonged protraction to avoid acute reactions altogether and to carry the radiation dose to very high levels, but at the expense of severe late normal-tissue injury (Andrews, 1965).

Radiation Quality

As explained earlier, there is little effect of dose fractionation when radiation is given with high-LET beams. Because with conventional x-rays or gamma rays, late-reacting normal tissues are preferentially spared by dose fractionation, it follows that these tissues will be more vulnerable than acutely reacting tissues to injury following high-LET irradiation. Thus, with neutron therapy schedules based on the same overall duration as photon treatments, acute reactions are mild to minimal with doses that cannot be exceeded for late normal-tissue injury. Since total doses are therefore predicated on tolerance of late-reacting normal tissues, the duration of neutron therapy treatments can be foreshortened without exceeding acceptable levels of acute normal-tissue reactions.

Concomitant Chemotherapy

Chemotherapeutic agents may interact with radiation therapy in a variety of ways to modify the radiation dose response. The complexity of the interactions and dosage uncertainties of systemically administered drugs at the cellular level make accurate prediction of normal-tissue reactions very difficult. The administration of cytotoxic drugs—either before, during, or after irradiation—has a potential for significant exacerbation of normal-tissue reactions, both acute and late (Phillips and Fu, 1978). This is particularly true with concomitant administration; under these circumstances, radiation and drug schedules must be determined empirically for each combination.

Trauma

Many irradiated normal tissues can sustain their functional integrity while intact, yet break down when subjected to trauma. Examples of trauma that may precipitate breakdown after radiation therapy include dental extractions, aggressive biopsies, thermal injury, chemical irritation from cigarette smoke or alcohol, and mechanical trauma from, for example, poorly fitting dentures. Any traumatic event that breaches mucosal integrity in the head and neck area also adds the element of infection to compound the basic radiation injury. Infected radionecrotic lesions are extremely difficult to heal with conservative management, and every effort should be taken to prevent their occurrence.

Nutritional Status

As with healing following surgery, the healing of acute radiation reactions is compromised in patients with negative nitrogen balance and poor caloric intake. This can, under certain circumstances, lead to acute mucosal necrosis. Any patient whose nutritional intake is compromised by acute reactions during radiotherapy should have supplemental nasogastric feeding.

THE CONCEPT OF NORMAL-TISSUE TOLERANCE AND THE THERAPEUTIC RATIO

The tolerance of normal tissues within a radiation treatment field determines the maximum dose that can safely be given. Because the probability of normal-tissue injury is dose related, the tolerance of a tissue must be specified in terms of the probability of acceptable injury under a given clinical circumstance. This will clearly vary according to the severity of the complications and the gravity of the disease being treated. For some normal tissues—e.g., the cervical spinal cord—radiation injury is so devastating as to be totally unacceptable, and tolerance levels are therefore set well below the dose expected to produce any incidence of this complication, with the corollary that tumors in very close proximity to the spinal cord can usually not be treated adequately with radiation therapy except with highly sophisticated particle beams that produce ex-

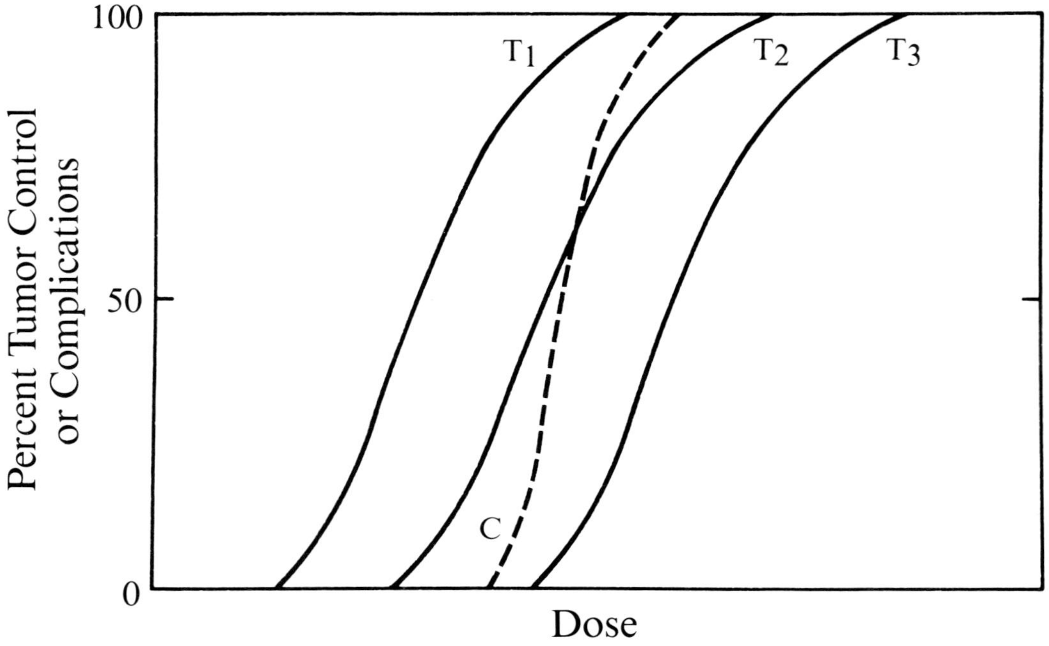

Figure 7–14. The therapeutic ratio relates the probability of tumor control to that of a treatment complication for a given dose of radiation. If curve C represents the dose response relationship for an unacceptable normal tissue injury, and curves T_1, T_2, and T_3 represent tumor control probabilities for, say, three increasing stages of the same tumor, the therapeutic ratio would be strongly positive for T_1, with a high percentage of uncomplicated cures possible; marginally positive for T_2, with a maximum of 20 to 25 percent of uncomplicated cures possible; and negative for T_3, for which curative treatment by radiotherapy would be contraindicated. (Reprinted with permission from Peters, 1985a, in press.)

tremely tight dose localization. For less serious normal-tissue injuries, tolerance will depend on the clinical circumstance and the philosophy of the radiation oncologist. Most physicians treating cancers of the head and neck region would regard a serious complication rate of about 5 percent to 10 percent (provided the cancers did not involve the central nervous system) as being acceptable in determining total dose limits.

For the majority of head and neck cancers, the dose-response curves defining tumor control and normal-tissue injury overlap. If the curve for tumor control lies to the left of that for dose-limiting normal-tissue injury (Figure 7–14), the therapeutic ratio is said to be positive; if it lies to the right of that for normal-tissue injury, the therapeutic ratio is negative, and radiotherapy is generally contraindicated except for palliation. The possible outcomes of radiation therapy with respect to tumor control and normal-tissue injury are tumor control without complications, tumor control with complications, failure of tumor control with complications. The therapeutic ratio is maximized when the greatest number of patients experience the first of these outcomes. The use of radiation treatments that are too conservative will unduly increase the number of patients experiencing failure of tumor control, whereas excessive escalation of the dose will increase the proportion of severe complications. The ultimate goal of all radiotherapy research is to increase the therapeutic ratio either by rendering tumors more susceptible to cure by ionizing radiation or by making normal tissues more resistant to injury.

REFERENCES

Anderson, R. E., and Warner, N. L.: Ionizing radiation and the immune response. *Adv. Immunol.,* 24:215–335, 1976.

Andrews, J. R.: Dose-time relationships in cancer radiotherapy: A clinical radiobiology study of extremes of dose and time. *Am. J. Roentgenol.,* 93:56–74, 1965.

Bacq, Z. M., and Alexander, P.: *Fundamentals of Radiobiology*, 2nd ed., p. 1. Pergamon Press, New York, 1961.

Barkley, H. T., Jr., and Fletcher, G. H.: The significance of residual disease after external irradiation of squamous cell carcinoma of the oropharynx. *Radiology*, 124:493–95, 1977.

Bataini, J. P., Bernier, J., Brugere, J., Jaulerry, C., Brunin, F., and Picco, C.H.: Approche radiothérapique des adenopathies cervicales secondaires aux cancers epidermiques du larynx et du pharynx. In Pinel, J., and Leroux-Robert, J. (eds.): *Adenopathies Cervicales Malignes*, pp. 129–35. Masson Publishing Co., Paris, 1982.

Batterman, J. J., Breuer, K., Hart, G. A., and van Peperzeel, H. A.: Observations on pulmonary metastases in patients after single doses and multiple fractions of fast neutrons and ^{60}Co gamma rays. *Eur. J. Cancer*, 17:539–48, 1981 (A).

Battermann, J. J., Hart, G. A. M., and Breur, K.: Dose-effect relations for tumor control and complication rate after fast neutron therapy for pelvic tumours. *Br. J. Radiol.,* 54:899–904, 1981 (B).

Bush, R. S., Jenkin, R. D. T., Allt, W. E. C., Beale, F. A., Bean, H., Dembo, A. J., and Pringle, J. F.: Definitive evidence for hypoxic cells influencing cure in cancer therapy. *Br. J. Cancer*, 37 (Suppl. III): 302–6, 1978.

Charbit, A., Malaise, P., and Tubiana, M.: Relation between the pathological nature and the growth rate of human tumors. *Eur. J. Cancer*, 7:307–15, 1971.

Cox, J. D.: Large-dose fractionation. *Cancer*, 55:2105–11, 1985.

Deacon, J., Peckham, M. J., and Steel, G. G.: The radioresponsiveness of human tumours and the initial slope of the cell survival curve. *Radiother. Oncol.*, 2:317–23, 1984.

Deegan, M. J., Coulthard, S. W., Quslman, S. J., and Schork, M. A.: A correlative analysis of *in vitro* parameters of cellular immunity in patients with squamous cell carcinomas of the head and neck. *Cancer Res.*, 37:4475–81, 1977.

Elkind, M. M., and Whitmore, G. F.: *The Radiobiology of Cultured Mammalian Cells*, Gordon and Breach, New York, 1967.

Elkind, M. M., and Sutton, H.: X-ray damage and recovery in mammalian cells in culture. *Nature*, 184:1293–6, 1959.

Fletcher, G. H.: Clinical dose-response curves of human malignant epithelial tumors. *Br. J. Radiol.*, 46:1–12, 1973.

Fletcher, G. H.: *Textbook of Radiotherapy*, 3rd ed., p. 228. Lea & Febiger, Philadelphia, 1980.

Fletcher, G. H.: Keynote address: The scientific basis of the present and future practice of clinical radiotherapy. *Int. J. Radiat. Oncol. Biol. Phys.*, 9:1073–82, 1983.

Fletcher, G. H.: Lucy Wortham James Lecture: Subclinical disease. *Cancer*, 53:1274–84, 1984.

Fletcher, G. H., Withers, H. R., and Peters, L. J.: Boost in radiotherapy: Rationale and technique. In Chu, F. C. H., Laughlin, J. S. (eds.): *Proceedings of the Symposium on Electron Beam Therapy*, pp. 107–12. Memorial Sloan-Kettering Cancer Center, New York, 1981.

Griffin, T. W., Davis, R., Laramore, G. E., Maor, M. H., Hendrickson, F. R., Rodriquez-Antunez, A., and Davis, L.: Mixed beam radiation therapy for unresectable squamous cell carcinomas of the head and neck. The results of a randomized RTOG Study. *Int. J. Radiat. Oncol. Biolol. Phys*, 10:2211-18, 1984.

Hall, E. J.: Radiation dose-rate: A factor of importance in radiobiology and radiotherapy. *Br. J. Radiol.*, 45: 81-97, 1972.

Henk, J. M.: Does hyperbaric oxygen have a future in radiation therapy? *Int. J. Radiat. Oncol. Biol. Phys.*, 7:1125-28, 1981.

Henk, J. M., and James, K. W.: Comparative trial of large and small fractions in the radiotherapy of head and neck cancer. *Clin. Radiol.*, 29:611-16, 1978.

Jesse, R. H., Ballantyne, A. J., and Larson, D.: Radical or modified neck dissection: A therapeutic dilemma. *Am. J. Surg.*, 136:516-19, 1978.

Kerr, J. F. R., and Searle, J.: Apoptosis: Its nature and kinetic role: In Meyn, R. E., and Withers, H. R. (eds.): *Radiation Biology in Cancer Research*, pp. 367-84. Raven Press, New York, 1980.

Knee, R., Fields, R. S., and Peters, L. J.: Concomitant boost radiotherapy for advanced squamous cell carcinoma of the head and neck. *Radiother. Oncol.*, 4:1-7, 1985.

Little, J. B.: Repair of potentially lethal radiation damage in mammalian cells: Enhancement by conditioned medium from stationary cultures. *Int. J. Radiat. Biol.*, 20:87-92, 1971.

Mason, J. M., Kitchens, G. G., Eastham, R. J., and Jennings, B. R.: T-lymphocytes and survival of head and neck squamous cell carcinoma. *Arch. Otolaryngol.*, 103:223-7, 1977.

Mossman, K. L.: Quantitative radiation dose-response relationships for normal tissues in man. II. Response of the salivary glands during radiotherapy. *Radiat. Res.*, 95:393-98, 1983.

Otkowski, Z. L., and Wilkins, S. A., Jr.: T-lymphocyte levels in the peripheral blood of patients with cancer of the head and neck. *Am. J. Surg.*, 130:440-4, 1975.

Parsons, J. T., Bova, F. J., and Million, R. R.: A reevaluation of split-course technique for squamous cell carcinoma of the head and neck. *Int. J. Radiat. Oncol. Biol. Phys.*, 6:1645-52, 1980.

Paterson, R.: *The Treatment of Malignant Disease by Radium and X-ray*, Williams & Wilkins, Baltimore, 1949.

Peters, L. J.: Biology of radiation therapy. In Thawley, S. E., Panje, W. R. (eds.): *Comprehensive Management of Head and Neck Tumors*, W. B. Saunders, Philadelphia, 1985a, in press.

Peters, L. J.: Biology of modern radiotherapy for head and neck cancer. In Chretien, P., et al. (eds.), *Head and Neck Cancer*, pp. 37-47. B. C. Decker, Inc., Publishers, Philadelphia and Toronto, 1985b.

Peters, L. J., Withers, H. R., and Fletcher, G. H.: Alternatives to radical neck dissection: The M. D. Anderson approach. *Aust. Radiol.*, 24:303-6, 1980.

Peters, L. J., Withers, H. R., Thames, H. D., Jr., and Fletcher, G. H.: Keynote address: The problem: Tumor radioresistance in clinical radiotherapy. *Int. J. Radiat. Oncol. Biol. Phys.*, 8:101-8, 1982.

Peters, L. J., Brock, W., and Johnson, T.: Predicting radiocurability. *Cancer*, 55:2118-22, 1985.

Peters, L. J., and Ang, K. K.: Unconventional fractionation schemes in radiotherapy. In Devita, V., Hellman, S., and Rosenberg, S. A., (eds.): *Important Advances in Oncology*, pp. 269-86. Lippincott, Philadelphia, 1986.

Phillips, T. L., and Fu, K. K.: The interaction of drug and radiation effects on normal tissues. *Int. J. Radiat. Oncol. Biol. Phys.*, 4:59-64, 1978.

Puck, T. T., and Marcus, P. I.: Action of x-rays on mammalian cells. *J. Exp. Med.*, 103:653-7, 1956.

Read, J.: The effect of ionizing radiation on the broad beam root, Part X. *Br. J. Radiol.*, 25:89, 154, 1952.

Searle, J., Kerr, J. F. R., and Bishop, C. J.: Necrosis and apoptosis: Distinct modes of cell death with fundamentally different significance. *Pathol. Annu.*, 17: 229-59, 1982.

Schantz, S., Poisson, L., Romsdahl, M. M., and Byers, R. M.: Natural killer cell activity and head and neck surgery. (Abstract #1214), In *Proceedings of the American Asosciation of Cancer Research*, Vol. 26, 1985, p. 308.

Sinclair, W. K.: Dependence of radiosensitivities upon cell age. In *Time and Dose Relationships in Radiation Biology as Applied to Radiotherapy*, p. 97. Brookhaven National Laboratory Report 50203 (C-57), 1969.

Stefani, S., Kerman, R., and Abbate, J.: Serial studies of immunocompetence in head and neck cancer patients undergoing radiation therapy. *Am. J. Roentgenol.*, 126:880-6, 1976.

Sutherland, R. M., and Durand, R. E.: Radiation response of multicell spheroids and *in vitro* tumour model. *Curr. Top. Radiat. Res.*, 11:87-139, 1976.

Taskinen, P. J.: Radiotherapy and TNM classification of cancer of the larynx. A study based on 1447 cases seen at the Radiotherapy Clinic of Helsinki during 1936-1961. *Acta Radiologica*, Suppl. 287:1-120, 1969.

Thames, H. D., Jr., Peters, L. J., Spanos, W., and Fletcher, G. H.: Dose response of squamous cell carcinomas of the upper respiratory and digestive tract. *Br. J. Cancer*, 41 (Suppl IV):35-8, 1980.

Thames, H. D., Withers, H. R., Peters, L. J., and Fletcher, G. H.: Changes in early and late radiation responses with altered dose fractionation: Implications for dose-survival relationships. *Int. J. Radiat. Oncol. Biol. Phys.*, 8:219-26, 1982.

Thames, H. D., Jr., Peters, L. J., Withers, H. R., and Fletcher, G. H.: Accelerated fractionation vs. hyperfractionation: Rationales for several treatments per day. *Int. J. Radiat. Oncol. Biol. Phys.*, 9:127-38, 1983.

Thomlinson, R. H., and Gray, L. H.: The histological structure of some human lung cancers and possible implications for radiotherapy. *Br. J. Cancer*, 9:539-49, 1955.

Tucker, S. L., and Thames, H. D., Jr.: Flexure dose: The low-dose limit of effective fractionation. *Int. J. Radiat. Oncol. Biol. Phys.*, 9:1373-83, 1983.

Vaeth, J. M. (ed.): Radiation effect and tolerance, normal tissue; basic concepts in radiation pathology. *Fron. Radiat. Ther. Oncol*, 6:1-526, 1972.

Vikram, B., Strong, E. W., Shah, J., and Spiro, R. H.: Elective postoperative radiation therapy in stages III and IV epidermoid carcinoma of the head and neck. *Am. J. Surg.*, 140:580–4, 1980.

Wanebo, H. J., Jun, M. Y., Strong, E. W., and Oettgen, H.: T-cell deficiency in patients with squamous cell cancer of the head and neck. *Am. J. Surg.*, 130:445–51, 1975.

Weichselbaum, R. R., and Little, J. B.: The differential response of human tumors to fractionated irradiation may be due to a postradiation repair process. *Br. J. Cancer*, 46:532–7, 1982.

Weichselbaum, R. R., Schmit, A., and Little, J. B.: Cellular repair factors influencing radiocurability of human malignant tumours. *Br. J. Cancer*, 45:10–16, 1982.

Williams, M. V., Denekamp, J., and Fowler, J. F.: A review of α/β ratios for experimental tumors: Implications for clinical studies and altered fractionation. *Int. J. Radiat. Oncol. Biol. Phys.*, 11:87–96, 1985.

Withers, H. R., and Peters, L. J.: The application of RBE values to clinical trials of high-LET radiation. In *High-LET Radiation in Clinical Radiotherapy*. A supplement to *Eur. J. Cancer*, 1979, 257–61.

Withers, H. R., Thames, H. D., Jr., and Peters, L. J.: Biological bases for high-RBE values for late effects of neutron irradiation. *Int. J. Radiat. Oncol. Biol. Phys.*, 8:2071–76, 1982.

CHAPTER 8

Head and Neck Cancer: Radiotherapeutic Precepts in the Management of the Neck

Rodney R. Million, Nicholas J. Cassisi, James T. Parsons, and William M. Mendenhall

EDITORS' COMMENT

Dr. Million and his coauthors provide us with a series of statements regarding the use of radiotherapy and surgery for metastatic squamous cancer to the neck. Some of these precepts are established facts requiring no additional documentation—for example, the combination of radiation and neck dissection for effective treatment of N2B neck disease or for subclinical disease, depending on extracapsular spread. Other precepts of Dr. Million are not as generally accepted by head and neck surgeons, such as the mandatory staging of neck dissections following curative radiation therapy or the routine use of computerized tomography (CT) to confirm pathologic adenopathy.

Most of Dr. Million's precepts are supported by a combination of his own personal clinical experience and hard data from the University of Florida, Gainesville. By studying his oncologic caveats, we can certainly add to our clinical skills in deciding the most appropriate use of combining radiation therapy and surgery.

INTRODUCTION

Over the past two decades, there have been considerable modifications and refinements in the management of squamous cell carcinoma that arises in the upper aerodigestive tract and is metastastic to regional lymph nodes in the neck. This chapter outlines the basic precepts that we currently follow in the radiotherapeutic management of neck disease. Although these are basic precepts, we never hesitate to individualize the neck treatment based on many patient-related factors that cannot be detailed in a short chapter. In particular, management of cancer at the primary site often dictates management of nodal disease, and the patient's wishes may also be decisive. We have no experience with the use of chemotherapy for nodal disease in the neck and will confine our remarks to the use of surgery and radiation therapy.

Basic Precepts

Precept 1. Both irradiation and neck dissection are at least 95 percent efficient in eradicating subclinical or occult disease in the neck.

There is voluminous literature, as noted elsewhere in this book, indicating that both elective irradiation of the neck and elective neck dissection, whether radical or functional, are highly efficient means for controlling occult disease in the neck. Surgery becomes less efficient when multiple nodes are found in the specimen or extracapsular spread has occurred, so these findings may indicate the addition of postoperative radiation therapy.

Patients with early-stage lesions and clinically negative neck nodes should usually have both the primary site and potential neck involvement managed initially by either surgery or radiation therapy, but not both. Specifically, we do not recommend surgical excision of a small primary lesion and then radiation therapy just for the clinically negative neck, as the morbidity of combined treatment is not justified, unless there are unsuspected findings in the operative specimen that signal use of postoperative irradiation.

In spite of the effectiveness of radiation therapy for subclinical disease, there are occasional failures, and these can usually be explained by one of several causes. Most of our failures of elective node irradiation have occurred at the edge or just outside the field of irradiation, indicating that irradiation failed to include all the disease. In addition, doses less than 4500 to 5000 cGy in 5 weeks, or its equivalent, predict an increased risk of failure. The approximate efficiency for increasing doses is shown in Table 8–1. Occasionally, the wrong radiation beam energy is selected. We have observed failures to control subclinical disease that appear to be due to selection of a high-energy photon beam (e.g., 8 or 17 MV). As a result, the lymph nodes are probably underdosed, particularly if the patient has a very thin neck and minimal subcutaneous fat. For this reason, cobalt 60 and 4 to 6 MV radiotherapy are used for subclinical disease in the neck.

For technical reasons, there is a greater risk of failure in the management of oral cavity cancers than in oropharynx, larynx, and nasopharynx cancers. The reason appears to be that in the latter group, the portals are larger, the lymph nodes lie in the center of the treat-

Table 8–1. Efficiency of Elective Neck Irradiation (ENI) for Subclinical Disease by Dose of Irradiation

				PERCENTAGE OF PATIENTS WITH N0 → N+ CONVERSION FOLLOWING TREATMENT		
AUTHOR	TUMOR SITE	NO. OF PATIENTS	DOSE TO NECK	*No ENI (%)*	*ENI (%)*	*Efficiency* (%)*
Fletcher (1973)	Oral cavity with N1–N2 ipsilateral neck disease	99	3000–4000 cGy/3–4 weeks to contralateral neck	35†	10†	71
Horiuchi and Adachi (1971)	Oral tongue	37	4000 cGy/3.5–4 weeks	37	5	86
Mendenhall et al. (1980)	Oral cavity	40	4500–5000 cGy/5 weeks	26	0‡	100
Fletcher (1973)	Faucial arch with N1–N2 ipsilateral neck disease	82	5000 cGy/5 weeks to contralateral neck	30†	0†	100

*Efficiency (%) = (1.00 – [failure rate following ENI/failure rate without ENI]) × 100%.
†Failure rate in contralateral N0 neck.
‡Excludes one out-of-field failure.
Credit line: From Parsons, J.T.: Time-dose-volume relationships in radiation therapy. In Million, R.R., and Cassisi, N.J. (eds.): *Management of Head and Neck Cancer: A Multidisciplinary Approach*, pp. 137–72. Philadelphia, J.B. Lippincott, 1984 (Table 13-3, p. 142).

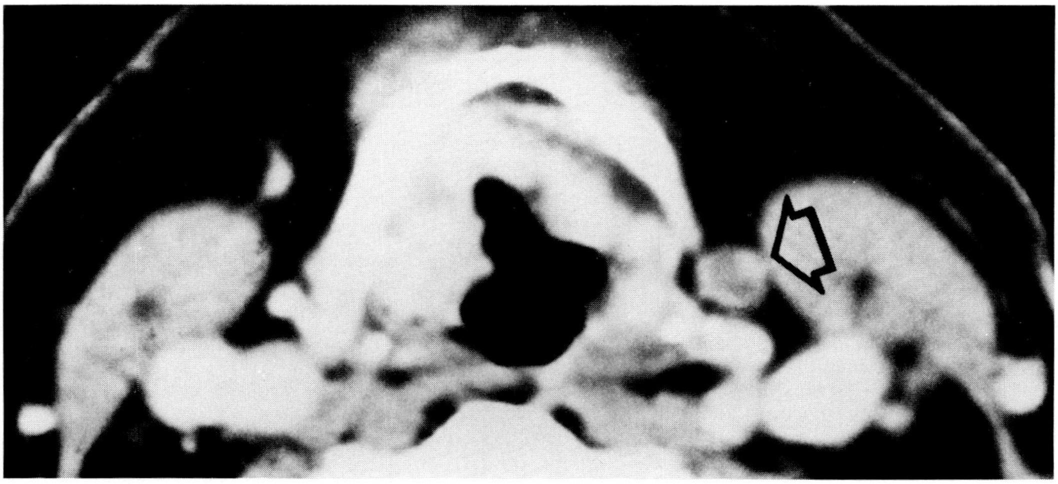

Figure 8–1. CT scan at the level of the hyoid bone. There is a large squamous cell carcinoma of the epiglottis. Physical examination of the neck by several examiners revealed no tumor involvement. CT scan shows a 1.5-cm lymph node with rim enhancement and a necrotic center (arrow) that was diagnosed as typical of metastatic carcinoma. The neck was reexamined, but the lymph node could not be felt. The patient was managed by total laryngectomy and neck dissection. The lymph node that was visualized on CT scan had been replaced by tumor. One additional lymph node that was approximately 5 mm in diameter also contained tumor, but could not be seen on the CT scan, even on retrospective review.

ment portals, and the high-risk nodes almost always receive 6000 cGy or more because of the dose required for the primary lesion. For elective node irradiation in patients with oral cavity cancers, the lymph nodes are frequently nearer the edge of the field and the external beam dose is equivalent to 4500 to 5000 cGy given in 5 to 6 weeks before an interstitial implant. Therefore, the site-related failures result from a combination of lower dose and a geographic miss.

It is likely that some of the failures to control subclinical disease by irradiation occur because lymph nodes larger than 1 cm are occasionally not detected, evey by experienced physical examiners, and nodal disease recurs after a dose of 5000 cGy or less (Figure 8–1). This detection failure occurs particularly in patients whose necks are difficult to examine. It may also occur in patients who are irradiated postoperatively when the incision extends into the contralateral neck and postoperative induration makes detection of positive nodes quite difficult.

In our experience, computed tomography has proved to be highly efficient for detecting small, clinically positive lymph nodes.

Elective neck surgery is highly efficient for control of neck disease, but there are also occasional failures for the following reasons:

1. Lymphadenectomy may fail to remove all the lymph nodes at risk. Lymphangiograms of the neck before and after neck dissection may show residual lymph nodes, particularly at the upper end of the operative field (Fisch, 1968; Million and Cassisi, 1984a).

2. Primary tumors at some anatomic sites are likely to have a greater number of occult positive nodes; thus, there is a greater risk of failure after elective neck dissection than with tumors at sites with a low risk for multiple occult metastases. For example, a base of tongue or pyriform sinus cancer would present a risk for multiple occult nodes in the neck, and thus a higher risk for failure of an elective neck dissection than a floor of mouth or oral tongue cancer, which would more often have only one or two occult positive nodes (Table 8–2).

3. There are no data to support the concept that functional neck dissection has a higher failure rate than radical neck dissection for subclinical disease, although the concept seems logical. There is a tendency to do more limited neck surgery (e.g., supraomohyoid

Table 8-2. Failure of Initial Neck Treatment in 596 Patients with Carcinoma of the Tonsillar Fossa, Base of Tongue, Supraglottic Larynx, or Hypopharynx

	STAGE							
	N0			N1 (%)	N2a (%)	N2b (%)	N3a (%)	N3b (%)
Treatment	*No Treatment*	*Partial*	*Complete*					
Irradiation		15%	2%	15	27	27	38	34
Surgery	55% (16/29)	35%	7%	11	8	23	42	41
Combined		1/5	0/6	0	0	0	23	25

*The University of Texas M.D. Anderson Hospital and Tumor Institute data for patients treated from 1948 to 1967.
Credit Line: Adapted with permission from Barkley H.T., Jr, Fletcher G.H., Jesse, R.H., Lindberg R.D.: Management of cervical lymph node metastases in squamous cell carcinoma of the tonsillar fossa, base of tongue, supraglottic larynx, and hypopharynx. *Am. J. Surg.* 124:462–67, 1972 (Table VI, p. 464).

neck dissection) for the clinically negative neck in oral cavity lesions than for oropharynx, larynx, and hypopharynx lesions. Therefore, failures may occasionally be related to residual subclinical disease beyond the limits of the neck dissection.

Precept 2. Radical neck dissection or radiation therapy used independently is equally effective (i.e., 85–95%) for N1 disease (Tables 8-2 and 8-3). When the enlarged lymph node is single and up to 3 cm in size, radical neck dissection or radiotherapy is quite efficient. There are occasions when a 3-cm node has extended beyond the capsule and is fixed, even though it is judged to be approximately 3 cm in diameter. In these cases, it is wise to perform a neck dissection after radiation therapy if regression during treatment is incomplete. Similarly, when neck dissection is done for a single clinically positive lymph node, but multiple nodes are found in the neck or there is extension through the capsule, postoperative radiation therapy is indicated.

If a primary lesion of the floor of the mouth or the oral tongue is to be treated by external beam radiation plus interstitial implant, the external beam dose may be limited to 3000 cGy in 2 weeks or 5000 cGy in 5 weeks, since the time factor seems to be critical in achieving local control by irradiation (Mendenhall et al., 1981). If a 2- to 3-cm mass is present, we prefer to limit the external beam dose and perform a neck dissection later rather than jeopardize control of disease at the primary site by extending the overall treatment time.

Radical neck dissection is highly effective for a single first-level lymph node 3 to 6 cm in diameter (N2a), provided cancer has not grown through the capsule into adjacent tissues and multiple positive lymph nodes are not found in the specimen (Table 8-2). Radiation therapy alone is not usually adequate

Table 8-3. Control of Clinically Positive Neck Nodes with Radiation Therapy Plus Surgery Versus Radiation Therapy Alone*

NO. OF NODES	NODE SIZE (CM)	RT + SURGERY	RT ALONE†
Single	<3	10/11 (91%)	59/64 (92%)
	3–4	17/21 (81%)	15/23 (65%)
	5–6	9/12 (75%)	4/5
Multiple	<3	4/4	24/32 (75%)
	3–4	13/17 (76%)	10/22 (45%)
	5–6	11/12 (92%)	5/7 (71%)
Single or multiple	7–8	11/17 (65%)	0/4
	≥9	3/6	0/4

*91 patients, 100 heminecks; primary sites (oral cavity, oropharynx, nasopharynx, hypopharynx, supraglottic larynx, lip, unknown head and neck primary lesion, multiple head and neck primary lesions) treated with radiation therapy alone. (No. heminecks with disease controlled/no. heminecks treated).
†Data for "RT Alone" from Mendenhall et al. (1984).
Credit Line: From Mendenhall W.M., Million R.R., Cassisi N.J.: Squamous cell carcinoma of the head and neck treated with radiation therapy: the role of neck dissection for clinically positive neck nodes. *Int. J. Radiat. Oncol. Biol. Phys.*, May 1986 (in press) (Table 1).

treatment for N2a disease, but these cases may be individualized. Patients with lymph nodes that are ≥3 cm and "fixed" should probably always have a neck dissection added after radiation therapy. If there is rapid and complete regression in mobile, 3- to 6-cm lymph nodes during the course of radiotherapy, one may wish to observe the neck and use surgery only in case of recurrence.

Precept 3. A combination of radiation therapy and neck dissection consistently provides a higher rate of disease control in the neck for patients with multiple clinically positive nodes or larger-diameter neck masses (N2b, N3a) (Tables 8–2 and 8–3). Management of N3b disease must be individualized, as each side of the neck is considered separately. Table 8–3 compares radiation therapy plus surgery with radiation therapy alone for control of disease in each affected half of the neck when the primary lesion is treated with radiation therapy. When the neck specimen was negative, the control rate by side of the neck was ≥95 percent regardless of the node diameter or whether there were single or multiple clinically positive lymph nodes. When the specimen was positive, the risk of treatment failure was substantial (Table 8–4). The control rate with radiation therapy plus surgery was considerably better when the nodes were considered mobile or tethered compared with fixed (Table 8–5). A dose-response analysis suggests that a higher dose reduced the number of positive specimens, especially in clinically fixed nodes (Mendenhall et al., 1986).

Precept 4. Radiation therapy in combination with less-than-radical neck dissection is effective when properly selected by the surgeon and when the dose of irradiation is adequate to control subclinical disease. This technique better preserves patient function (Jesse et al., 1977; Lingeman et al., 1977; Roy and Beahrs, 1969; Bocca and Pignataro, 1967). The decision to save the 11th nerve, the sternocleidomastoid muscle, and the jugular vein is based on the location of the involved lymph nodes, tumor regression following irradiation, node mobility prior to irradiation, the dose of irradiation to the mass, the wishes of the patient and, most important, the skills and judgment of the surgeon.

Table 8–4. Control of Clinically Positive Neck Nodes as a Function of Pathologic Findings in Neck Dissection Specimen

NODE SIZE (CM)	NO. HEMINECKS CONTROLLED/ NO. TREATED	
	Negative specimen	*Positive specimen*
<3–6	51/52 (98%)	27/42 (64%)
7–9	10/11 (91%)	6/16 (38%)

Data from Mendenhall et al., 1986.

Table 8–5. Control of Clinically Positive Neck Nodes as a Function of Node Mobility

NODE SIZE (CM)	FIXED	MOBILE/TETHERED
<3–6	9/14 (64%)	69/80 (86%)
7–9	6/13 (46%)	10/14 (71%)

Data from Mendenhall et al., 1986.

Precept 5. It is our observation that appropriate doses of radiation therapy followed by neck dissection result in less late morbidity than attempts to cure lymph-node involvement with higher doses of irradiation. Patients in whom a large lymph node has been successfully treated by irradiation alone generally have more fibrosis in the neck than patients who have received equivalent doses of irradiation but in whom a neck dissection was also performed. This seeming paradox is likely due to the fact that the fibrous stroma of the lymph node contributes to the overall fibrosis in the neck when it is not surgically removed. Unilateral or bilateral 12th cranial nerve palsy secondary to nerve entrapment by dense fibrosis is sometimes seen in this setting. In addition, early detection of neck recurrence following high-dose irradiation is made difficult by the presence of accompanying fibrosis so that salvage of neck failure is often long-delayed and fraught with wound complications.

Precept 6. It is possible to convert inoperable neck disease to operable disease with radiation therapy. The doses must often be quite high (in the 7000 to 8000 cGy range), but we have observed many cases of invasion of the skin, fixation to bone, or encasement of the neurovascular bundle in which the neck disease could be controlled with high-dose preoperative irradiation. The radiation therapy should be given first in these situations, and the surgeon must have considerable experience in operating after these high doses. These are not cases for the beginner. There are many technical "tricks" that are necessary on the part of the surgeon and radiation therapist to carry out these high-dose combined procedures.

Precept 7. Incisional or excisional biopsy of metastasis in a lymph node *does not* increase the treatment failure rate in the neck or decrease the cure rate when radiation therapy is the initial step in the definitive treatment. If incisional biopsy is performed, radiation therapy may be followed by neck dissection, and resection of the primary tumor may be added as indicated.

Parsons et al. (1985) studied the question of therapy following biopsy at the University of Florida. In 25 patients with no gross residual disease after excisional biopsy (NX), the referring surgeons' and pathologists' reports showed that a single, clinically positive lymph node had been totally excised. These patients received irradiation to the primary site and neck. No other clinically positive lymph nodes were found upon referral, and no neck dissections were performed for this group of patients. The absolute 5-year disease-free survival in the NX group was 79 percent, the 5-year determinate survival was 88 percent, and the rate of neck-disease control was 96 percent (Table 8–6). These results are quite good, considering that all patients had stage III or IV disease.

Fifty-five patients had gross residual neck disease after biopsy (Parsons et al., 1985). In some patients, only an incisional biopsy of a very large mass had been performed; in others, only one of several lymph nodes had been removed. The absolute 5-year disease-free survival in this group of patients was 31 percent, the 5-year determinate survival was 38 percent, and the rate of neck disease control was 64 percent. All but three of these patients had stage IV disease. The more consistent addition

Table 8–6. Control of Neck Disease in Heminecks After Neck Node Biopsy, According to Treatment Technique

N STAGE	RT ALONE	RT PLUS NECK DISSECTION
NX	23/24 (96%)	0/0
N1–N2	13/20* (65%)	6/7† (86%)
N3a	2/7 (29%)	5/8 (63%)

*Includes 3 patients with N1, 2 with N2a, and 15 with N2b disease.
†Includes 3 patients with N2a and 4 with N2b disease.
Credit line: From Parsons, J.T., Million, R.R., and Cassisi, N.J.: The influence of excisional or incisional biopsy of metastatic neck nodes on the management of head and neck cancer. *Int. J. Radiat. Oncol. Biol. Phys.,* 11:1447–54. Copyright 1985, Pergamon Press, Ltd. (Table 4, p. 1450).

of a neck dissection in recent years has resulted in an improved neck-disease control rate in this group (Table 8–6).

Open biopsy of a neck mass has the potential to disseminate cancerous cells into tissues not removed by a classical neck dissection. When a patient who has recently undergone excisional or incisional biopsy of a metastatic lymph node is referred to us, we prefer that the next step be irradiation in order to sterilize the areas of potential microscopic contamination. If an operation is performed first, tumor cells may be spilled into the tissues adjacent to the biopsy site and may not be removed. These cells may be scattered further throughout the surgical bed, resulting in a higher rate of treatment failure in the neck and, thus, distant metastases. Cobalt 60 or 4 to 6 MV irradiation will usually result in a better dose distribution than higher energy beams for this group of patients. We advise that the scar be bolused to ensure an adequate dose to this high-risk site. If the primary lesion is to be resected, we generally favor administering preoperative irradiation to both the primary site and neck.

Since the normal lymphatic pathways have been surgically interrupted by the open biopsy procedure, shunting of lymph to the contralateral side of the neck may occur, placing it at risk of treatment failure even when it would not normally be at risk (Fisch, 1968; Million and Cassisi, 1984a).

When a neck node has been subjected to incisional biopsy, we recommend radiation therapy as the initial treatment regardless of the eventual management of the primary lesion. If the primary lesion is to be treated with radiation therapy, neck dissection should be added in a majority of cases.

The 21 percent incidence of distant metastases in Parsons' series was identical to the incidence in the historical control group of the Iowa series, in which open-neck biopsy had not been performed. Although not directly comparable, the University of Florida series showed a distant metastatic rate half that of the Iowa series, in which open-neck biopsy preceded surgical therapy. The overall incidence of distant metastasis was approximately 50 percent in the series reported by Razack et al. (1977).

The rates of control for disease above the clavicles and survival do not differ significantly for patients who underwent open biopsy at the University of Florida compared with similarly staged patients with head and neck cancer in whom open biopsy did not precede definitive treatment. We do not recommend open-neck biopsy when it can be avoided—when the primary lesion can be found or needle biopsy is appropriate—but, when necessary, node biopsy does not significantly change the cure rate when our outlined plan of management is followed. Ill-advised and ill-placed incisional or excisional biopsy scars, however, create additional morbidity for the patient, and sometimes make neck dissection necessary when it might not otherwise have been indicated. One patient's disease became incurable following incisional biopsy because of a 2-month delay between incisional biopsy and start of radiation therapy, during which time the mass grew out of the incision (Figure 8–2). It is certainly preferable to start

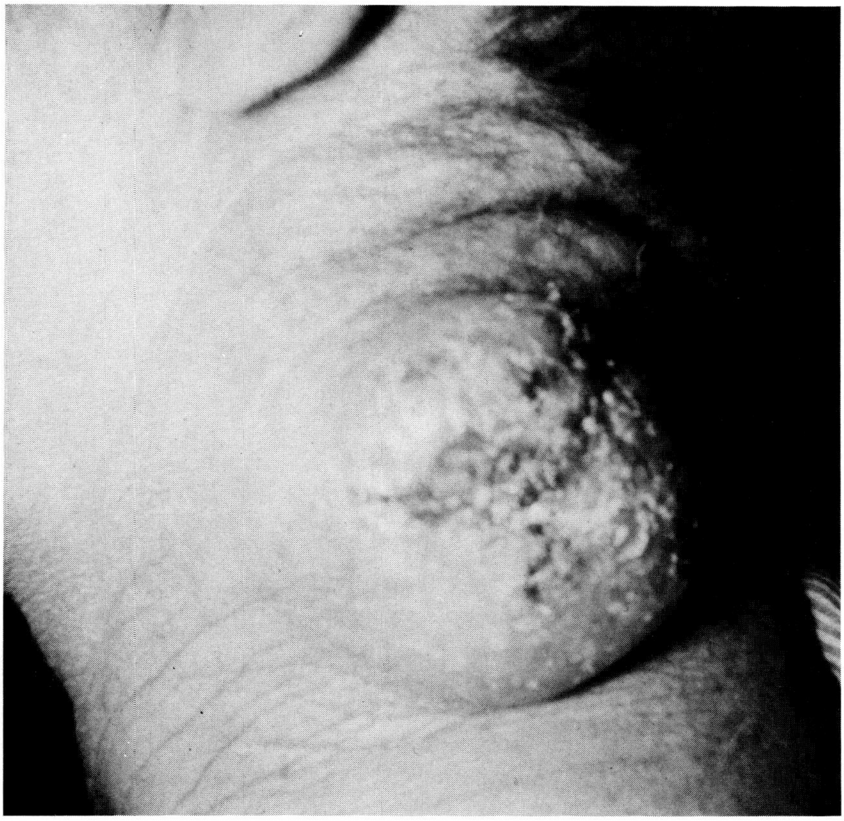

Figure 8–2. This patient had an incisional biopsy of a neck node at an outside hospital 2 months prior to starting radiation therapy. He had an obvious lesion in the nasopharynx. The photograph shows the large tumor mass extending from the incision site. Treatment failed because of inability to control the neck disease.

Table 8–7. Control of Clinically Positive Neck Nodes as a Function of Interval to Surgery*

NODE SIZE (CM)	INTERVAL FROM RT TO SURGERY	
	< 6 weeks	*> 6 weeks*
< 3–4	32/39 (82%)	23/28 (82%)
5–9	33/45 (73%)	6/9 (67%)

*University of Florida, 10/64–12/82; analysis 12/84 by W. M. Mendenhall, M.D. No. heminecks with disease controlled/no. treated.

radiation therapy as soon as possible following incisional biopsy.

Precept 8. When radiation therapy is added after operation, it is important to initiate treatment as soon as possible—within 4 to 6 weeks, if possible (Vikram et al., 1984). The dose we use at the University of Florida for patients with negative surgical margins is 6000 cGy in 6 weeks to 6500 cGy in 7 weeks to the primary tumor and upper neck portal (Parsons, 1984). The dose is higher if the surgical margins were positive. The dose to the lower neck is 5000 cGy in 5 weeks, but is increased to 6000 to 6500 cGy if the risk of nodal metastasis is judged to be greater. It is preferable to begin treatment within 4 to 6 weeks even if healing is incomplete.

Precept 9. When neck dissection follows radiation therapy, the interval between them is not critical for neck disease control (Table 8–7). It is more important that the patient have healed skin and mucosa and be in positive nitrogen balance. It should be noted, though, that operative complications doubled when there was a delay in surgery of more than 6 weeks for patients receiving more than 6000 cGy (Mendenhall et al., 1986).

Precept 10. When bilateral neck dissection is to follow irradiation, staged neck dissection is preferred in order to reduce complications (Table 8–8).

Precept 11. A high-quality CT scan of the head and neck is essentially equivalent to pathologic confirmation for masses ≥2 cm (Mancuso and Hanafee, 1982).

Precept 12. There is a dose-volume response for squamous cell carcinoma metastatic to the neck lymph nodes (Mendenhall et al., 1984). The general time-dose-volume guidelines used at the University of Florida are shown in Table 8–9. There is also a time-dose-volume response when radiation therapy is combined with surgery (Mendenhall et al., 1986).

Precept 13. If the patient has a primary lesion that can be treated equally well by surgery or radiation therapy, the management indicated for neck disease may dictate therapy for the primary lesion. For example, a patient with a small primary lesion of the supraglottic larynx or pyriform sinus and major disease in nodes on one or both sides of the neck would have a better functional result with radiation therapy followed by one or two neck dissections than with supraglottic laryngectomy or partial laryngopharyngectomy, one or two neck dissections, and postoperative irradiation (Figure 8–3).

Precept 14. A neck incision, whether recent or not, may lead to eventual lymph obstruction, so the risk for unusual and contralateral metastasis must be considered in management (Figure 8–4).

DISCUSSION

Although there are still a significant number of patients in whom it is not possible to

Table 8–8. Postoperative Complications Following Radiation Therapy Plus Neck Dissection (Radiation Therapy Alone to Primary Site)

	NUMBER OF PATIENTS	COMPLICATION RATE (%)	SECOND OPERATION RATE (%)	OPERATIVE DEATH RATE (%)
Unilateral neck dissection	143	23	12	2.7
Bilateral neck dissection				
Simultaneous	12	58	42	0
Staged	6	33	17	0

Data from Mendenhall et al., 1986.

Table 8–9. Lymph-Node Control Using Continuous-Course Irradiation

SIZE (CM)	1000 CGY/WEEK		900 CGY/WEEK	
	Dose range (cGy)	*Control*	*Dose range (cGy)*	*Control*
≤2.0	6250–7000	28/28	6500–7000	5/6
2.5–3.0	6250–7500	9/9	6500–7500	?
3.5–6.0	7000–7500	3/3	7000–8500	4/6

Data from Mendenhall et al., 1984.

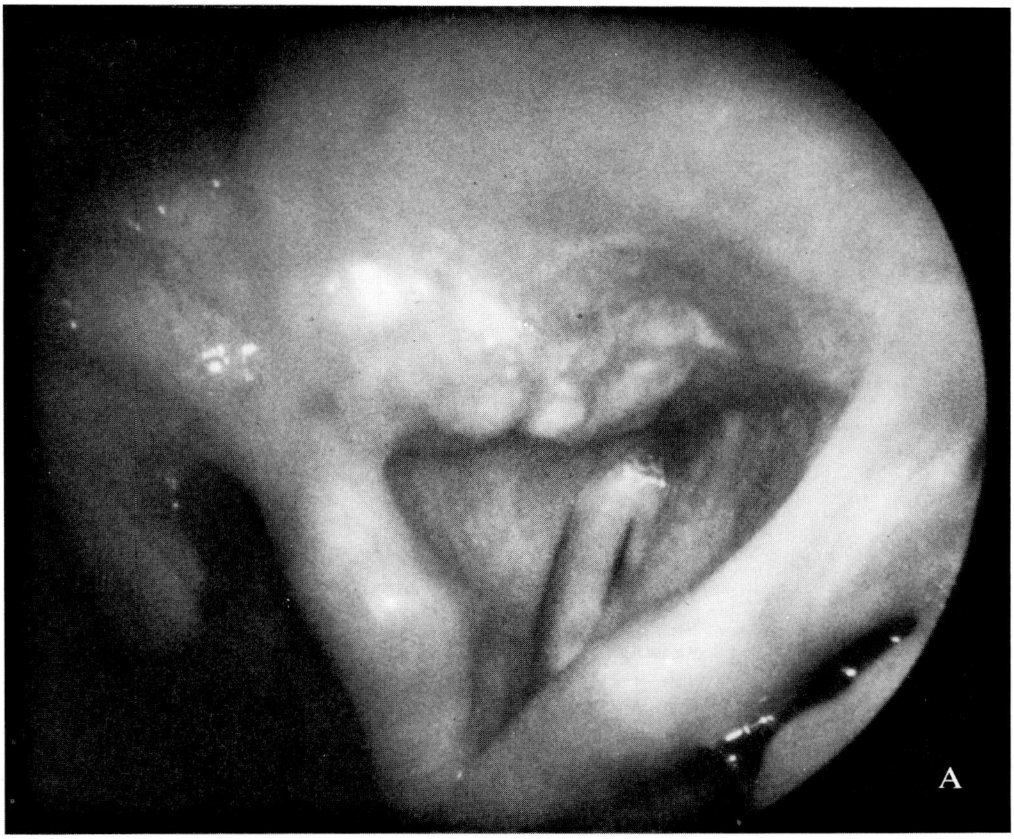

Figure 8–3. A 68-year-old man who was admitted for a lens implant was noted to have a mass in the left upper neck. Examination revealed a squamous cell carcinoma of the infrahyoid epiglottis with multiple bilateral neck nodes (T2N3b). The largest lymph note on the left was 5 × 3 cm, and the largest lymph node on the right was 3 × 2 cm. All of the lymph nodes were mobile. (*A*) Lesion of the infrahyoid epiglottis, with minimal extension to the aryepiglottic fold and pharyngoepiglottic fold. We elected to treat the primary lesion with radiation therapy because of the desirability of combining radiation therapy and neck dissection for management of neck disease. High-energy x-rays (17 MV) were selected in view of the planned bilateral neck dissection. The radiation treatment plan included 7000 cGy/7 weeks, 17 MV x-rays to the primary lesion and upper neck. The lower neck received 5000 cGy/5 weeks, 8 MV x-rays. The posterior upper neck received 1000 cGy, 10 MeV electrons. Staged neck dissections followed at 1 month and 2 months after radiation therapy.

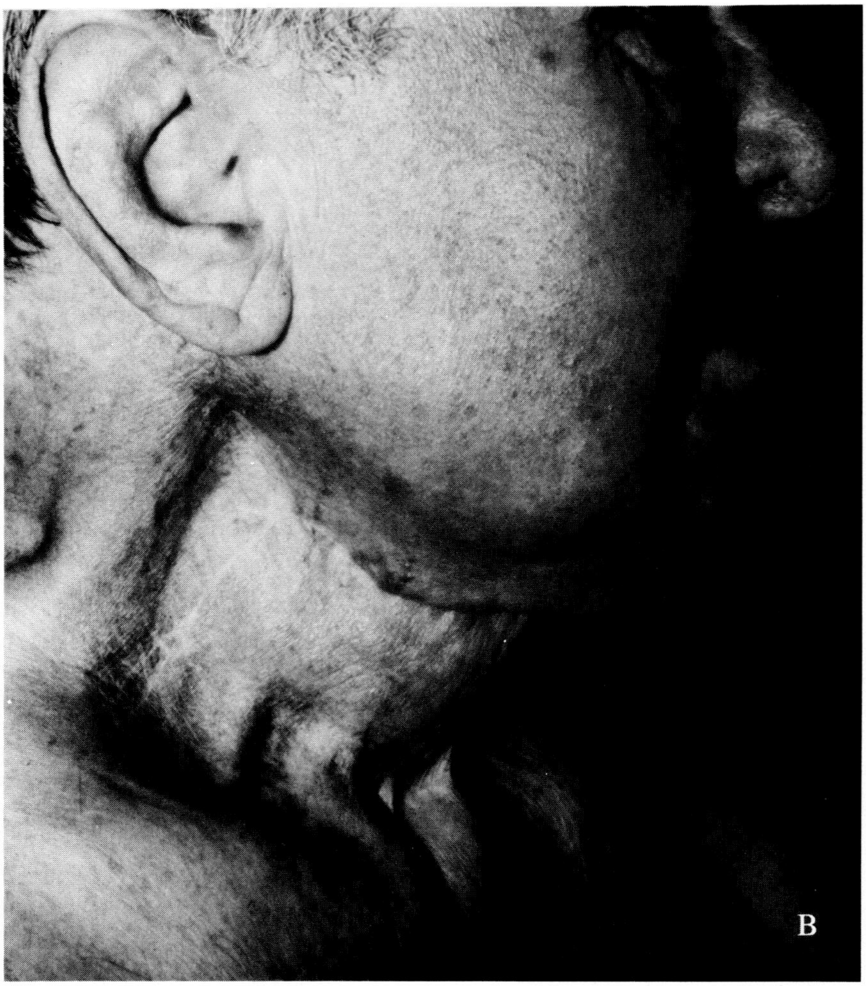

Figure 8-3 (cont.) (*B*) Appearance of the right side of neck after radical neck dissection; no tumor was found in 16 lymph nodes. (*C*) Appearance of left side of neck after radical neck dissection; no tumor was found in 44 lymph nodes. There were no postoperative wound complications. Moderate facial and submental lymphedema slowly subsided over the next 3 months. (*D*) At 20 months, there was essentially no edema. The patient was free of disease at 24 months. From Million, R.R., and Cassisi, N.J. Larynx. In Million, R.R., and Cassisi, N.J. (eds.): *Management of Head and Neck Cancer: A Multidisciplinary Approach*, J.B. Lippincott, Philadelphia, 1984, FIg. 19-26, p. 346, with permission.)

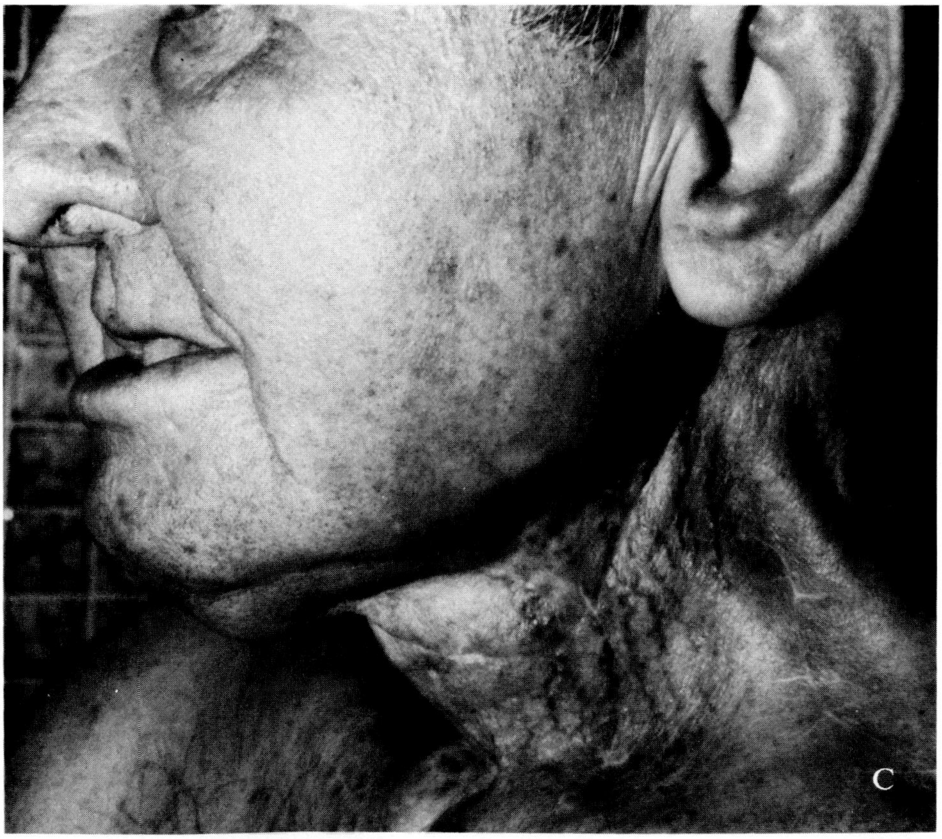
C

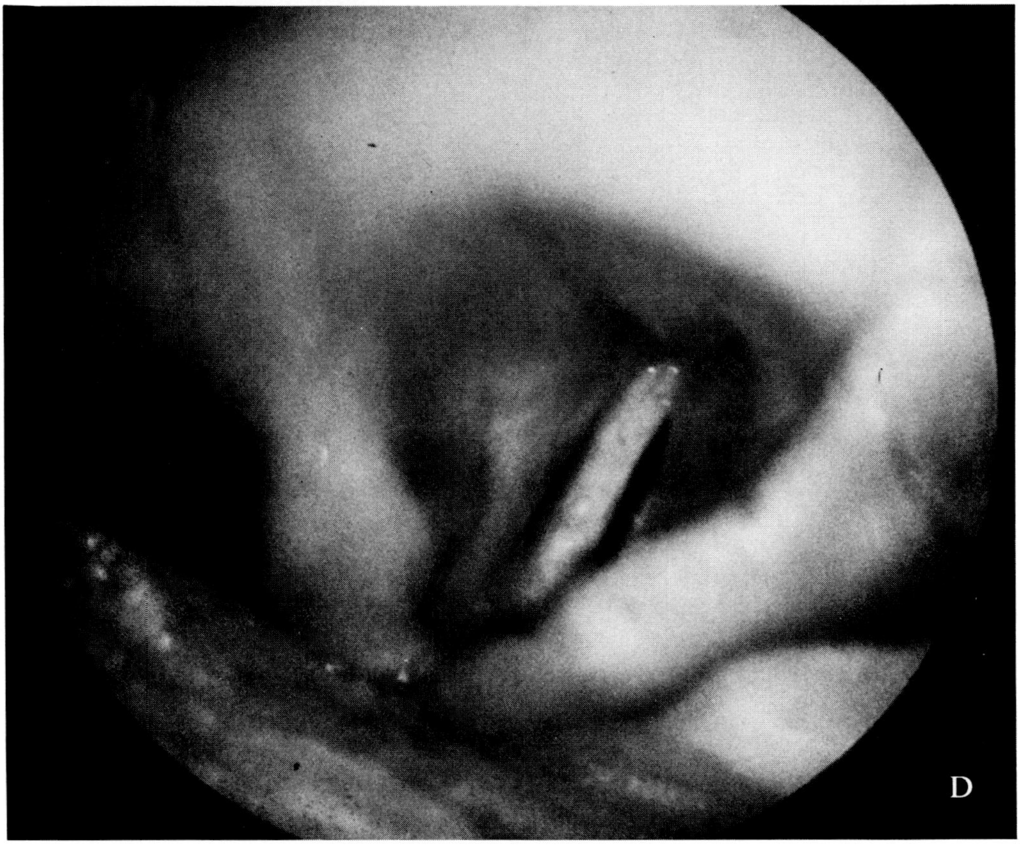
D

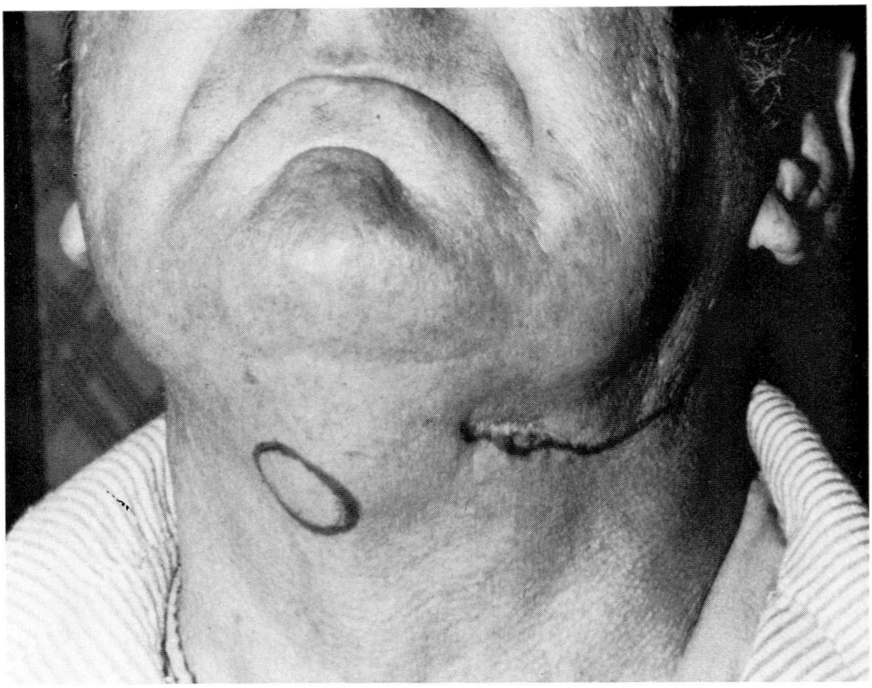

Figure 8–4. This 59-year-old man underwent an open drainage procedure for a suppurative infection of the left submandibular gland in 1943. In November 1983, he presented with a 6-week history of a sore in the left side of his mouth. Examination revealed a 3 × 2 cm lesion of the left retromolar trigone, with minimal extension to the left anterior tonsillar pillar and soft palate. Biopsy showed squamous cell carcinoma. A single clinically positive lymph node was present in the submental region just to the right of midline at the level of the hyoid bone (T2N3C). The scar from the prior surgical procedure on the left side and the clinically positive right submental lymph node have been outlined with ink on the patient's skin. The patient underwent a left partial mandibulectomy, left suprahyoid neck dissection, and an excision of the contralateral submental lymph node. Pathologic findings revealed bone invasion at the retromolar trigone site; the only positive lymph node was the contralateral submental lymph node. Postoperative irradiation was administered. (Reprinted with permission from *Int. J. Radiat. Oncol. Biol. Phys.*, 11:1447–54. Parsons, J. T.; Million, R. R.; and Cassisi, N. J.: The influence of excisional or incisional biopsy of metastatic neck nodes on the management of head and neck cancer. Copyright 1985; Pergamon Press, Ltd.)

control the primary lesion by any combination or method of treatment, it should be possible to control a very high percentage of disease metastatic to the neck if the proper sequence of radiation therapy and surgery is used in an interdisciplinary method.

REFERENCES

Barkley, H. T., Jr., Fletcher, G. H., Jesse, R. J., and Lindberg, R. D.: Management of cervical lymph node metastases in squamous cell carcinoma of the tonsillar fossa, base of tongue, supraglottic larynx, and hypopharynx. *Am. J. Surg.*, 124:462–67, 1972.

Bocca, E., and Pignataro, O.: A conservation technique in radical neck dissection. *Ann. Otol. Rhinol. Laryngol.*, 76:975–87, 1967.

Fisch, U.: *Lymphography of the Cervical Lymphatic System*, pp. 142–46. W.B. Saunders, Philadelphia, 1968.

Fletcher, G. H.: Clinical dose-response curves of human malignant epithelial tumors. *Br. J. Radiol.*, 46:1–12, 1973.

Horiuchi, J., and Adachi, T.: Some considerations on radiation therapy of tongue cancer. *Cancer*, 28:335–39, 1971.

Jesse, R. H., Ballantyne, A. J., and Larson, D.: Radical or modified neck dissection: A therapeutic dilemma. *Am. J. Surg.*, 136:516–19, 1977.

Lingeman, R. E., Helmus, C., Stephens, R., and Ulm, J.: Neck dissection: Radical or conservative. *Ann. Otol. Rhinol. Laryngol.*, 86:737–44, 1977.

Mancuso, A. A., and Hanafee, W. N.: *Computed Tomography of the Head and Neck*, pp. 204–43. Williams & Wilkins, Baltimore, 1982.

Mendenhall, W. M., Million, R. R., and Bova, F. J.: Analysis of time-dose factors in clinically positive neck nodes treated with irradiation alone in squamous cell carcinoma of the head and neck. *Int. J. Radiat. Oncol. Biol. Phys.*, 10:639–43, 1984.

Mendenhall, W. M., Million, R. R., and Cassisi, N. J.:

Elective neck irradiation in squamous cell carcinoma of the head and neck. *Head Neck Surg.*, 3:15–20, 1980.

Mendenhall, W. M., Million R. R., and Cassisi, N. J.: Squamous cell carcinoma of the head and neck treated with radiation therapy: the role of neck dissection for clinically positive neck nodes. *Int. J. Radiat. Oncol. Biol. Phys.*, May 1986 (in press).

Mendenhall, W. M., Van Cise, W. S., Bova, F. J., and Million, R. R.: Analysis of time-dose factors in squamous cell carcinoma of the oral tongue and floor of mouth treated with radiation therapy alone. *Int. J. Radiat. Oncol. Biol. Phys.* 7:1005–11, 1981.

Million, R. R., and Cassisi, N. J.: General principles for treatment of cancers in the head and neck: Selection of treatment for the primary site and for the neck. In Million, R. R., Cassisi, N. J. (eds.): *Management of Head and Neck Cancer: A Multidisciplinary Approach*, pp. 43–62. J.B. Lippincott, Philadelphia, 1984a.

Million, R. R., and Cassisi, N. J.: Larynx. In Million, R. R., Cassisi, N. J. (eds.): *Management of Head and Neck Cancer: A Multidisciplinary Approach*, pp. 315–64. J.B. Lippincott, Philadelphia, 1984b.

Parsons, J. T.: Time-dose-volume relationships in radiation therapy. In Million, R. R., Cassisi, N. J. (eds.): *Management of Head and Neck Cancer: A Multidisciplinary Approach*, pp. 137–72, J.B. Lippincott, Philadelphia, 1984.

Parsons, J. T., Million, R. R., and Cassisi, N. J.: The influence of excisional or incisional biopsy of metastatic neck nodes on the management of head and neck cancer. *Int. J. Radiat. Oncol. Biol. Phys.*, 11:1447–54, 1985.

Razack, M. S., Sako, K, and Marchetta, F. C.: Influence of initial neck node biopsy on the incidence of recurrence in the neck and survival in patients who subsequently undergo curative resectional surgery. *J. Surg. Oncol.*, 9:347–52, 1977.

Roy, P. H., and Beahrs, O. H.: Spinal accessory nerve in radical neck dissections. *Am. J. Surg.* 118:800–4, 1969.

Vikram, B., Strong, E. W., Shah, J. P., and Spiro, R.: Failure in the neck following multimodality treatment for advanced head and neck cancer. *Head Neck Surg.*, 6:724–9, 1984.

PART FOUR

NECK DISSECTION: ALTERNATIVES

CHAPTER 9

Radical Neck Dissection for Squamous Carcinoma of the Head and Neck

Elliot W. Strong and Larry J. Sheman

EDITORS' COMMENT

Dr. Elliot Strong and Dr. Larry Sheman, of the Head and Neck Service at Memorial Sloan-Kettering Cancer Center in New York City, have written this chapter on radical neck dissection from an insider's point of view in an institution rich in the heritage of head and neck cancer treatment. Following in the footsteps of Dr. Hayes Martin, the mentor of so many head and neck surgeons, Dr. Strong and Dr. Sheman succinctly document the history of the neck dissection with a well-annotated bibliography.

The importance of an accurate clinical evaluation of disease metastatic to the neck can be predicted in light of the size and location of the primary tumor. The authors' bias toward surgical treatment of any clinically positive neck by nothing less than a classic radical neck dissection is noted with appropriate documentation.

Indications in both the N0 and N+ neck are duly noted by the author, along with his rationale for the use of adjunctive radiation therapy. Additional applications for radical neck dissection are noted by the authors in patients who have previously disturbed or regionally recurrent neck disease. In addition to the information in the text, the reader will find the extensive bibliography valuable for future reference.

The polarization of opinions regarding the value of one operative procedure over another sometimes takes on strong emotional overtones. Dr. Strong and Dr. Sheman have produced an objective, clear, and practical assessment of a method of surgical control of cervical metastases. The radical neck dissection is a surgical procedure with definite indications. Given the complexity and multiplicity of possibilities in cervical metastases, no single technical solution would solve all the problems. The most successful surgeons will be those who are able to select the best treatment for each patient.

INTRODUCTION

The classic radical neck dissection has evolved from the procedure first described by George Crile, Sr., in 1906. He reasoned that close proximity of the deep cervical lymph nodes to the internal jugular vein and its branches demanded removal of the vein for adequate tumor resection. He advocated and practiced en bloc removal of the entire contents of the anterior and lateral triangles of the neck, including the sternocleidomastoid muscle, the internal jugular vein, the spinal accessory nerve, and facial envelopes enclosing fat, lymphatics, and cervical lymph nodes. He did not routinely remove the submandibular salivary gland unless clinically involved lymph nodes were adjacent to it.

Crile's remarkable report serves as the beginning of the systematic treatment of regional lymph-node metastases from head and neck cancer. The indications, anatomy, technique, and complications of radical neck dissection were amplified by Martin et al. (1951) based on their experience with 1450 patients. Other authors have since confirmed the usefulness and limitations of radical neck dissection (Barkley et al., 1972; Beahrs and Barber, 1962; De Santo et al., 1982; Kalnins et al., 1977; Naham et al., 1977; Spiro et al., 1974). Extension of the procedure to more adequately encompass regional lymph nodes at risk because of unusual primary tumors and disease entities has been described (Bocca and Pignataro, 1967; Canley, 1970; Pressman, 1955; Wander and Chaudhuri, 1976).

The effectiveness of radical neck dissection has been questioned (Brandenberg and Lee, 1981; Carenfelt and Eliasson, 1980; Jesse et al., 1978; Lingeman et al., 1977; Schuller et al., 1981), but the procedure still stands as the benchmark against which to measure other surgical procedures for the treatment of cervical lymph nodes potentially or actually involved by metastatic cancer.

IMPORTANCE OF REGIONAL METASTASES

The clinical significance of cervical lymph-node metastases from head and neck squamous carcinoma has been well documented (Bocca and Pignataro, 1967; Martin, 1941; Schuller et al., 1980). Marino et al. (1977) have also emphasized the relationship between the cervical lymph-node tumor burden (N stage) and the incidence of distant metastases, which correlates better than with the T-stage of the primary tumor.

The likelihood of regional lymph node metastases and their distribution in the cervical lymph nodes can generally be predicted based on the site and stage of the primary cancer (Lindberg, 1972; McGavran et al., 1961; Shah and Tollefson, 1974; Shear et al., 1976; Spiro and Strong, 1971). Recent experience with floor-of-mouth cancer (Shaha et al., 1984) showed that of those patients with involved cervical lymph nodes, 60 percent had multiple levels of tumor involvement. Only 29 percent had metastases in the submandibular triangle only, whereas 42 percent had metastases in those lymph nodes in the upper third of the jugular chain, 40 percent in the middle third of the jugular chain, and 23 percent in the lower third of the jugular chain; 5 percent had positive nodes in the posterior triangle.

Of the 110 patients with N0 neck disease who were merely observed, only 16 (14.5%) later developed evidence of nodal involvement, and most of these patients had T_2 or T_3 primary cancers. Local and/or regional recurrence occurred mostly in patients with large tumors (T_3 or T_4) or advanced neck disease (N2 or N3).

The detection of nodal metastases is based on clinical assessment of deviation from expected normal size and a firmer-than-normal consistency of regional lymph nodes at risk. Unfortunately, the assessment of minimal involvement is imperfect, with errors ranging from 15 to 35 percent in the estimate of the presence or absence of metastatic tumor (Bocca and Pignataro, 1967; Carenfelt and Eliasson, 1980; McGavran et al., 1961).

Other methods of assessment of lymph-node involvement are equally unsuccessful. Evaluation of cervical lymph-node status by lymphangiography is too cumbersome and unreliable (Mendenhall et al., 1984). Although needle aspiration biopsy is highly reliable in the diagnosis of disease in involved lymph nodes (Young et al., 1981), its use in screening patients with clinically negative nodes is limited, and its false-negative rate is significant. Computed tomographic (CT) scanning is of value, but is probably not sufficiently accurate in the assessment of lymph nodes 1 cm or less in diameter. Thus, it is of limited value in the detection of minimal cervical lymph-node metastases (Friedman et al., 1984). The choice of who should undergo treatment of the neck is therefore made largely on clinical grounds.

Although some may find radiotherapy helpful for the treatment of cervical lymph-node metastases (Mendenhall et al., 1984), its major role appears to be as an adjunct to the surgical removal of involved cervical lymph nodes (Barelink et al., 1983; Jesse and Lindberg, 1975; Snow et al., 1980; Vikram et al., 1984) or in the eradication of occult metastatic tumor (Schuller et al., 1981). Because the microscopic extent of metastatic disease in cervical lymph nodes is not predictable with certainty, it seems imperative that the entire neck at risk be treated (Chu and Strawitz, 1978; Donegan et al., 1982; Schuller et al., 1978; Schuller et al., 1981). Supraomohyoid neck dissection may be of value as a staging procedure, but it is accompanied by an excessive risk of local recurrence, with subsequent lessened survival in patients with involved cervical lymph nodes compared with more radical resection (Chu and Strawitz, 1978; Donegan et al., 1982).

INDICATIONS FOR DISSECTION IN THE N0 NECK

The indications for radical neck dissection as part of the management of squamous carcinoma of the head and neck are controversial. A modified procedure for the management of N0 and even N1 neck disease is being advocated by some (Bocca and Pignataro, 1967; Jesse et al., 1978; Lingeman et al., 1977); they would reserve radical neck dissection for patients with obvious metastatic disease. The dilemma of the appropriate treatment of N0 neck disease remains unresolved. The debate over elective neck dissection versus observation only continues to rage, with little factual basis on which to make a valid decision (Beaver et al., 1982; Lee and Krause, 1975; Spiro and Strong, 1973; Volterrani et al., 1982). Clearly, the smaller the tumor burden in the neck, the better the prognosis (Farr et al., 1982; Kalnins et al., 1977), but documentation of improved survival following elective dissection of the neck for pathologically staged N0 disease over disease that is clinically N0 but minimally pathologically N+ is lacking (Spiro and Strong, 1971; 1973).

It would seem obvious that adequate removal of minimal disease would optimize local control and perhaps lessen the incidence of distant metastases. For patients with N0 neck disease, the indications for elective neck dissection may include: (1) 20 percent or greater risk of regional lymph-node metastases based on historical data; (2) difficult-to-evaluate neck disease due to short, fat stature (endomorph), muscular hypertrophy, or previous surgical scarring; (3) CT scan suggestion of involved cervical lymph nodes for clinically staged N0 disease; (4) necks that must be entered surgically in order to adequately resect the primary tumors; (5) unwillingness or inability of the patient to remain under constant and continuing postoperative observation; and (6) unwillingness or inability of the patient to tolerate radiation therapy should it be required. Clearly, patients with significant risk of lymph-node metastases from other than squamous cancers for which no other effective treatment is available would benefit from elective treatment of the neck at risk.

INDICATIONS FOR DISSECTION IN THE N+ NECK

The treatment for clinical N+ neck disease is less controversial. The prognosis of head and neck cancer is directly related to the stage of the disease at the time of treatment (Callery et al., 1984; DeSanto et al., 1982; Farr et al., 1980; Kalnins et al., 1977; Shaha et al., 1984; Spiro et al., 1974; Stell et al., 1983). The prognostic significance of the extent of cervical nodal metastatic tumor has been well documented. In the study reported by Kalnins et al. (1977), 340 radical neck dissection specimens were cleared, the nodes accurately identified, their location recorded, and at least three pathologic sections taken from each node. When the lymph nodes were histologically uninvolved, the 5-year survival was 75 percent. When one lymph node was involved by metastatic tumor, the 5-year survival was 49 percent; when two nodes were involved, it was 30 percent; and when three or more nodes contained metastatic cancer, it was only 13 percent. In this last group of patients, the incidence of recurrent disease was 72 percent and of distant metastases, 70 percent.

Clearly, the prognosis significantly worsened with an increasing number of involved nodes, with involvement of nodes lower in the neck, in the presence of extracapsular invasion, and in the presence of extranodal soft tissue involvement. The authors concluded that the presence or absence of histologically confirmed cervical lymph-node metastases was of vital prognostic significance in patients treated surgically for squamous cancer of the oral cavity and oropharynx.

Johnson et al. (1981) confirmed the significance of extracapsular spread of lymph-node metastases. They found that 65 percent of involved nodes less than 2.9 cm in diameter and 75 percent of those more than 3 cm in diameter demonstrated extracapsular spread. They also showed that failure to control cervical nodal metastases was more common in patients with extracapsular spread, and that those patients had significantly poorer overall survival.

On the basis of this information, it seems imperative to adequately treat N+ neck disease, even that with only a solitary lymph-node metastasis less than 3 cm in diameter; if the physician relies on surgery alone, radical neck dissection appears to be indicated. With more than minimal metastatic tumor burden (i.e., with bulky nodal metastases more than 3 cm in diameter, with more than two involved lymph nodes, or with involved lymph nodes low in the neck) or with extracapsular or extranodal soft-tissue spread, adjunctive radiation therapy appears to be most appropriate, beginning no later than 6 weeks postoperatively whenever possible, and delivering at least 5000 cGy in 5 weeks to the primary site and entire neck, generally bilaterally, with boosts to the areas of original gross-tumor involvement (Sako et al., 1964; Schuller et al., 1978; Vikram et al., 1984). The most ominous late complication of the treatment of cervical lymph node metastases is local recurrence in the neck. The likelihood of control of such a recurrence in the previously dissected neck is very small (Pearlman, 1979).

It also seems appropriate to perform radical neck dissection on patients who have recurrent metastatic squamous cancer after radiotherapy; on patients who have significant scarring of the neck from previous minimal surgery that obliterates the tissue planes; and on patients in whom adjunctive irradiation for microscopic residual tumor would be impossible or unavailable. Patients who cannot or will not stop their tobacco and alcohol abuse will tolerate external radiotherapy poorly; for them, surgery is the major treatment modality for the eradication of metastatic tumor. It may also be inappropriate to irradiate patients with multifocal precancerous mucosal abnormalities within the potential field of radiation lest that radiation enhance the mucosal abnormalities or accelerate malignant degeneration.

The safety and efficacy of anything less than radical neck dissection for the removal of cervical lymph node metastases from squamous cancer of the head and neck, with or without adjunctive irradiation, has yet to be documented by prospective randomized study. Although the spinal accessory nerve may run for three-quarters of its course in the posterior triangle where regional lymph-node metastases are relatively uncommon, its upper quarter lies in immediate juxtaposition to the uppermost internal jugular lymph nodes. If the nerve is preserved in this area, en bloc excision of regional nodes at risk may be incomplete.

MORBIDITY OF RADICAL NECK DISSECTION

The loss of spinal accessory nerve function is the major morbidity following radical neck dissection. The disability resulting from that sacrifice, which will be covered elsewhere in this book, affects shoulder function, making the patient unable to actively abduct the arm beyond 90°. This inability results from loss of innervation of the trapezius muscle, but since that innervation is variable, not all patients suffer gross shoulder disability.

Morbidity can be lessened with appropriate postoperative physiotherapy. On the basis of pre- and postoperative evaluations, Liepzig et al. (1983) concluded that 40 percent of those who underwent radical neck dissection demonstrated "minimal" shoulder disability compared with 60 percent of those who had a modified neck dissection; disability in both cases was documented by objective and subjective criteria. Thus, it is apparent that even though the spinal accessory nerve may be preserved in a modified neck dissection, function may be impaired and subsequent shoulder pain may occur.

Long-term studies with objective measurement of shoulder function before and after radical and modified neck dissection are necessary to definitively answer this question.

Unless the modified operation is as effective in the control of metastatic tumor—as radical neck dissection—equivalence usually requires combination with postoperative radiotherapy and is less morbid in its postoperative sequelae, its advantages are lost. In that case, the radical operation may be the more logical therapeutic approach to the management of cervical lymph nodes containing metastatic squamous carcinoma.

DISCUSSION

Head and neck cancer is a devastating disease. The sequelae of its treatment are usually obvious and have profound impact on the patient's psychological, functional, social and occupational status. Nevertheless, foremost among physician and patient goals is the eradication of the cancer wherever possible. For most patients with advanced disease, multidisciplinary therapy may be necessary for optimum results. The components and sequencing of such therapy are currently under active clinical investigation.

Appropriate surgical modifications to lessen the cosmetic and functional impact on the patient are wise, provided they do not compromise the adequacy of tumor resection. There appears to be adequate justification for advising radical neck dissection for patients with clinically involved regional lymph nodes and for the treatment of patients with minimal disease by surgeons inexperienced or unfamiliar with the technically more demanding modified procedure. Whenever modified radical neck dissection removes histologically positive cervical lymph nodes, serious consideration of adjunctive postoperative irradiation appears mandatory if excessive lcoal recurrence rates are to be avoided.

REFERENCES

Barkley, H. T., Fletcher, G. H., and Jesse, R. J., and Lindberg, R. D.: Management of cervical lymph-node metastases in squamous carcinoma of the tonsillar fossa, base of tongue, supraglottic larynx, and hypopharynx. *Am. J. Surg.,* 124:462–67, 1972.

Bartelink, H., Breur, J., Hart, G., Annyas, B., van Slooten, E., and Snow, G.: The value of postoperative radiotherapy as an adjunct to radical neck dissection. *Cancer*, 52:1008–13, 1983.

Beahrs, O. H., and Barber, K. W.: The value of radical dissection of structures of the neck in the management of carcinoma of the lip, mouth and larynx. *Arch. Surg.,* 85:49–56, 1962.

Beaver, B., Ferrara, J., Young, D., and James, A. G.: Primary procedure in carcinoma of the tongue: Local resection versus combined local resection and radical neck dissection. *Curr. Surg.,* 39:405–7, 1982.

Bocca, E., and Pignataro, O.: A conservative technique in radical neck dissection. *Ann. Otol. Rhinol. Laryngol.,* 76:975–87, 1967.

Brandenberg, J. H., and Lee, C. Y. S.: The eleventh nerve in radical neck surgery. *Laryngoscope*, 91:1851–8, 1981.

Callery, C. D., Spiro, R. H., and Strong, E. W.: Changing trends in squamous carcinoma of the tongue. *Am. J. Surg.,* 148:449–54, 1984.

Carenfelt, C., and Eliasson, K.: Cervical metastases following radical neck dissection that spared the spinal accessory nerve. *Head Neck Surg.,* 2:181–4, 1980.

Chu, W., and Strawitz, J. G.: Results in suprahyoid, modified radical, and standard radical neck dissection for metastatic squamous cell carcinoma: Recurrence and survival. *Am. J. Surg.,* 136:512–5, 1978.

Conley, J. J.: *Concepts in Head and Neck Surgery*. Grune and Stratton, New York, 1970.

Crile, G., Sr.: Excision of cancer of the head and neck with special reference to the plan of dissection based upon 132 operations. *J.A.M.A,* 47:1780–86, 1906.

DeSanto, L. W., Holt, J. J., Beahrs, O. H., and O'Farron, W. M.: Neck dissection: Is it worthwhile? *Laryngoscope*, 92:502–9, 1982.

Donegan, J. O., Gluckman, J. L., and Crissman, J. D.: The role of suprahyoid neck dissection in the management of cancer of the tongue and floor of mouth. Head Neck Surg., 4:209–12, 1982.

Farr, H. W., Goldfarb, P. M., and Farr, C. W.: Epidermoid carcinoma of the mouth and pharynx at Memorial Sloan Kettering Cancer Center 1965–1969. *Am. J. Surg.,* 140:563–7, 1980.

Fisch, U. P., and Sigel, M. E.: Cervical lymphatic system as visualized by lymphography. *Ann. Otol.,* 73:869–83, 1964.

Friedman, M., Shelton, V. K., Mafee, M., Bellity, P., Grubauskas, V., and Skolnick, E.: Metastatic neck dis-

ease: Evaluation by computed tomography. *Arch. Otolaryngol.*, 110:443–7, 1984.
Jesse, R. H., Ballantyne, A. J., and Larson, A.: Radical or modified neck dissection: A therapeutic dilemma. *Am. J. Surg.,* 136:516–9, 1978.
Jesse, R. H., and Lindberg, R. D.: The efficacy of combining radiation therapy with a surgical procedure in patients with cervical metastases from squamous cancer of the oropharynx and hypopharynx. *Cancer*, 35: 1163–6, 1975.
Johnson, J. T., Barnes, E. L., Myers, E. N., Schramm, V. L., Jr., Borochovitz, D., and Siegler, B. A.: The extracapsular spread of tumor in cervical node metastasis from squamous cancer of the oropharynx and hypopharynx. *Cancer*, 35:1163–6, 1975.
Kalnins, I. K., Leonard, A. G., Sako, K., Razack, M. S., and Shedd, D. P.: Correlation between prognosis and degree of lymph-node involvement in carcinoma of the oral cavity. *Am. J. Surg.,* 134:450–4, 1977.
Lee, J. G., and Krause, C. J.: Radical neck dissection: Elective, therapeutic, and secondary. *Arch. Otolaryngol.*, 101:656–9, 1975.
Leipzig, B., Suen, J. Y., English, J. L., Barnes, J., and Hooper, M.: Functional evaluation of the spinal accessory nerve after neck dissection. *Am. J. Surg.,* 146:526–30, 1983.
Lindberg, R.: Distribution of cervical lymph-node metastases from squamous cell carcinoma of the upper respiratory and digestive tracts. *Cancer*, 29:1446–9, 1972.
Lingemann, R. E., Helmus, C., Stephens, R., and Ulm, J.: Neck dissection: Radical or conservative. *Ann. Otol. Rhinol. Laryngol.*, 86:737–44, 1977.
Lingeman, R. E., Helmus, C., Stephens, R., and Ulm, J.: Neck dissection: Radical or conservative. *Ann. Otol. Rhinol. Laryngol.*, 86:737–44, 1977.
Martin, H. E., Del Valle, B., Ehrlich, H., and Cahan, W. G.: Neck dissection. *Cancer*, 4:441–99, 1951.
McGavran, M. H., Bauer, W. C., and Ogwa, J. H.: The incidence of cervical lymph-node metastases from epidermoid carcinoma of the larynx and their relationship to certain characteristics of the primary tumor. *Cancer*, 14:55–66, 1961.
Mendenhall, W. H., Million, R. R., and Bova, F. J.: Analysis of time-dose factors in clinically positive neck nodes treated with irradiation alone in squamous cell carcinoma of the head and neck. *Int. J. Radiat. Oncol. Biol. Phys.,* 10:639–43, 1984.
Mendenhall, W. M., Millioin, R. R., and Cassisi, N. J.: Elective neck irradiation in squamous cell carcinoma of the head and neck. *Head Neck Surg.,*
Merino, O. R., Lindberg, R. D., and Fletcher, G. A.: An analysis of distant metastases from squamous cell carcinoma of the upper respiratory and digestive tracts. *Cancer*, 40:145–51, 1977.
Nahma, A. A., Bone, R. C., and Davidson, T. M.: The care for elective prophylactic neck dissection. *Trans. Am. Acad. Opthalmol. Otol.,* 82:603–12, 1977.
Pearlman, N.: Treatment outcome in recurrent head and neck cancer. *Arch. Surg.*, 114:39–42, 1979.
Pressman, J. J.: Extended retrohyoid radical neck dissection for cancer of the oral cavity. *Surg. Gynecol. Obstet.*, 100:329–44, 1955.
Sako, K., Pradier, R. N., Marchetta, F. C., and Pickren, J. W.: Fallibility of palpation in the diagnosis of metastases to cervical nodes. *Surg. Gynecol. Obstet.*, 188: 989–90, 1964.
Schuller, D. E., McGuirt, W. F., McCabe, B. F., and Young, D.: The prognostic significance of metastatic cervical lymph nodes. *Laryngoscope*, 88:439–50, 1978.
Schuller, D. E., Platz, C. E., and Drause, C. J.: Spinal accessory lymph nodes: A prospective study of metastatic involvement. *Laryngoscope*, 88:439–50, 1978.
Schuller, D. E., Saunders, W. H., Miglets, A. W., and Kelley, D. R.: Conservative neck dissection. Radical approach? *Arch. Otololaryngol.*, 107:642–5, 1981.
Shah, J. P., and Tollefson, H. R.: Epidermoid carcinoma of the supraglottic larynx: Role of neck dissection in initial surgical treatment. *Am. J. Surg.,* 128:494–9, 1974.
Shaha, A. R., Spiro, R. H., Shah, J. P., and Strong, E. W.: Squamous carcinoma of floor of the mouth. *Am. J. Surg.,* 148:455–9, 1984.
Shear, M., Hawkins, D. M., and Farr, H. W.: The prediction of lymph-node metastases from oral squamous carcinoma. *Cancer*, 37:1901–7, 1976.
Snow, J. B., Gelbert, R. D., Kramer, S., Davis, L. W., Marcial, V. A., and Lowry, L. D.: Randomized preoperative and postoperative radiation therapy for patients with carcinoma of the head and neck. Preliminary report. *Laryngoscope*, 90:930–45, 1980.
Spiro, R. H., Alfonso, A. E., Farr, H. W., and Strong, B. W.: Cervical lymph-node metastases from epidermoid carcinoma of the oral cavity and oropharynx. *Am. J. Surg.,* 128:562–7, 1974.
Spiro, R. H., and Strong, E. W.: Epidermoid carcinoma of the mobile tongue: Treatment by partial glossectomy alone. *Am. J. Surg.,* 122:707–10, 1971.
Sprio, R. H., and Strong, E. W.: Epidermoid carcinoma of the oral cavity oropharynx: Elective vs therapeutic radical neck dissection as treatment. *Arch. Surg.,* 107:382–4, 1973.
Stell, P. M., Morton, R. P., and Singh, S. D.: Cervical lymph-node metastases: The significance of the level of the lymph node. *Clin. Oncol.*, 9:101–7, 1983.
Strong, E. W.: Head and neck cancer: Meaning of lymph-node metastases and their effective treatment. In Weiss, Gilbert, Ballon (eds.): *Lymphatic System Metastases*, pp. 461–76. G.K. Hall, Boston, 1980.
Toker, C.: Some observations on the distribution of metastatic squamous carcinoma within cervical lymph nodes. *Am. Surg.,* 157:419–26, 1963.
Vikram, B., Strong, B. W., Shah, J. P., and Spiro, R. H.: Failure in the neck following multimodality treatment for advanced head and neck cancer. *Head Neck Surg.,* 6:724–9, 1984.
Volterrani, F., Chiesta, F., and Molinar, R.: Arguments in favor of precautional treatment of cervical nodes in clinically N0 oral cancer. *Tumori*, 68:241–5, 1982.
Wander, J. V., and Chaudhuri, P. K.: Dissection of the posterior part of the neck. *Surg. Gynecol. Obstet.,* 143:97–100, 1976.
Young, J. E. M., Archibald, S. D., and Shier, K. J.: Needle aspiration cytologic biopsy in head and neck masses. *Am. J. Surg.,* 142:484–89, 1981.

CHAPTER 10

Indications for Modified Neck Dissection in Squamous Cancer of the Neck

Robert M. Byers, Patricia F. Wolf, and Rick Shallenberger

EDITORS' COMMENT

Dr. Robert Byers, known for his advocacy of the modified neck dissection in the tradition of Ballantyne and Jesse at the University of Texas M.D. Anderson Hospital and Tumor Institute at Houston presents the counterarguments for neck surgery other than the classic radical neck dissection. Drawing on knowledge gained over two decades by Strong, Fletcher, Jesse, Ballantyne, and Lindberg, Dr. Byers "sets the stage for a conceptual revolution" in the surgical treatment of metastatic cancer to the neck.

After dispensing with the possibility, because of "ethical considerations," of ever having a truly randomized prospective study comparing the classic and modified dissections, the senior author presents his classification of modifications of the neck dissection; then outlines the rationale for applying each operation to a specific disease process.

Dr. Byers reports on the "largest series of patients (967) treated by modified neck dissections (1372) available in the world's literature." This feat demonstrates, as well as a retrospective study can, that, in selected cases, cervical metastases from head and neck cancer can be treated with equal effectiveness by modified neck dissection compared with radical neck dissection. The author then outlines the thought process involved in the adjunctive use of radiation therapy after pathologic evaluation of the lymphadenectomy specimen is complete.

This chapter is in obvious contrast to Dr. Strong's thoughts on the indications for radical neck dissection. We do not feel that the two authors are very far apart if one considers that both believe there are definite indications for the other's advocated neck-dissection technique, and that radiation therapy is noted by both to be an integral part of the definitive treatment of the patient with extracapsular spread of metastatic cancer to the head and neck.

INTRODUCTION

Since the early 1960s, the surgeons at The University of Texas M.D. Anderson Hospital (UTMDAH) have been performing modifications of the classic radical neck dissection. During the 1970s, the operation was refined and perfected, so that today the procedure is a well-defined and reproducible technique.

When the literature began to show that

there was a high recurrence rate in the necks of patients with extracapsular nodal disease treated by surgery only (Johnson et al., 1981); that moderate doses of preoperative radiation significantly reduced the incidence of regional recurrence in stage N2 and N3 neck disease treated by a radical neck dissection (Strong, 1969); and that 5000 cGy in 5 weeks sterilized subclinical microsocpic metastases (Fletcher, 1972), the stage was set for a conceptual revolution in the surgical treatment of cervical metastases from squamous carcinoma of the head and neck.

With these selective modifications, the nodal groups at highest risk for metastatic disease are removed, preserving most of the functional and cosmetic structures within the neck (Lindberg, 1972). Many times, a less-than-radical neck dissection can be performed but, occasionally, the proper resection requires that additional nodal groups, such as the retropharyngeal, the suboccipital, the paratracheal, and the intraparotid, be removed.

Criteria for the use of the modified neck dissection alone or combined with perioperative radiation therapy were developed (Jesse and Fletcher, 1977). Because of ethical considerations, a prospective randomized study comparing the modified and radical neck dissections will never be undertaken. Therefore, this study was designed to review retrospectively the largest series of patients (967) treated by modified neck dissections (1372) available in the world's literature in order to give an appropriate perspective to the procedure's indications with and without adjunctive radiation therapy.

METHODS AND MATERIALS

During the years 1970 to 1980, the surgeons at UTMDAH were performing modified neck dissections with and without radiation for most cases in which squamous carcinoma had metastasized or was suspected of having metastasized to cervical nodes. The surgeon selected the type of dissection in a nonrandomized manner and, using the results of pathologic examination of the specimen and certain criteria, decided if postoperative radiation was indicated.

The four major primary sites selected were the oral cavity, oropharynx, larynx, and hypopharynx. The types of modified neck dissections performed were the suprahyoid, functional, anterior, supraomohyoid, posterior, and lower. Each of the modifications was defined by the nodal groups included in the resection: the suprahyoid—the submental and submaxillary nodes; the supraomohyoid—the submental, submaxillary, subdigastric, upper posterior cervical, and the midjugular; the anterior—the subdigastric, midjugular, and lower jugular; the posterior—the upper, middle, and lower posterior cervical; the lower—the lower posterior cervical, the lower jugular, and the supraclavicular; and the functional—the submental, submaxillary, subdigastric, upper, middle, and lower posterior cervical, and mid and lower jugular.

Location of the primary tumor dictated which type of neck dissection was selected. For example, the suprahyoid was performed for primary tumors of the lip, the supraomohyoid for oral cavity and oropharynx primary tumors, and the anterior for larynx and hypopharynx primary tumors. Many of the dissections were bilateral and in various combinations, such as a bilateral anterior, anterior and functional, bilateral supraomohyoid, or supraomohyoid and functional neck dissection.

The patient's disease was classified according to the 1979 American Joint Committee TNM staging classification (ASC, 1979). The recurrence rate was correlated only with the pathologic staging. All the patients were previously untreated. The postoperative radiation dose was at least 5000 cGy in 5 weeks given between 3 and 12 weeks after surgery. A patient who had a recurrence in the dissected neck was included in the study only if the primary at the time of the failure was under control. Operative death was defined as death from any cause within 30 days postoperatively. The neck was considered as having a right and left side, and each side was analyzed separately. Follow-up information was obtained from routine clinic visits, autopsy material, and correspondence with the patient, the patient's family, or the referring physician. Nine hundred sixty-seven patients were eligible for evaluation.

RESULTS

Nine hundred sixty-seven patients had a modified neck dissection on at least one side of the neck. Four hundred fifty-eight patients had unilateral modified dissection, 405 had bilateral modified dissection, and 104 had modified dissection on one side and radical dissection on the other. Thus, 1372 modified neck dissections were performed (Table 10–1). There were 455 supraomohyoid neck dissections, 441 functional neck dissections, 419 anterior dissections, 53 suprahyoid dissections, 2 lower neck dissections, and 2 posterior neck dissections.

Four hundred forty-eight patients had primary tumors in the oral cavity (Table 10–2), 142 in the oropharynx, 265 in the larynx, and 112 in the hypopharynx. Five hundred and seven patients had surgery only, and 351 had surgery and postoperative radiation. A smaller number of patients (109) had preoperative radiation and a modified neck dissection.

Table 10–1. Types of Modified Neck Dissections

TYPE	PRIMARY TUMOR	HEMINECKS
Supraomohyoid	Oral cavity	336
	Oropharynx	76
	Larynx	29
	Hypopharynx	14
	Subtotal	455
Functional radical	Oral cavity	161
	Oropharynx	87
	Larynx	141
	Hypopharynx	52
	Subtotal	441
Anterior	Oral cavity	3
	Oropharynx	17
	Larynx	301
	Hypopharynx	98
	Subtotal	419
Suprahyoid	Oral cavity	52
	Oropharynx	0
	Larynx	1
	Hypopharynx	0
	Subtotal	53
Posterior	Oral cavity	1
	Oropharynx	1
	Larynx	0
	Hypopharynx	0
	Subtotal	2
Lower	Oral cavity	0
	Oropharynx	0
	Larynx	2
	Hypopharynx	0
	Subtotal	2
	Total	1372

Table 10–2. Site of the Primary Tumors

SITE		NO. OF PATIENTS	
Oral cavity	Oral tongue	110	
	Floor of mouth	137	
	Buccal mucosa	23	
	Lower gum	62	
	Retromolar trigone	46	
	Hard palate	8	
	Upper gum	6	
	Upper lip	7	
	Lower lip	49	
	Subtotal	488	(46%)
Oropharynx	Base of tongue	56	
	Tonsil	23	
	Pharyngeal wall	37	
	Soft palate	11	
	Faucial arch	15	
	Subtotal	142	(15%)
Hypopharynx	Pyriform sinus	108	
	Postcricoid	4	
	Subtotal	112	(12%)
Larynx	Supraglottic	185	
	Glottic	80	
	Subtotal	265	(27%)

Based on the number of involved sides of the neck, the incidence at presentation of clinically and pathologically N0 disease was 51.2 percent, whereas for clinically N0 but pathologically N+ disease it was 12.9 percent and for clinically and pathologically positive disease it was 24. 9 percent (Tables 10–3, 10–4, and 10–5). The operative mortality was 2 percent. The 11th cranial nerve (spinal accessory) was dissected and preserved in 837 cases. The incidence of local failure in which the nerve was dissected and preserved with surgery alone was 7.9 percent. If radiation was included, the local failure rate was 6.8 percent. If the local control versus treatment was analyzed according to the pathologic findings in the neck, however, adjunctive radiation therapy reduced the local failure by 50 percent in necks with multiple positive nodes or nodes of over 3 cm in diameter. The 2- and 5-year vital status for the entire group of patients is shown in Tables 10–6 and 10–7.

CONCLUSION

The analysis of the data produced from this retrospective study of 967 patients shows that

Table 10-3. Nodal Status by Heminecks

CLINICAL STAGE	PATHOLOGIC STAGE				TOTAL
	N0		N+		
	No.	*%*	*No.*	*%*	
N0	703	79.9	177	20.1	840
N+	150*	30.5	342	69.5	492
Total	843	62.2	519	37.8	1372

*Includes 7 NX, of whom 1 had pre-op XRT; 101 N1, of whom 27 had pre-op XRT; 12 N2A, of whom 12 had pre-op XRT; 26 N2B, of whom 8 had pre-op XRT; 4 N3A of whom 4 had pre-op XRT.

in selected instances, cervical metastases from squamous carcinoma of the oral cavity, oropharynx, larynx, and hypopharynx can be effectively treated with a modification of the classic radical neck dissection. A radical neck dissection is not necessary as elective treatment for any patient with clinically staged N0 neck disease because a modification of the radical neck dissection—which preserves the sternocleidomastoid muscle, the external and internal jugular veins, the great auricular nerve, the cervical roots, and the spinal accessory nerve—produces very little cosmetic functional alteration and no compromise in cancer control.

When an elective dissection is indicated, the nodal groups most likely to be involved pathologically (which depends on the primary site) are removed. If, on pathologic examination of the dissected specimen, multiple positive nodes are discovered, the use of adjunctive postoperative radiation is indicated. If only one pathologically positive node is revealed from a modified neck dissection of clinically staged N0 neck disease, combined treatment is not necessary as long as the surgical treatment of the primary tumor is also adequate. If the primary tumor is a midline tumor or it approaches the midline, if the nodal status is clinically N0, and if an elective neck dissection is indicated, a bilateral modified neck dissection is the proper therapeutic strategy. Again, if only one pathologically positive node is found on either one or both sides without extracapsular invasion, no radiation is indicated.

It is obvious from this approach that adequate sampling and thorough examination of the nodes is critical to determine the patients who truly have N0 or N+ disease. A unilateral radical neck dissection removes an average of 44 nodes, compared with the 31 nodes removed by a modified neck dissection. The sampling difference of 13 nodes is not significant because the modified dissection removes only the nodes predictably at highest risk. Very rarely are the nodes in the posterior cervical triangle involved in a patient with clinically staged N0 neck disease and a primary tumor in the oral cavity, oropharynx, hypopharynx, or larynx. The thoroughness and competency with which the pathologist examines the nodes, however, is very crucial. To help the pathologist, the surgeon must orient the specimen so that the location of the nodes are properly identified; if necessary, a frozen section examination of any clinically suspicious node or groups of nodes can be performed.

Table 10-4. Clinically Determined Nodal Status for Both Sides of Neck

STAGE RIGHT SIDE	STAGE LEFT SIDE						TOTAL
	Nx	*N0*	*N1*	*N2a*	*N2b*	*N3a*	
NX	0	6	0	0	0	0	6
N0	4	446	96	32	48	11	637
N1	1	128	21	5	11	0	166
N2a	0	45	3	1	1	0	50
N2b	0	66	9	0	17	1	93
N3a	0	12	3	0	0	0	15
Total	5	703	132	38	77	12	967

Table 10-5. Pathologically Determined T and N Status (by Hemineck)

NODAL STATUS	TUMOR STAGE					TOTAL
	Tx	*T1*	*T2*	*T3*	*T4*	
N0	58	61	191	350	193	853
N1	10	16	36	63	34	159
Multiple nodes	14	16	44	72	54	200
Extracapsular invasion	36	18	37	41	28	160
Total	118	111	308	526	309	1372

It is important for the surgeon to know intraoperatively the exact location of the pathologically involved node because if a supraomohyoid dissection has been performed and the single metastatic node is in the submaxillary triangle, no further treatment is indicated. If the node is at the midjugular level, however, the operation must be extended to include the lower jugular nodes in case of their involvement.

A supraomohyoid neck dissection removes the nodes at highest risk for a primary tumor originating in the oral cavity or oropharynx. For a primary in either the glottic or supraglottic larynx, however, a bilateral anterior modified neck dissection is better because the bilateral removal of the subdigastric, midjugular, and lower jugular nodes, as well as the paratracheal nodes, gives an adequate sampling of the highest-risk nodal groups. The submental and submaxillary nodes are not at risk.

The same concept is used for selecting the kind of neck dissection for patients with N0 neck status and a primary tumor of the hypopharynx, except that the retropharyngeal nodes are also included. If a single retropharyngeal node is positive at the base of the skull, postoperative radiation is probably necessary, although there are not enough cases to analyze and substantiate this statement statistically.

If neck disease is staged N1 unilaterally or bilaterally, it is important to define where the nodal disease is located and to consider the features of the primary tumor in order to select the proper surgical treatment. Stage T_3 and T_4 primary tumors probably require combined treatment regardless of the status of the neck nodes. Any clinically positive node less than 3 cm in diameter in the submaxillary tri-

Table 10-6. Patient Status 2 Years After Treatment

STATUS		NO. OF PATIENTS	
Living	No evidence of disease	599	
	Primary disease only	6	
	Neck disease only	7	
	Distant metastases only	16	
	Primary and neck disease	2	
	Neck disease and distant metastases	2	
	Not available for follow-up	11	
	Subtotal	643	(66.5%)
Dead	Complications of treatment	31	
	Head and neck cancer	184	
	Non-head and neck cancer	20	
	Intercurrent disease	49	
	Unknown causes	32	
	Other causes	8	
	Subtotal	324	
	Total	967	(33.5%)

Table 10-7. Patient Status 5 Years After Treatment

STATUS		NO. OF PATIENTS	
Living	No evidence of disease	365	
	Primary disease only	6	
	Neck disease only	1	
	Distant metastases only	5	
	Primary and neck disease	1	
	Not available for follow-up	104	
	Subtotal	482	(49.8%)
Dead	Complications of treatment	33	
	Head and neck cancer	255	
	Non-head and neck cancer	37	
	Intercurrent disease	86	
	Unknown causes	55	
	Other causes	19	
	Subtotal	485	(50.2%)
	Total	967	

angle in a patient with a primary tumor in the oral cavity or oropharynx has a high potential of being pathologically negative (33 percent). This high rate may be due to confusion of nodal disease with an inflammatory node secondary to poor oral hygiene, or even with direct extension of a primary tumor. In these cases, a unilateral or bilateral supraomohyoid neck dissection is selected depending on whether or not the enlarged nodes ares unilateral or bilateral.

If unilateral or bilateral nodes are negative pathologically or positive without extracapsular invasion, the resection of the primary tumor is adequate. If no adverse pathologic criteria such as perineural invasion are evident, postoperative irradiation is unnecessary. If the primary tumor is in the larynx or hypopharynx and the clinically positive node is in the jugular chain, a bilateral anterior modified neck dissection is preferred. If the N1 node is adjacent to the 11th nerve, either before it enters the sternocleidomastoid muscle (most commonly) or after it exits the sternocleidomastoid muscle in the posterior cervical triangle (rarely), the nerve can be preserved with no compromise in cancer control. If the N1 node is adherent to the nerve but can be peeled off, it is better to do so and give postoperative radiation than to resect the nerve or resect and graft it. If the nodal disease completely encases the nerve, the nerve must be resected and preferably grated. Postoperative radiation, however, is still necessary in this situation because the nodal disease has invaded outside the capsule.

Whenever there is connective tissue involvement, combined treatment is indicated; however, less-than-radical neck dissection can usually be performed as long as all the gross disease is removed.

In patients whose necks contain a clinically positive node more than 3 cm in diameter or multiple positive nodes (N2A, N3A, N2B), the surgical objective is to remove the gross disease with as little cosmetic or functional defect as possible, obtain good wound healing (usually within 6 weeks), and give postoperative radiation (at least 5000 cGy in 5 weeks, but preferably 6000 cGy in 6 weeks). Often, this can also be accomplished with a modification of the radical neck dissection. If preoperative radiation has been given to the neck for clinically positive nodes, a modified neck dissection can usually be performed 5 weeks after completion of radiation therapy if the primary tumor is under control. If the nodal disease was unresectable before irradiation and becomes resectable after radiation, a radical neck dissection is preferable.

REFERENCES

American Joint Committee for Cancer Staging and End Results Reporting. *Manual for Staging of Cancer*, 1979. American Joint Committee, Chicago, 1979.

Fletcher, G. H.: Elective irradiation of subclinical disease in cancers of the head and neck. *Cancer*, 29:1450, 1972.

Jesse, R. H., and Fletcher, G.: Treatment of the neck in patients with squamous cell carcinoma of the head and neck. *Cancer*, 39:868–72, 1977.

Johnson, J. T., Barnes, E. L., Muers, E. N., Schramm, V. L., Borochovita, D., and Sigler, B.: Extracapsular spread of tumors in cervical node metastasis. *Arch. Otolaryngol.*, 107:725–29, 1981.

Lindberg, R. D.: Distribution of cervical lymph-node metastases from squamous cell carcinoma of upper respiratory and digestive tracts. *Cancer*, 29:1446–49, 1972.

Strong, E. W.: Preoperative radiation and radical neck dissection. *Surg. Clin. North Am.*, 49:271–76, 1969.

CHAPTER 11

Morbidity of Radical Neck Dissection

David E. Schuller

EDITORS' COMMENT

Coming from the same surgical school as Dr. Strong, Dr. Schuller generally notes the same sources as Strong to justify use of the radical neck dissection of Crile. Citing the fact that "though the lymphatics are not present in muscle, they extensively involve the fascial planes overlying the muscle," Dr. Schuller concludes that they must be removed in any surgical procedure of the neck.

Dr. Schuller begins by outlining the attempts by other surgeons to lessen the morbidity from loss of the 11th nerve and resultant denervation of the trapezius muscle. These attempts include mechanically immobilizing the scapula, grafting the 11th nerve, or preserving the 11th nerve intraoperatively. In the middle third of the chapter, Dr. Schuller outlines the importance of the 11th nerve and the lymphatics associated with it. Though acknowledging the work of McGavran et al. (1961) and Skolnik (1976), he cites his own 1978 study as justification for removal of the 11th nerve and its adjacent lymphatic tissue in all neck dissections, regardless of the site of the primary tumor. The author also makes the assumption that almost all modified neck dissections require adjunctive radiation therapy to be as effective as the more radical procedure. This is not necessarily so, as the reader saw in the last chapter.

The last portion of the chapter reports the results of a survey of neck dissection patients performed at a variety of institutions. The patients were asked to subjectively evaluate the morbidity related to their neck surgery (both radical and modified dissections). Dr. Schuller found no significant difference between the two procedures according to the patients' own reporting. Although this study gives us a unique evaluation of the morbidity from the results of a patient-documented questionnaire, flaws inherent in the study include its multiinstitutional bias, its obvious subjectivity, and the difficulty of separating the effects of neck surgery when, in many cases, it has been combined with an operation on the primary site.

Despite the problems with the questionnaire, Dr. Schuller has given us another perspective from which we can view both removal of the 11th nerve in the neck dissection and its resultant morbidity.

Supported by the Ohio State University Comprehensive Cancer Center (Head and Neck Oncology Program) and the Bremer Foundation.

INTRODUCTION

The cervical lymphatics play an important role in head and neck oncology, and represent the organ system most frequently involved by metastatic disease from epidermoid carcinoma arising in the upper aerodigestive tract. This tumor–nodal interaction has the potential for affecting the biologic behavior of the malignancy, and should certainly be considered in the development of treatment approaches.

Almost 40 percent of the lymph nodes in the human body are located in the neck region (Hellstrom et al., 1971). The cervical lymphatic system, including the lymph nodes and lymphatic channels, is intimately involved with all tissues except for muscle and the central nervous system (Feind, 1972). Even though the lymphatics are not present in muscle, they extensively involve the fascial planes overlying the muscle. This extensive involvement of components of the lymphatic system with other structures in the neck is critical to the discussion that follows.

Another important consideration is the degree of metastatic involvement of the cervical lymphatic system. With the exception of carcinomas arising on the true vocal cords, almost all the other possible sites of epidermoid carcinoma within the head and neck reveal frequent metastasis to neck nodes. Although there is some discussion about the prognostic importance of certain features of metastasis to neck nodes, it is clear that there is general agreement on others.

There is no question that the presence of metastatic nodal disease in the neck drastically alters the patient's prognosis. It used to be generally agreed that the increasing size of metastatic nodes or increasing number of metastatic nodes also reflected a worse prognosis. Although these factors are now being challenged, there is no doubt that some means of quantitating the magnitude of the cancer's impact on the lymphatic system will probably reflect a worsening prognosis. When the anatomic extensiveness of the cervical lymphatic system is considered along with its propensity for being frequently involved by metastatic disease, the therapeutic challenge to the clinician becomes obvious.

Radical neck dissection, originally described by Crile in 1906, represented the first surgical attempt to meet this challenge. The operation was designed as a means of removing all the cervical lymphatic system. In an effort to be complete, certain anatomic structures are intentionally excised, rather than removing just the tissue involved by direct cancerous extension. Therefore, some structures are routinely removed because they are intimately related to the lymphatic structures that may contain metastatic disease. The submandibular gland, internal jugular vein, cervical sensory plexus, spinal accessory nerve, and sternocleidomastoid muscle are removed as a means of totally excising lymphatic-containing tissue.

The removal of this amount of tissue, however, creates potential morbidity. "Shoulder syndrome" (Nahum et al., 1961) is a term reflecting the fact that the primary contributor to this morbidity is the loss of the sternocleidomastoid muscle and the spinal accessory nerve, with a resultant denervation of the trapezius. This denervation and muscle excision can result in a shoulder that is weakened and painful on movement and has a decreased range of motion. Scapular depression and rotation also occurs, resulting in a cosmetic deformity. Numerous approaches have been described to deal with rehabilitating a patient following radical neck dissection. One approach has been to try to prevent the shoulder syndrome.

PREVENTION OF RADICAL NECK DISSECTION MORBIDITY

The shoulder syndrome develops after a patient has had a radical neck dissection and the scapula moves out of its normal anatomic position. This lack of scapular stability is one of the primary contributors to the syndrome. Anything that prevents that scapular movement might help minimize the morbidity.

One approach has been to prevent the scapular movement by fixing it into its usual position. In 1950, DeWar and Harris described an approach to decrease this handicap by fixing the root of the spine of the scapulae to the vertebral processes of the second and third dorsal vertebrae. This was done with fascial slings. After this was completed, the levator scapula was released from its inferior point of attachment and transplanted to the outer end of the scapular spine.

In 1965, Harris and Dickey described another approach. They advocated taking a greater auricular nerve graft and placing it between the proximal and distal stumps of the severed spinal accessory nerve as a means of reinnervating the trapezius muscle. They reported excellent results with this technique.

Still another approach for avoiding the morbidity of radical neck dissection is to preserve the sternocleidomastoid muscle, the spinal accessory nerve, or both. If the motor innervation to the trapezius muscle is intact, the mechanism for maintaining normal scapular position would be undisturbed and morbidity would be minimized. There has been considerable debate, however, about the advisability of preserving the spinal accessory nerve in terms of cancer control. Critical to this discussion is understanding the anatomy and frequency of involvement of the portion of the cervical lymphatic system related to the spinal accessory nerve.

RATIONALE FOR SPINAL ACCESSORY NERVE PRESERVATION

If the spinal accessory nerve were anatomically distinct from the surrounding structure, this separation might provide a basis for attempting its preservation in a cancer operation. In 1967, Bocca and Pignataro reported on an anatomic description of the neck contents. Their paper provided a precise description of the aponeurotic system of the neck. The aponeurotic compartments were filled with connective tissue and the lymphatic system. They appeared to be distinct from other critical structures, such as muscles, vessels, and nerves. The in-continuity removal of these aponeurotic compartments could theoretically be accomplished with the preservation of the other distinct structures. The study revealed, however, that the spinal accessory nerve is not segregated throughout its entire course. It does transect one of the aponeurotic compartments that contains lymphatic tissue in the superior portion of the neck.

Another approach to justifying preservation of the spinal accessory nerve has been the attempts to demonstrate that it is only rarely involved by metastatic neck-nodal disease. Critical to this discussion is the determination of whether a distinct spinal accessory node chain exists in the neck. A prospective study in 1978 by Schuller et al. in cancer patients demonstrated a distinct separate spinal accessory nodal chain. The primary question, then, is whether that lymph-node chain is involved frequently enough to justify always removing the nerve.

Some studies suggested it is rarely involved. McGavran, Bauer, and Ogura (1961) found no evidence of metastatic nodes in the posterior neck triangle of patients with squamous carcinoma of the larynx. Skolnik et al. (1976) found no evidence of metastatic nodal disease in the posterior triangle in a group of patients with a variety of primary tumor sites undergoing both therapeutic and elective neck dissections. Their conclusion, based on this study, was that the posterior triangle did not have to be dissected in elective neck dissections, not even in some selected therapeutic dissections.

In the study previously described, Schuller et al. (1978) also evaluated the matter of spinal nerve and metastatic nodal involvement. This analysis demonstrated no statistically significant difference between the frequency of metastatic disease in the nodes from the entire neck specimen compared with the nodes in the spinal accessory node chain. The same study demonstrated that the spinal accessory lymph nodes could be involved by metastatic disease independent of the jugular nodal chain. There was no predilection for this metastatic involvement of the spinal accessory nodes from one particular primary tumor site. The study also demonstrated that the spinal accessory nodal chain could be involved by occult metastases as the only location of metastatic disease in the entire neck.

The study involved the evaluation of neck nodes adjacent to the spinal accessory nerve for the entire course of the nerve from the posterior triangle to the skull base, where it is adjacent to the upper end of the internal jugular vein. This fact may reflect the apparent differences in results from this study compared with those previously published. The inferior end of the spinal accessory nerve—namely, the portion of the nerve that coursed through the posterior cervical triangle—was only rarely involved (4.8%) by metastatic disease. It was the superior end that was the sole location of metastases in the overwhelming majority (90.5%) of patients. Therefore, it is not possible to claim that the spinal accessory nerve is infrequently involved by lymphatic-containing tissue. By contrast, it is commonly involved by metastatic disease.

Irrespective of whether or not the spinal accessory nerve is anatomically segregated or is infrequently involved by metastases, an important consideration is whether or not there is a reduction in local neck-disease control rates for patients whose nerves are preserved in a modified neck dissection, compared with the rates for patients who have undergone a radical neck dissection. The literature contains several reports that document comparable survival rates. Lingeman et al. (1977) showed that in a group of patients with N0 nodal status, none of those who had modified dissection had neck recurrences, compared with 14 percent of those who had traditional neck dissection. Their failure rate for N1 or N2 groupings for the two operations was also similar. In a later report, Jesse et al. (1978) also demonstrated no statistical difference in neck-disease recurrence rates in patients undergoing modified versus radical neck dissection.

It is important to understand that most surgeons using modified neck dissection include it as part of a combined therapy program with radiation therapy, either preoperatively or postoperatively. In spite of the absence of any anatomic or other means of justifying the safety of preserving the spinal accessory nerve, there is information in the literature to support its preservation in combination procedures with radiation therapy that do not result in a worsening of the local control rates.

DESCRIPTION OF MORBIDITY: RADICAL NECK DISSECTION VERSUS MODIFIED NECK DISSECTION

Combined therapy programs became popular in the mid-1960s. They incorporated the use of surgery and radiation therapy as a means of improving the local and regional control of the disease for advanced-stage lesions. Combined therapy has continued to be popular, and is now undergoing investigation to evaluate the role of chemotherapy.

Most discussions concerning morbidity are preoccupied with the impact of the surgical treatment. The previous discussion dealt with the impact of severing the spinal accessory nerve by radical neck dissection, and how patients with that particular surgically created problem can be rehabilitated. But the popularity of combined therapy, especially the widespread use of surgery and radiation therapy when modified neck dissection is used, requires an assessment of the entire program rather than just one particular phase to gain an appreciation of the overall impact on the patient. The assumption has always been that the modified neck dissection, because it preserves the spinal accessory nerve and sometimes even the sternocleidomastoid muscle, creates no shoulder syndrome, and hence fewer problems, for the patient.

The paucity of information in the medical literature about this subject provided the stimulus for a multiinstitutional study (Schuller et al., 1983) intended to characterize the impact of the total treatment program. Information was obtained on patient job status, social activities, psychosocial adjustment, and esthetic reaction to treatment. The study was designed so that the information obtained dealt only with the stress from the neck surgery, and not that related to the primary tumor excision.

The impact on the patients' job status is shown in Table 11-1. There were 203 patients who were employed prior to treatment. Following completion of the entire treatment pro-

Table 11–1. Distribution of Reasons for Not Returning to Usual Job (n = 90)

REASON	PERCENT OF PATIENTS WITH POSITIVE RESPONSE TO		SIGNIFICANCE
	Radical neck dissection (%)	*Modified neck dissection (%)*	
Limitation of shoulder movement	55.2	59.1	NS*
Pain, limitation related to removal of tumor	62.1	76.2	$p<0.05$
Reasons other than treatment	53.3	50.0	NS

*NS = not significant.

gram, a surprisingly high percentage (51.2%) returned to their jobs. More than half of those who had radical neck dissection (50.3%) and 54.0% of those who had modified neck dissection returned to their jobs. There was no statistically significant difference between the two groups. Table 11–1 also shows that in those individuals who did not return to their jobs, there was no difference between the two groups in terms of limitation of shoulder movement. These results will be surprising to those who assumed there would be no dysfunction following modified neck dissection.

The type of employment is characterized according to how strenuous it is as it relates specifically to shoulder movement. Table 11–2 shows there is no direct relationship between the type of surgery, the strenuousness of the job, or the patient's ability to return to work.

When the impact of treatment on the patient's social activities was assessed, however, it was found that in a greater proportion (45.1%) of patients who underwent radical neck dissection treatment did have an adverse affect on social acitivities compared with those who had a modified neck dissection (30.6%). This difference was attributable to the type of surgery. When the esthetic impact by treatment was assessed, it was apparent that patients undergoing radical neck dissection were bothered more frequently than the modified neck patients. But the scientific factors that caused them to be bothered were not identified in the study. It did not relate to either flattening of the neck or scarring.

Surprising findings were noted in the psychosocial evaluation of these patients. It was found that radiation therapy appeared to have a significant impact on patients, irrespective of whether the patients had undergone radical or modified neck dissections. A number of analyses were done to determine if the stage of disease or magnitude of surgery created this psychosocial impact, but none identified any factors other than radiation therapy.

The preceding discussion emphasizes the need for assessing the impact of a total treatment rather than focusing on one particular aspect. There is no question that a radical neck dissection that cuts the spinal accessory nerve will invariably cause some degree of pain, deformity, and functional impairment of the shoulder. But another important question is the assessment of the entire treatment on morbidity. The preceding analyses suggest that the dissection that preserves the spinal acces-

Table 11–2. Relationship of Surgery, Strenuousness of Occupation, and Return to Job

	NOT STRENUOUS (74 PATIENTS)		MODERATELY STRENUOUS (74 PATIENTS)		VERY STRENUOUS (49 PATIENTS)	
	RND (%)	*MND (%)*	*RND (%)*	*MND (%)*	*RND (%)*	*MND (%)*
Returned to usual job	32/59 (54.2)	8/15 (53.3)	29/55 (52.7)	15/19 (78.9)	15/36 (41.7)	4/13 (30.8)
Did not return to usual job	27/59 (45.8)	7/15 (46.7)	26/55 (47.3)	4/19 (21.1)	21/36 (58.3)	9/13 (69.2)
Not significant	$p<0.05$			$p<0.05$		

RND = radical neck dissection; MND = modified neck dissection.

sory nerve during modified neck dissection may compromise its vascularity to the point where postoperative radiation therapy impairs nerve function, resulting in shoulder movement limitation.

TREATMENT OF MORBIDITY

After a radical neck dissection has been performed, therapeutic intervention can help to minimize the symptoms associated with trapezius denervation and the shoulder dysfunction. The key to the effectiveness of any treatment program is whether or not it will permit adequate patient compliance. A practical physical therapy program cannot be dependent on the patient's receiving regular frequent treatment at a physical therapy facility, or require the use of expensive exercise equipment that has to be rented or purchased.

It is possible to develop an effective home physical therapy program for patients that does not require expensive equipment, a great deal of time, or patient discomfort. Saunders and Johnson outlined such a program in 1975. Instituting therapy as early after surgery as possible is helpful. The essence of the program involves range-of-motion exercises that are easy for the patient to understand. Often these exercises can be more effectively accomplished if they are preceded by the application of local heat to the shoulder. The exercises similarly require the patient to stand at arm's length from a wall, facing parallel to it, and use the fingers to elevate the shoulder girdle as high as possible. Doing this several times a day will help to maintain the mobility of the shoulder joint and decrease the restricted range of motion and pain. Patient motivation is the key to the success of this or any physical therapy program.

OTHER CONSIDERATIONS

The intent of radical neck dissection is to remove as much of the cervical lymphatic system as possible. It reflects our current inability to determine preoperatively which tissue is contaminated by cancerous deposits. Without this ability, it is necessary to remove all tissue in an attempt to minimize the possibility of residual cancer. This surgical eradication of a significant amount of the body's lymphatic system, whether it be with radical or modified neck dissection, obviously has an impact on the host's immune response. In fact, the three conventional modalities of treating malignancies (surgery, radiation therapy, and chemotherapy) are all immunosuppressive (Schuller, 1984).

The recent demonstration of regional immunoreactivity by lymph nodes to head and neck cancer (Schuller et al., 1985) suggests that these nodes may have a therapeutic potential. The present inability of diagnostic tests to identify cancerous tissue mandates a nonspecific form of treatment that eradicates nodes that indeed might be helpful in therapy. Hopefully, diagnostic sophistication will improve so that greater use of tumor-specific treatment will become a reality. Discussions such as this of morbidity from radical or modified neck dissection will then become a part of medical history.

REFERENCES

Bocca, E., and Pignataro, O.: A conservation technique in radical neck dissection. *Ann. Otol. Rhinol. Laryngol.*, 74:975–87, 1965.

Crile, G.: Excision of cancer of the head and neck. *J.A.M.A.*, 47:1780–86, 1906.

DeWar, F. P., and Harris, R. I.: Restoration of function of the shoulder following paralysis of the trapezius by fascial sling fixation and transplantation of the levator scapulae. *Ann. Surg.*, 132:1111–15, 1950.

Feind, C. R.: The head and neck. In Haagensen, C. D. (ed.): *The Lymphatics in Cancer*, pp. 60–230. W.B. Saunders, Philadelphia, 1972.

Harris, H. H., and Dickey, V. R.: Nerve grafting to restore function of trapezius muscle after radical neck dissection. *Ann. Otol. Rhinol. Laryngol.*, 74:880–86, 1965.

Hellstrom, K. E., and Hellstome, I.: Immunologic defenses against cancer. In Good, R. A., and Fisher, D. W. (eds.): *Immunobiology*, pp. 209–18. Sinauer Associates, Stanford, CT, 1971.

Jesse, R. H., Ballantyne, A. J., and Larson, D.: Radical or modified neck dissection: A therapeutic dilemma. *Am. J. Surg.*, 136:516–24, 1978.

Lingeman, R. E., Helmus, E., Stephens, R., et al.: Neck dissection: Radical or conservative. *Ann. Otol. Rhinol. Laryngol.*, 86:737–41, 1977.

McGavran, M. H., Bauer, W. C., and Ogura, J. H.: The incidence of cervical lymph-node metastases from epidermoid carcinoma of the larynx, and their relationship to certain characteristics of the primary tumor. *Cancer*, 14:55–66, 1961.

Nahum, A. M., Mullally, W., and Marmor, L.: A syndrome resulting from radical neck dissection. *Arch. Otolaryngol.,* 74:424–34, 1961.

Saunders, W. H., and Johnson, E. W.: Rehabilitation of the shoulder after radical neck dissection. *Ann. Otol. Rhinol. Laryngol.*, 84:812–16, 1975.

Schuller, D. E.: An assessment of neck-node immunoreactivity in head and neck cancer. *Laryngology*, 94 (suppl. 35) November, 1984.

Schuller, D. E., Libby, D. H., Rinehart, J. J., and Milo, G. G.: Immunomodulation of nodal lymphocytes in head and neck cancer. *Arch. Otolaryngol.*, 111:465–68, 1985.

Schuller, D. E., Platz, C. E., and Krause, C. J.: Spinal accessory nodes: A prospective study of metastatic involvement. *Laryngoscope*, 88:439–59, 1978.

Schuller, D. E., Reiches, N. A., Hamaker, R. C., et al.: Analysis of disability resulting from treatment including radical neck dissection or modified neck dissection. *Head Neck Surg.,* 6:551–58, 1983.

Skolnik, E. M., Yee, K. F., Friedman, M., and Golden, T. A.: The posterior triangle in radical neck surgery. *Arch. Otolaryngol.,* 102:1–4, 1976.

CHAPTER 12

Morbidity of Modified Neck Dissection

Daniel Remmler, Jan Scheetz, Robert Byers, Georgia White, Stuart Zimmerman, Barbara Shell, and Helmuth Goepfert

EDITORS' COMMENT

Daniel Remmler and his colleagues review the experience of The University of Texas M.D. Anderson Hospital and Tumor Institute at Houston with 11th nerve function after modified neck dissection because, as the authors first note, this is a point of contention in the literature. In an attempt to clarify the possibility of shoulder dysfunction from either 11th nerve sparing and 11th nerve sacrifice, a prospective, longitudinal study was conducted over a 12-month period. Ninety patients undergoing 103 neck dissections were enrolled in the study. Operations in 94 cases spared the 11th nerve; in nine it was sacrificed. Careful preoperative and postoperative evaluation by unbiased physical therapists was carried out at regular intervals over the ensuing 12 months. This resulted in 59 patients evaluable at 6 months and only 25 patients at 12 months.

The results of this study showed, as expected, a loss of upper and middle trapezius function by both individual muscle testing and electromyographic means in patients with known loss of the 11th nerve; the nerve sparing group maintained their trapezius muscle function. The range of motion, however, was the same in both groups.

In this study, the authors have established beyond any doubt that there is significant muscle loss with division of the 11th nerve. They also show the importance of adequate, early initiation of a good physical therapy program regardless of the type of neck dissection performed. We routinely give our patients active and passive range-of-motion exercises after any neck dissection because of the possibility that neurapraxia may accompany nerve sparing. Dr. Remmler and his coauthors seem to confirm the value of this routine with their data.

INTRODUCTION

Historically, surgeons have accepted the shoulder dysfunction and discomfort resulting from sacrifice of the spinal accessory nerve in the classic radical neck dissection. Beginning in the later part of the 1960s, however, this disability motivated the development of alternative neck-dissection procedures to clear the neck of metastatic cancer yet preserve the spinal accessory nerve and, if possible, spare the sternocleidomastoid muscle and internal jugular vein (Bocca and Pignataro, 1967; Bocca, 1975; Jesse et al., 1978; Lingeman et al., 1977; Becker and Parell, 1979). The appropriate selection from these neck-dissection procedures depends on the site of the primary cancer, the probability of lymphatic metastasis, and lymph-node staging.

Although much progress has been achieved in the use of modified, nerve-sparing dissections, uncertainty remains about the superiority of these operations in predictably avoiding shoulder disability. Notably, several clinical studies have reported varying degrees of trapezius dysfunction in patients undergoing these modified procedures despite anatomic preservation of the spinal accessory nerve (Gordon et al., 1977; Carenfelt and Eliasson, 1980; Schuller et al., 1983; Leipzig et al., 1983). Therefore, to clarify any functional advantages related to spinal accessory nerve preservation, we recently conducted a prospective longitudinal study at UTMDAH that evaluated the postoperative course of shoulder dysfunction following various modified and radical neck-dissection procedures (Remmler et al., 1985).

In this chapter, we briefly review the related anatomy and function of the shoulder girdle mechanism, and discuss our experience with shoulder dysfunction following both nerve-sparing and nerve-sacrificing neck-dissection procedures. This chapter is intended to provide the practicing head and neck surgeon with a more complete understanding of the course and severity of shoulder dysfunction associated with such operations.

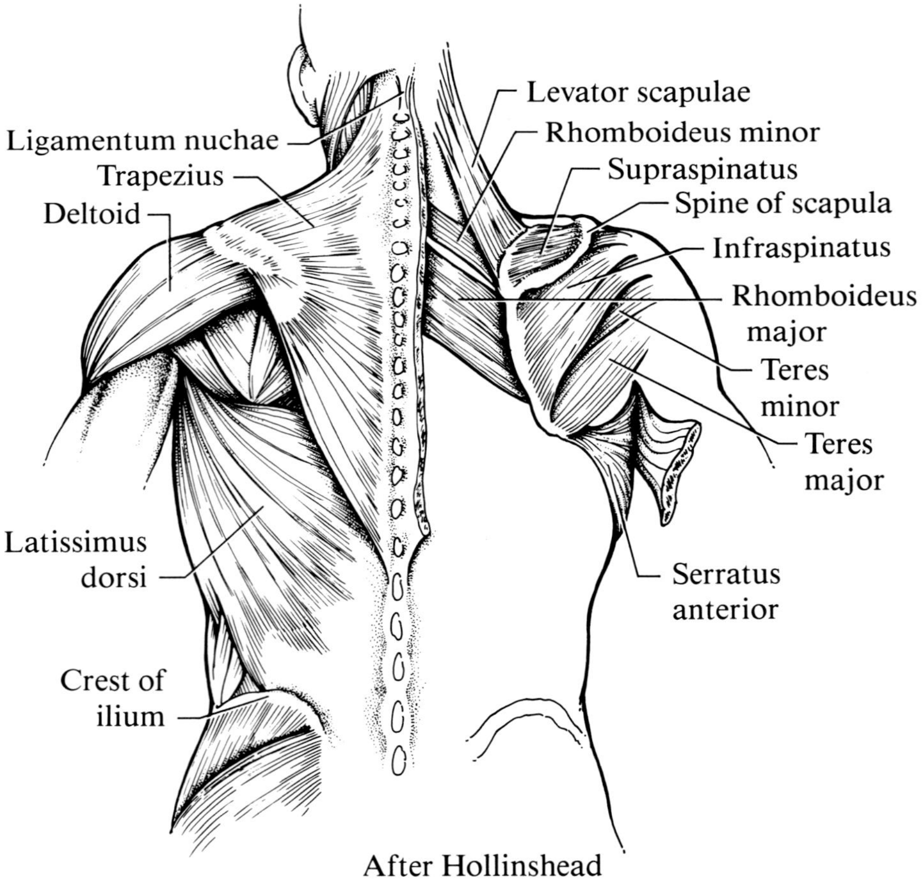

Figure 12–1. Posterior view of muscles of the shoulder. The trapezius, latissimus, and deltoid have all been removed from the right side.

ANATOMIC CONSIDERATIONS

The trapezius muscle is of major functional importance because it provides the primary supportive and rotatory actions of the shoulder girdle mechanism (Hollingshead, 1968; Inman et al., 1944; Warwick, 1971). Anatomically, the trapezius is a large, flat, triangular muscle that arises from broad vertebral and occipital attachments and converges laterally to its scapular and clavicular insertions (see Figure 12–1). Both functionally and topographically, the trapezius is divided into three parts—upper, middle, and lower—each serving different but complementary roles. Furthermore, these muscular divisions participate with other muscles that are also attached to the scapula in steadying and controlling the shoulder girdle during active use of the upper limb. In this respect, the levator scapulae acts with the upper trapezius to elevate the scapula, the major and minor rhomboids assist the middle trapezius in retracting and stabilizing the scapula against the posterior thoracic cage, and the serratus anterior contributes to scapular rotation (Hollinshead, 1968; Inman et al., 1944; Warwick, 1971).

It is also important to recognize that the simultaneous and combined actions of the upper and lower parts of the trapezius muscle cooperate to exert a unique upward rotatory action on the scapula (see Figure 12–2). The function of the upper trapezius is crucial, however, since it is the only muscle that lifts up the lateral angle of the shoulder—an action that is necessary to produce full upward rotation of the scapula. Fundamentally, this full upward rotation of the scapula occurs simultaneously with abduction of the arm at the

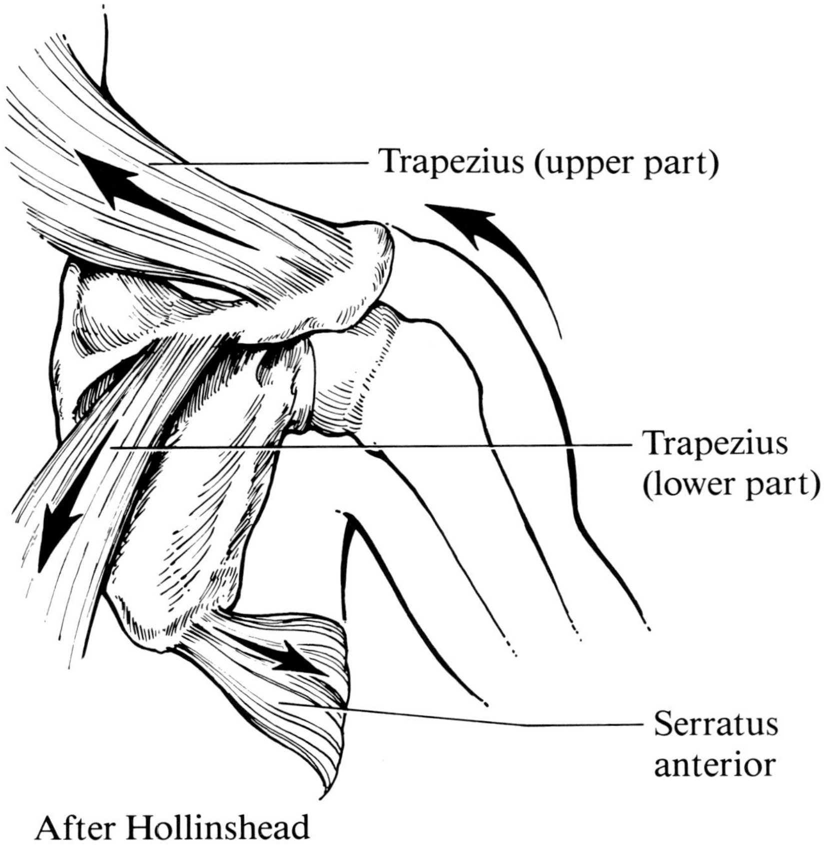

Figure 12–2. Upward rotators of the scapula.

glenohumeral joint to produce complete elevation of the arm above shoulder level (Hollinshead, 1986; Inman et al., 1944).

The trapezius muscle is innervated by the spinal accessory nerve, which extends from the foramen jugulare to the lateral border of the upper trapezius and is vulnerable to operative injury from procedures involving either the anterior or posterior cervical triangles. It is not widely appreciated that the accessory nerve is usually joined by nerve branches of the second cervical nerve at or just prior to the point where it penetrates the sternocleidomastoid muscle (Hollinshead, 1968; Hill and Olson, 1979). More posteriorly, the accessory nerve may receive further communications from the 3rd and 4th cervical nerve; alternatively, these cervical nerve branches may proceed directly across the posterior triangle to supply the middle and lower parts of the trapezius (Hollinshead, 1968; Warwick, 1971) (see Figure 12–3).

The prevailing experimental and clinical evidence is still controversial, but it indicates that cervical nerves that innervate the trapezius contribute only sensory or proprioceptive fibers (Hollinshead, 1968, Warwick, 1971; Carbin and Harrison, 1939; Anderson and Flowers, 1969). Little disageement exists, however, that the upper trapezius, the most important part of the trapezius with respect to scapular rotation, receives motor fibers solely from the spinal accessory nerve (Hollinshead, 1968; Warwick, 1971).

SHOULDER DISABILITY RESULTING FROM TRAPEZIUS PARALYSIS

Surgical sacrifice of the spinal accessory nerve will result in a characteristic shoulder disability syndrome involving deformity, weakness, and pain of the shoulder-girdle mechanism (Ewing and Martin, 1952; Nahum et al., 1961; Mead, 1952; Saunders and Johnson, 1975). The configuration of the shoulder is altered, too, since paralysis of the trapezius muscle allows the scapula to be drawn inferiorly and laterally because of both the weight of the upper limb and the unbalanced action of the other shoulder muscles. Consequently, the entire shoulder girdle appears to drop downward and forward. Resultant atrophy of the trapezius muscle is particularly evident in its upper portion, where the normal profile is replaced by a notched appearance.

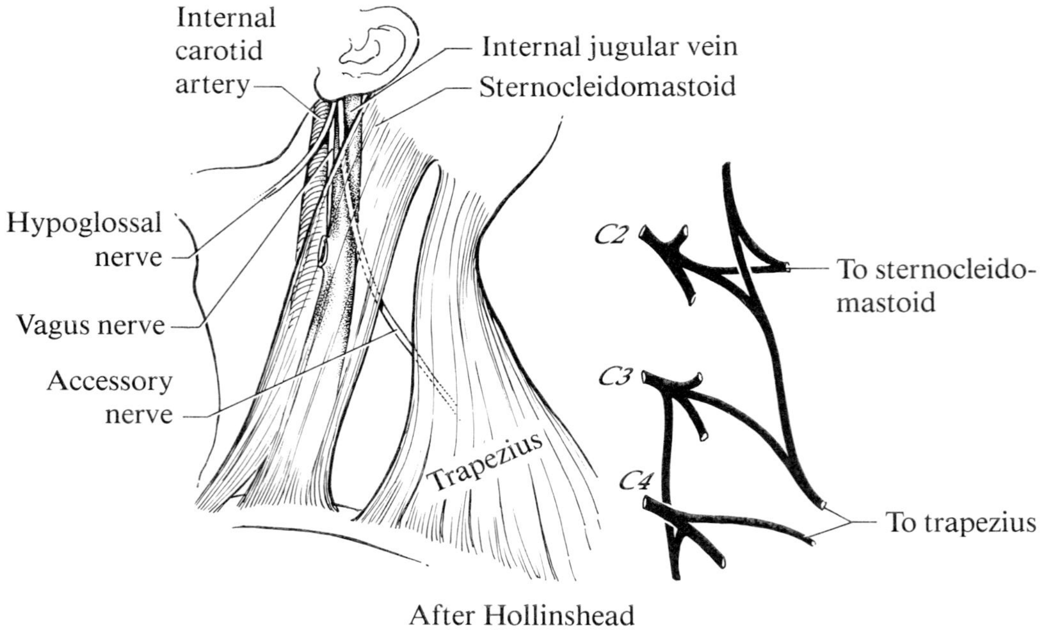

Figure 12–3. Diagram of the course of the accessory nerve in the neck (*A*) and of the cervical nerves to it (*B*).

Further wasting of the trapezius reveals the underlying bony margins of the scapula as well as the remaining supporting shoulder muscles, such as the levator and the rhomboids, which hypertrophy and become even more prominent. The shoulder discomfort that accompanies these changes is usually described as a dull ache along the upper margin of the scapula; it may radiate down the arm or up into the neck. This pain is attributed to increased supportive demands imposed on the levator scapulae and rhomboid muscles (Nahum et al., 1961; Saunders and Johnson, 1975).

Understandably, even greater pain and disability will occur if the nerves to the levator muscle are severed in the course of the neck dissection (Ballantyne and Buinn, 1962; Harris and Dickey, 1965). The most significant impairment, however, is the functional loss of full upward rotation of the scapula. Although some patients can compensate for this loss by bringing the shoulder forward and further elevating the arm by means of flexion, most complain that they can no longer perform tasks that involve overhead use of the arm, such as combing their hair or reaching for something on a shelf (Ewing and Martin, 1952; Saunders and Johnson, 1975; Ballantyne and Guinn, 1962).

CLINICAL MATERIAL AND METHODS

All patients scheduled to undergo a neck dissection at UTMDAH from June 1983 to June 1984 were eligible for the study and were evaluated preoperatively by a physical therapist. Patients found to have preexisting disease or injuries affecting the shoulder-joint mechanism were not included in the study. Ninety patients were enrolled. Their ages ranged from 19 to 82 years, with an average age of 56 years. Seventy patients were men, 20 were women. A total of 103 neck dissections were performed on the 90 patients (simultaneous bilateral dissections were performed on 13 of the them). Shoulder function on the operated side was evaluated by a physical therapist following each neck-dissection procedure. All patients were taught a program of physical therapy aimed at maintaining the range of motion at the shoulder joint. The pathology of the primary lesions related to the neck dissections is presented in Table 12–1.

Table 12–1. Pathology of Primary Lesion

HISTOLOGY	NUMBER OF NECK DISSECTIONS
Squamous cell carcinoma of upper aerodigestive tract	73
Melanoma	10
Salivary gland malignancy	6
Skin cancer	4
Thyroid cancer	3
Adenocarcinoma of upper aerodigestive tract	3
Other	4
Total	103

The 103 neck dissections evaluated in this study consisted of nine standard radical neck dissections in which the spinal accessory nerve was sacrificed (nerve-sacrifice group) and 94 dissections in which the spinal accessory nerve was preserved (nerve-spared group). Four types of modified neck dissection procedures were included in the nerve-spared group (see Table 12–2).

In a *supraomohyoid dissection*, the upper, middle, and (occasionally) the lower jugular nodal groups were removed, and the sternocleidomastoid muscle, the internal jugular vein, and the spinal accessory nerve were preserved.

In a *posterior triangle neck dissection*, the upper, middle, and lower posterior cervical nodes were removed and the spinal accessory nerve was preserved.

In a *functional neck dissection*, all the nodal groups of the anterior and posterior cervical

Table 12–2. Distribution of Neck Dissections According to Management of Spinal Accessory Nerve

EXTENT OF DISSECTION	MANAGEMENT OF NERVE	
	Preserved	*Sacrificed*
Supraomohyoid	76	—
Posterior	7	—
Functional	3	—
Modified radical	8	—
Standard radical	—	9
Total	94	9

Table 12–3. Distribution of Neck Dissections According to Nodal Staging

EXTENT OF DISSECTION	IPSILATERAL NODAL STAGING					TOTAL
	N0	*N1*	*N2*	*N3*	*NX*	
Supraomohyoid	43	27	5	0	1	76
Posterior	2	4	1	0	0	7
Functional	0	1	2	0	0	3
Modified radical	1	0	6	0	1	8
Standard radical	0	1	7	1	0	9
Total	46	33	21	1	2	103

triangles were removed, and the sternocleidomastoid muscle, the internal jugular vein, and the spinal accessory nerve were preserved.

In a *modified radical neck dissection*, the spinal accessory nerve was dissected out and preserved in an otherwise standard radical neck dissection. The clinical staging of disease in the dissected necks is summarized in Table 12–3 according to the type of dissection.

Shoulder function on the operated side was objectively evaluated by a physical therapist. Results were recorded preoperatively and 1, 3, 6, and 12 months postoperatively. Poor compliance with discharge instructions, various disease conditions, and recurrent cancer prevented some of the patients from returning for each scheduled measurement interval, and resulted in a decline in the number of shoulders available for study over the 12-month observation period (see Figure 12–4).

Shoulder function in both the nerve-spared and nerve-sacrificed groups was assessed with three types of tests: manual muscle testing, range-of-motion measurements, and electrodiagnostic testing. Trapezius muscle strength was tested according to techniques described

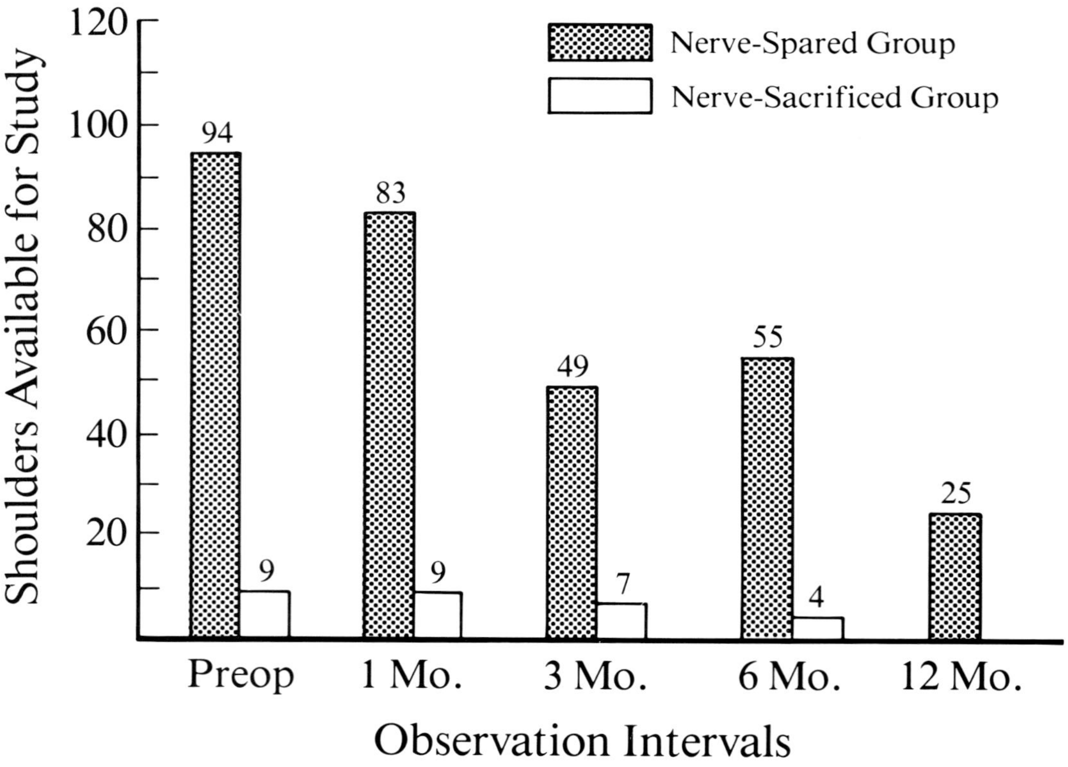

Figure 12–4. Profile of study population.

by Daniels and Worthingham (1972). Upper trapezius muscle function was measured by manually testing the strength of scapular elevation, and middle trapezius function was measured by manually testing the strength of scapular adduction. The muscle strength revealed in both tests was scored as follows: 5 indicated muscle strength that could be overcome only with strong manual resistance exerted by the examiner; 4 indicated muscle strength that could be overcome by moderate manual resistance; 3 indicated muscle strength that was only sufficient to hold a position against the force of gravity; 2 indicated muscle strength capable of producing action only when the upper limb was supported by the examiner; 1 indicated muscle strength only capable of producing a palpable muscle contraction. A score of 0 indicated no palpable evidence of muscle contraction.

Range-of-motion at the shoulder joint was measured with the patient actively abducting the arm while lying supine. Results were recorded in degrees. Standard noninvasive electrodiagnostic testing was performed on the upper trapezius muscle using a Teca CH3 Chronaxie Meter according to methods described by previous clinical investigators (Arief, 1948; Scott, 1975). Using these data, standard strength–duration curves reflecting the integrity of the nerve–muscle complex were formulated, then classified as representing either innervated or denervated muscle.

RESULTS

Results of upper trapezius muscle strength testing were averaged for both the nerve-spared and nerve-sacrificed groups over the 12-month postoperative period (see Figure 12–5). Average upper trapezius strength in the nerve-spared group dropped significantly, from 4.8 preoperatively to 3.7 at 1 month and 3.6 at 3 months postoperatively ($p < 0.05$). Thereafter, however, upper trapezius muscle strength recovered, with average scores increasing to 4.1 at 6 months and 4.0 at 12 months postoperatively. There was no statistically significant difference between the initial preoperative muscle-strength scores and those obtained following recovery at 6 and 12

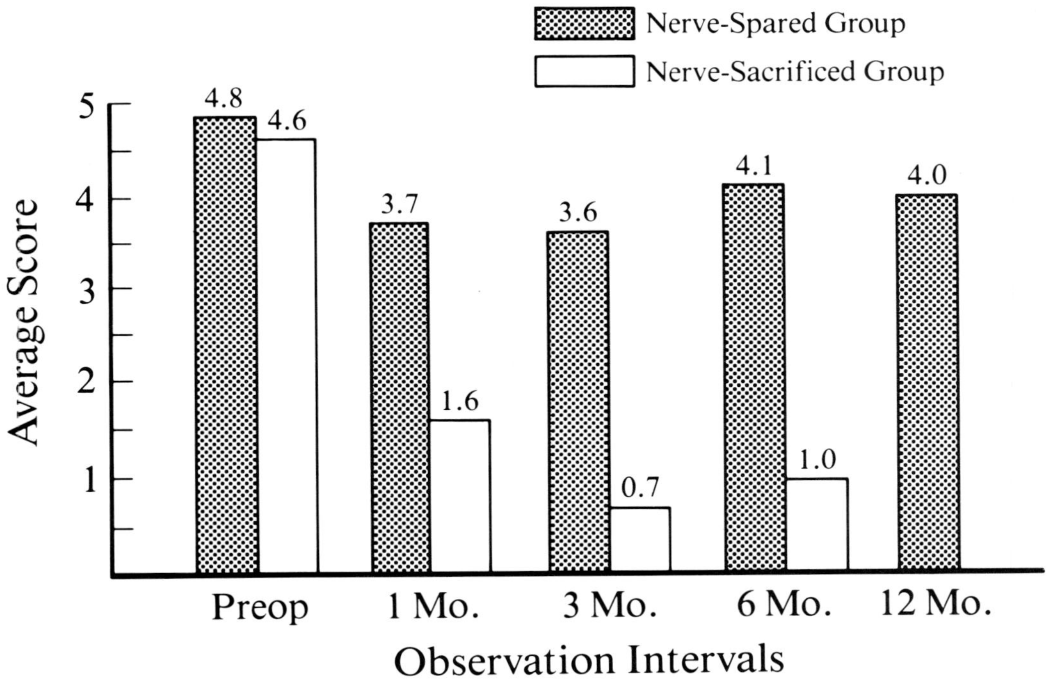

Figure 12–5. Profile of upper trapezius muscle strength.

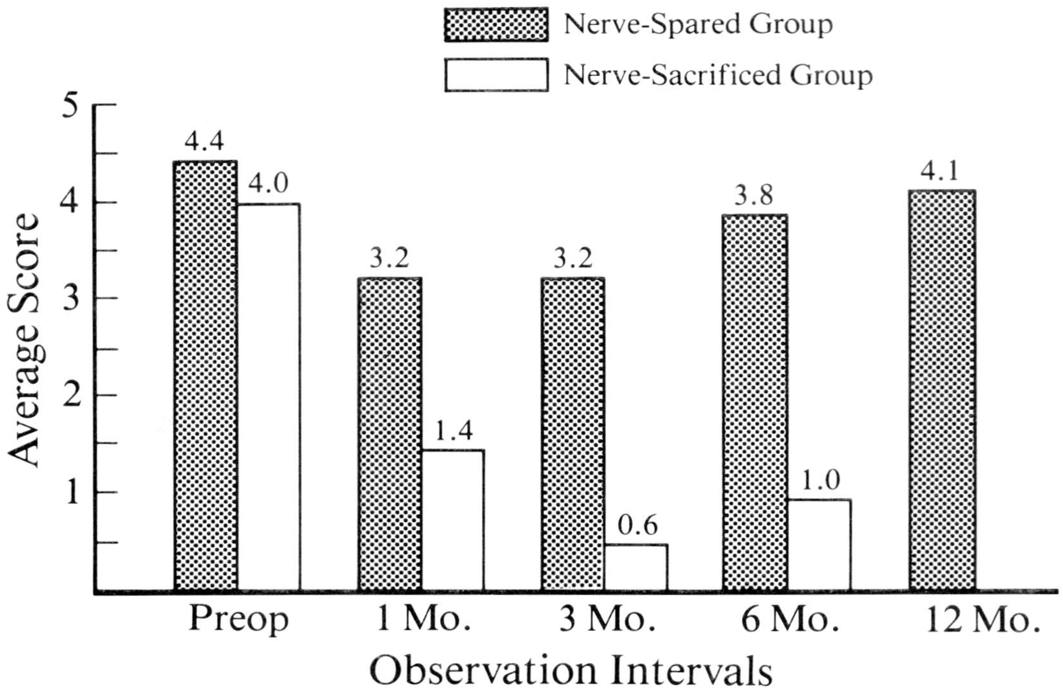

Figure 12–6. Profile of middle trapezius muscle strength.

months ($p<0.05$). In the nerve-sacrificed group, the average middle trapezius strength score dropped significantly, from 4.0 preoperatively to 1.4 at 1 month, 0.7 at 3 months, and 1.0 at 6 months postoperatively ($p<0.05$).

The results of middle trapezius muscle strength testing were similarly analyzed (see Figure 12–6). In the nerve-spared group, the average middle trapezius strength score dropped significantly, from 4.4 preoperatively to 3.2 at 1 month and 3.2 at 3 months postoperatively ($p<0.05$). Thereafter, however, middle trapezius muscle strength recovered, with average scores increasing to 3.8 at 6 months and 4.1 at 12 months postoperatively. As was found with upper trapezius muscle testing, there was no statistically significant difference between the initial preoperative muscle strength scores and those obtained following recovery at 6 and 12 months ($p>0.05$). In the nerve-sacrificed group, the average middle trapezius strength score dropped significantly from 4.0 preoperatively to 1.4 at 1 month, 0.6 at 3 months, and 1.0 at 6 months postoperatively ($p<0.05$).

The results of active supine range-of-motion testing for both the nerve-spared and -sacrificed groups are summarized in Figure 12–7. Range-of-motion measurements for the nerve-spared group did not differ significantly from those of the nerve-sacrificed group ($p<0.05$). Both groups showed a mild but significant reduction in range of motion 1 month postoperatively by comparison with the respective preoperative values ($p<0.05$). Thereafter, however, average range-of-motion in both groups returned to values that were not significantly different from the preoperative measurements ($p<0.05$).

Results of electrodiagnostic testing of the upper trapezius muscle for the nerve-spared and nerve-sacrificed groups are illustrated in Figures 12–8 and 12–9. The percentage of each group distributed in either electrodiagnostically innervated or denervated categories is presented for each observation interval over the 12-month observation period. For the nerve-spared group, 49 percent of the shoulders showed evidence of normal innervation 1 month and 3 months postoperatively. Im-

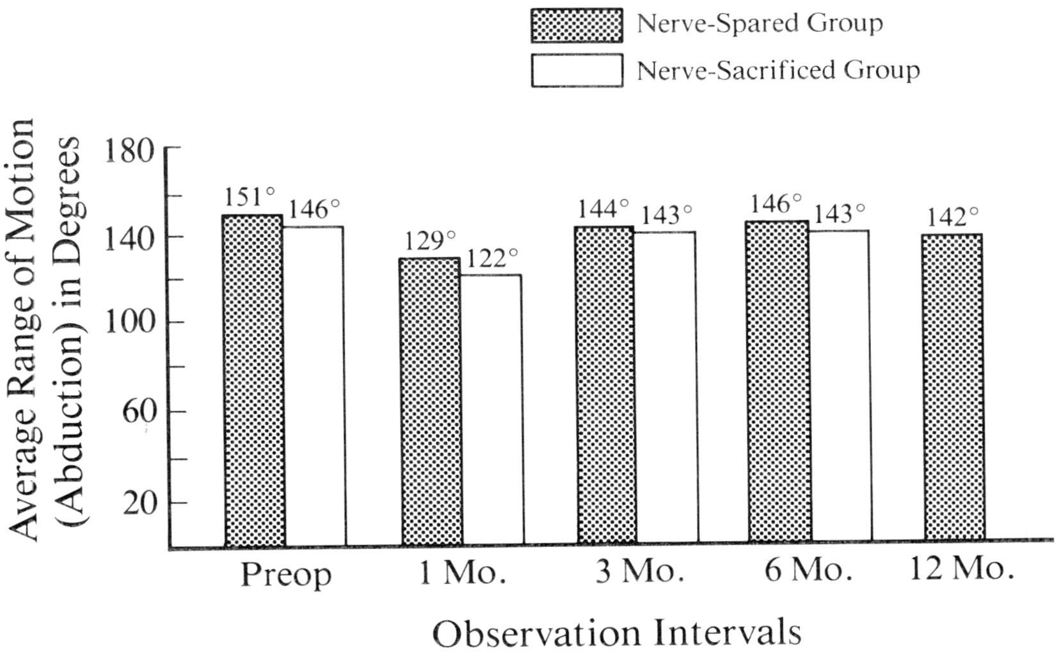

Figure 12-7. Results of active supine range-of-motion testing.

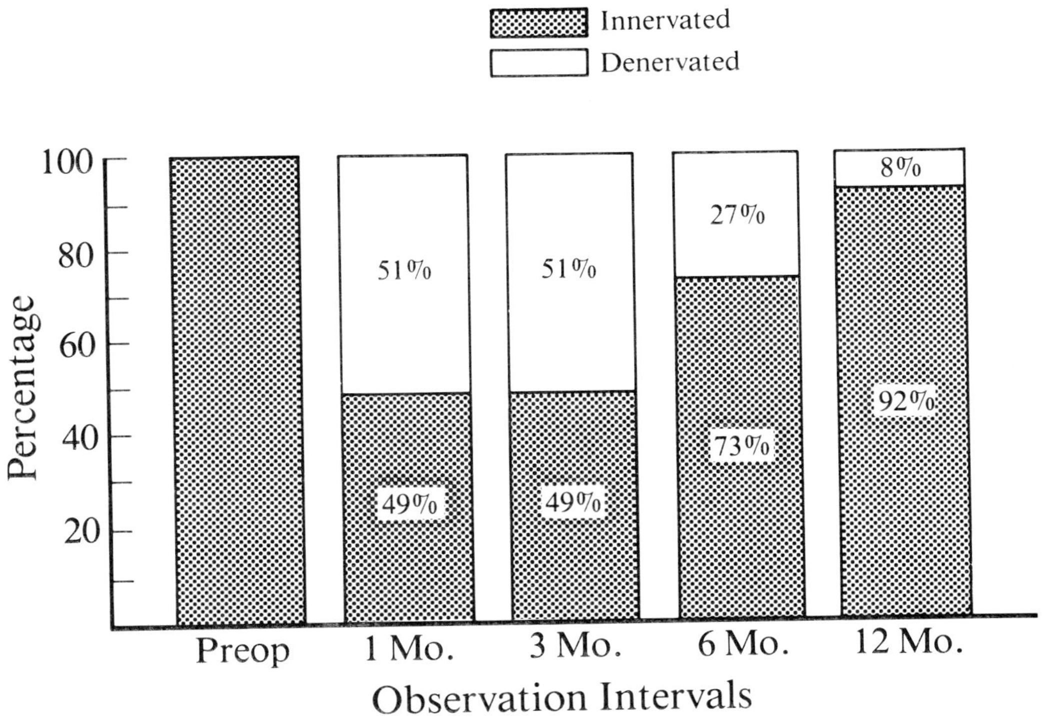

Figure 12-8. Results of electrodiagnostic testing of the nerve-spared group.

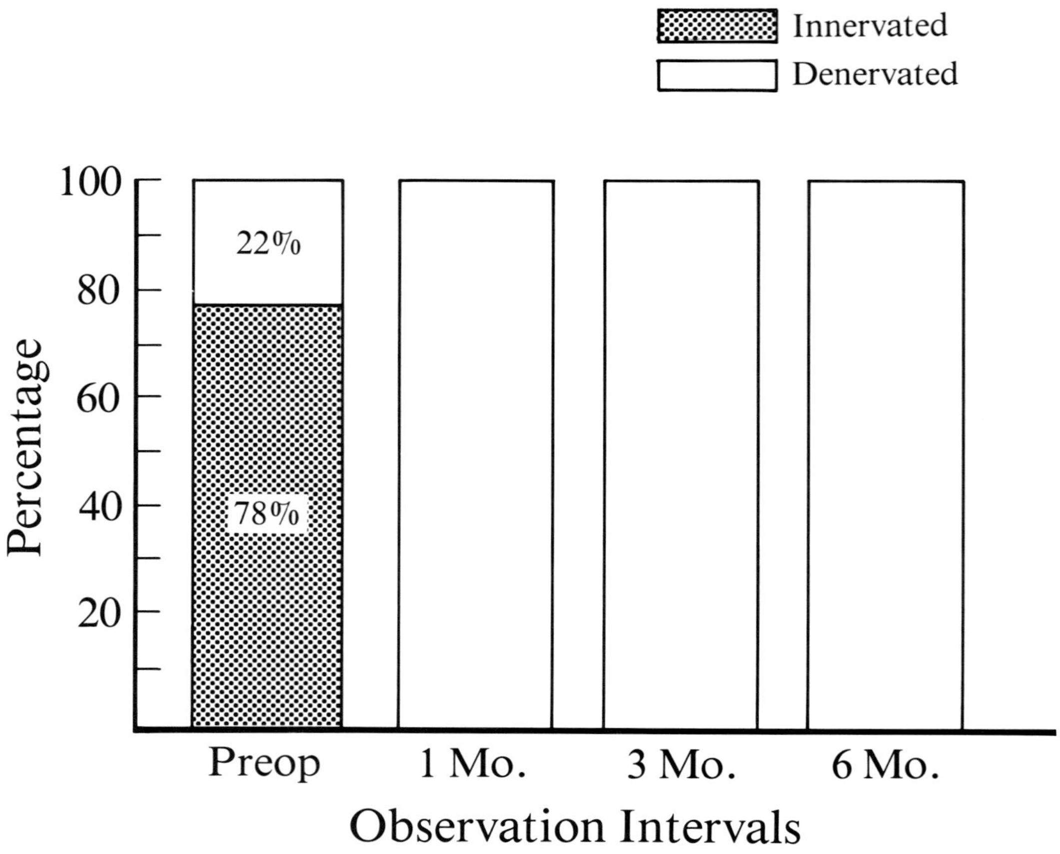

Figure 12–9. Results of electrodiagnostic testing of the nerve-sacrificed group.

provement occurred thereafter, with 73 percent of the nerve-spared group normally innervated at 6 months and 92 percent at 12 months. Postoperatively, virtually all of the nerve-sacrificed group demonstrated evidence of denervation at subsequent measurement intervals. Twenty-two percent of the nerve-sacrificed group showed electrodiagnostic evidence of denervation preoperatively. In these patients, lymph-node biopsies believed to have injured the spinal accessory nerve had been performed prior to their referral to UTMDAH.

DISCUSSION

Preservation of the spinal accessory nerve has gained acceptance because a number of studies have reported that the nodal-disease recurrence rate is not jeopardized with various modified neck-dissection procedures employed in appropriately selected patients (Jesse et al., 1978; Lingeman et al., 1977; Roy and Beahrs, 1969; Brandenberg and Lee, 1981; Skolnik et al., 1967; 1976). Moreover, shoulder function is improved over that observed following radical neck dissection (Leipzig et al., 1983; Short et al., 1984). Short and coworkers (1984) found that patients who undergo nerve-sparing dissections have significantly less shoulder pain, weakness, and disability than those who undergo radical neck dissection.

Nevertheless, several recent clinical studies have reported substantial degrees of shoulder disability and dysfunction in various modified procedures despite anatomic preservation of the spinal accessory nerve (Gordon et al., 1977; Carenfelt and Eliasson, 1980; Schuller et al., 1983; Leipzig et al., 1983). In a retrospective study on subjective questionnaires sent to patients who underwent treatment programs involving either radical or modified nerve-sparing dissections, Schuller and coworkers (1983) reported no advantage of modified neck dissection over radical neck dissection in patients returning to their preemployment status. Shortly thereafter, Leipzig and associates (1983) reported that 25 percent of patients in their study who underwent nerve-sparing dissections with preservation of the spinal accessory nerve, sternocleidomastoid muscle, and internal jugulare vein developed a permanent shoulder drop. Furthermore, they found that the incidence of shoulder drop increased to 50 percent in more extensive modified dissections, which differed from radical neck dissection only in that the spinal accessory nerve was preserved. They attributed this shoulder dysfunction to inadvertent transection of the spinal accessory nerve, or strong traction placed on the nerve during dissection of nodes underneath the sternocleidomastoid muscle.

By comparison, the results of our study indicate that careful preservation of the spinal accessory nerve in various modified neck-dissection procedures is usually followed by a temporary and reversible phase of trapezius muscle dysfunction. This phase is characterized by a mild but statistically significant reduction in both upper and middle trapezius muscle strength, as well as electrodiagnostic evidence of muscular denervation. Significant recovery of trapezius function in patients undergoing modified nerve-sparing procedures was found to occur within 6 months postoperatively. Further improvement in average upper and middle trapezius muscle function, however, was minimal after 6 months. This reversible phase of trapezius dysfunction was most likely related to mild traction placed on the nerve during dissection, or retraction of adjacent tissues in the course of the neck operation.

In contrast, we found that the shoulders of patients undergoing radical neck dissection uniformly demonstrated profound and unrecoverable loss of upper and middle trapezius muscle function that did not improve during the period of the study. Furthermore, none of the shoulders in this group demonstrated normal trapezius muscle strength or innervation at any point postoperatively.

In our study, range-of-motion testing indicated that the course of postoperative shoulder joint mobility was not significantly different between the nerve-spared and nerve-sacrificed neck-dissection groups. Both groups showed a similar reduction of shoulder-joint mobility 1 month postoperatively. This was most likely due to residual postoperative pain related to the neck dissection. Subsequently, however, recovery of joint mobility was achieved and maintained to much the same degree in both groups. It is important to recognize that despite the loss of trapezius innervation in the nerve-sacrificed group, patients lying supine could abduct their arms well beyond 90°. This is explained by the compensatory role of the seratus anterior in scapular rotation, which allows full abduction of the arm in a direction unopposed by the force of gravity (Hollinshead, 1968; Warwick, 1971).

In summary, the results of our study indicate that modified neck dissections involving preservation of the spinal accessory nerve are usually followed by a temporary and reversible phase of shoulder dysfunction. By comparison, radical neck dissection is followed by profound and permanent trapezius muscle weakness and denervation. The program of physical therapy was of probable benefit to both groups in maintaining and restoring range of motion at the shoulder joint; its value should not be underestimated even when the spinal accessory nerve is preserved.

REFERENCES

Anderson, R., and Flowers, R. S.: Free grafts of the spinal accessory nerve during radical neck dissection. *Am. J. Surg.*, 118:796–99, 1969.

Arief, A. J.: Newer concepts of electrodiagnosis in peripheral nerve injuries. *Arch. Phys. Med. Rehabil.*, 29:571–78, 1948.

Ballantyne, A. J., and Guinn, G. A.: Reduction of shoulder disability after neck dissection. *Am. J. Surg.*, 112:662–65, 1962.

Becker, G. D., and Parell, G. J.: Technique of preserving the spinal accessory nerve during radical neck dissection. *Laryngoscope*, 89:827–31, 1979.

Bocca, E.: Conservative neck dissection. *Laryngoscope*, 85:1511–15, 1975.

Bocca, E., and Pignataro, O.: A conservative technique in radical neck dissection. *Ann. Otol.,* 76:975–87, 1967.

Bradenburg, J. H., and Lee, C. Y. S.: The eleventh nerve in radical neck surgery. *Laryngoscope,* 91:1851–59, 1981.

Carenfelt, C., and Eliasson, K.: Occurrence, duration, and prognosis of unexpected accessory nerve paresis in radical neck dissection. *Acta Otolaryngol.,* 90:470–73, 1980.

Corbin, K. B., and Harrison, F.: The sensory innervation of the spinal accessory nerve and tongue musculature in the rhesus monkey. *Brain,* 62:191–97, 1939.

Daniels, L., and Worthingham, C., eds.: Muscle testings: In *Techniques of Manual Examination,* 3rd ed., pp. 78–82. W.B. Saunders, Philadelphia, 1972.

Ewing, M. R., and Maritn, H.: Disability following radical neck dissection. *Cancer,* 5:873–83, 1952.

Gordon, S. L., Graham, W. P., Black, J. T., and Miller, W. H.: Accessory nerve function after surgical procedures in the posterior triangle. *Arch. Surg.,* 112:264–68, 1977.

Harris, H. H., and Dickey, J. R.: Nerve grafting to restore function of the trapezius muscle after radical neck dissection. *Ann. Otol. Rhinol. Laryngol.,* 74:880–86, 1965.

Hill, J. H., and Olson, N. R.: The surgical anatomy of the spinal accessory nerve and the internal branch of the superior laryngeal nerve. *Laryngoscope,* 89:1935–42, 1979.

Hollinshead, W. H.: Pectoral region, axilla, and shoulder. In *Anatomy for Surgeons: Back and Limbs,* 3rd ed., pp. 263–348. Harper and Row, Hagerstown, Maryland, 1968.

Inman, B. T., Saunders, M., and Abbott, L. C.: Observations on the function of the shoulder joint. *J. Bone Joint Surg.,* 26:1–18, 1944.

Jesse, R. H., Ballantyne, A. J., and Larson, D.: Radical or modified neck dissection: A therapeutic dilemma. *Am. J. Surg.,* 136:516–19, 1978.

Leipzig, G., Suen, J. Y., English, J. L., Barnes, J., and Hooper, M.: Functional evaluation of the spinal accessory nerve after neck dissection. *Am. J. Surg.,* 146:526–30, 1983.

Lingeman, R. E., Stephens, R., Helmus, C., and Ulm, J.: Neck dissection: Radical or conservative. *Ann. Otol.,* 86:737–44, 1977.

Mead, S.: Posterior triangle operations and trapezius paralysis. *Arch. Surg.,* 64:752–55, 1952.

Nahum, A. M., Mullally, W., and Marmor, L.: A syndrome resulting from radical neck dissection. *Arch. Otol.,* 74:424–28, 1961.

Remmler, D., Byers, R., Scheetz, J., Shell, B., Zimmerman, S., Goepfert, H.: Head and neck surgery. *Surgery* 8:280–86, 1986.

Roy, P. H., and Beahrs, O.: Spinal accessory nerve in radical neck dissections. *Am. J. Surg.,* 118:800–4, 1969.

Saunders, W. H., and Johnson, E. W.: Rehabilitation of the shoulder after radical neck dissection. *Ann. Otol.,* 84:812–16, 1975.

Schuller, D. E., Reiches, N. A., Hamaker, R. C., Lingeman, R. E., Weisberger, E. C., Suen, J. Y., Conley, J. J., Kelly, D. R., and Miglets, A. W.: Analysis of total disability resulting from treatment programs including radical neck dissection and modified neck dissection. *Head Neck Surg.,* 6:551–58, 1983.

Scott, P. M.: Electrical reactions. In Scott, P. M. (ed.): *Clayton's Electrotherapy and Actinotherapy,* 7th ed., pp. 173–78. Williams and Wilkins, Baltimore, 1975.

Short, S. O., Kaplan, J. N., Laramore, G. E., and Cummings, C. W.: Shoulder pain and function after neck dissection with or without preservation of the spinal accessory nerve. *Am. J. Surg.,* 148:478–82, 1984.

Skolnik, E. M., Tenta, L. T., Wineinger, D. M., and Tardy, M. E.: Preservation of XI cranial nerve in neck dissections. *Laryngoscope,* 77:1304–14, 1967.

Skolnik, E. M., Yee, K., Friedman, M., and Golden, T. A.: The posterior triangle in radical neck surgery. *Arch. Otolaryngol.,* 102:1–4, 1976.

Warwick, R., and Williams, P. (eds.): *Gray's Anatomy,* 35th ed., pp. 532–38, 1024–25. W.B. Saunders, Philadelphia, 1973.

CHAPTER 13

Synchronous Bilateral Neck Dissection

Alando J. Ballantyne

EDITORS' COMMENT

In still another variation of neck dissection, Dr. Ballantyne, Senior Head and Neck Surgeon at the University of Texas M.D. Anderson Hospital and Tumor Institute at Houston gives us a unique chapter. After identifying the indications for synchronous bilateral neck dissection (tumors of midline structures), the author presents the results of the dissection of 700 patients who have undergone the procedure in a 10-year period. In answer to complaints that the results are tainted by exclusion of some patients, Dr. Ballantyne includes *every* patient who had a synchronous bilateral neck dissection in the 10-year period.

To make the data easier to interpret, the results are organized by primary site—cervical esophagus, glottis, oral tongue, base of tongue, pyriform sinus, pharyngeal wall, floor of mouth, oral cavity (not tongue), and unknown primary. There are subsets of patients within the larynx group separated by recurrence site (glottis, supraglottis, pyriform sinus) and by the role radiation therapy played in each of these groups. All of the categories noted have their individual figures stratified by the staging of the primary and neck disease, treatment of the primary and neck disease, adjunctive treatment, the fate of patients with histologically positive nodes bilaterally, recurrence rate, survival at 5 years, occurrence of a second primary, and a summary of the disease process with appropriate comments.

In this tour de force, Dr. Ballantyne has included a voluminous amount of material from which only general observations can be made with certainty (e.g., synchronous neck dissection can be a safe procedure, second primaries in the head and neck are frequent, recurrent pyriform sinus cancer is uniformly deadly). Other suggested conclusions are not so obvious (e.g., Is adjunctive radiotherapy of real benefit to the long-term survival of these patients?).

One of the obvious weaknesses of this series is that in an attempt to be all-inclusive, few solid conclusions can be reached because of stratification and substratification of exceptions to the rule. One fact demonstrated very clearly is the difficulty in objectively assessing any series conducted over a period of years by a variety of surgeons, even within the same institution. A corollary of this is the obvious problems that arise when comparing multiple multiinstitutional patients and making any meaningful conclusions from studies such as this.

INTRODUCTION

Since metastasis to the cervical lymph nodes is the single most important factor in determining the outcome of the treatment of head and neck cancer, any approach to treatment must take cognizance of the presence of cervical lymph nodes clinically positive for disease, and the possibility that subclinical metastases might exist. In cancers such as those of the nasopharynx, which are treated primarily by radiation therapy, surgery plays a minor role in the therapy of the cervical lymph nodes because neck dissections are infrequent. When surgery is the primary treatment modality, a neck dissection is mandatory if the nodes are clinically positive for disease. Neck dissection may be considered an elective part of the procedure if the expected incidence of cervical nodal metastases is greater than 20 percent.

The other approaches to treatment of the neck nodes clinically negative for disease are observation or irradiation. There are several drawbacks to the watchful waiting route: (1) the patient may not return for observation; (2) frequent follow-up visits for a patient coming from a long distance are an economic burden; and (3) neck nodes that contain clinically occult metastases at the time of the initial treatment may become large and difficult to treat in the patient whose neck is difficult to examine or who is uncooperative. Elective radiation entails a period of morbidity longer than that required for an elective neck dissection and has undesirable sequelae, such as dry mouth and other changes associated with the late sequelae of radiation therapy. In addition, the radiation must be given to fields in which second primary cancers are prone to develop.

In cancers that occur in midline structures, such as the floor of the mouth, the larynx, the pharynx, and the pharyngeal wall, metastases can occur in either side of the neck, and an elective neck dissection, to be a rational procedure, must be done bilaterally (Ballantyne, 1982). Also, if nodes clinically positive for disease are present in one side of the neck in midline cancers, the chance of occult metastasis to the opposite side of the neck is high. Bilateral neck dissections were performed in the early 1900s, as indicated by Crile (1906), but most of them were of the asynchronous variety. When the radical neck dissection proposed by Martin (1951) came to be the standard surgical treatment for overt or possible cervical metastases, Martin himself questioned the advisability of performing bilateral radical neck dissection as an elective procedure, so it was almost never done.

Synchronous bilateral radical neck dissections increased the morbidity and mortality because of the sacrifice of both internal jugular veins, which caused an increase in cerebral edema with possible serious consequences, and also edema of the face and neck structures that slowed wound healing. With the advent of the functional neck dissection, the synchronous bilateral neck dissection became a relatively frequent procedure, since it could be performed without an increase in morbidity or mortality and could be used both as an elective procedure and when nodes were clinically positive for disease (Ballantyne et al., 1982).

Although subject to question, bilateral neck dissection seems to be the logical procedure when cancers of the midline structures, such as the larynx, pharynx, or cervical esophagus, are being removed. More debatable is the role of elective neck dissection in the treatment of oral cavity cancer with nodes clinically negative for disease. This chapter reviews the experience at UTMDAH with synchronous bilateral neck dissections performed during the 10-year period between 1971 and 1980.

In any analysis of a large series of cases, a decision must be made about how much to include and how much to delete. In most series, the number of deletions leaves one wondering about the clinical presentation of patients and treatment results. Most survival figures are given as either determinate figures or figures derived by the use of some statistical method, such as Berkson-Gage. In the following presentation, there are no deletions, and all survival figures are expressed as absolute figures with no exclusions. Inclusion of all this detail makes for both cumbersome reading and a repetitive style, but the material is there for anyone who wishes to review it. Tables are included to summarize the voluminous data, and the discussion and conclusions summarize the pertinent points.

MATERIALS AND METHODS

The charts of 703 patients undergoing some type of synchronous bilateral neck dissection were reviewed to determine the efficacy of treating metastatic cervical nodes and to determine the toll of such a procedure in terms of morbidity and mortality. I hoped that some light might be shed on the value of adjunctive treatment such as postoperative irradiation in contributing to the success of the operative procedure, even though I realized that patients were not randomized. In addition, the numerous variables that are always difficult to quantitate in a retrospective study would probably make definitive statements of questionable validity.

I readily recognized at the beginning of the study that difficulties would be encountered in classifying the types of neck dissection, since it was frequently unclear, both in the operative report and in the pathologic report, exactly what had been accomplished. Neck dissections were done by a number of different surgeons and were not standardized. Pathologists were not always helpful in determining the exact location and number of lymph nodes removed. In general, the operations in which nodes were removed from both sides of the neck synchronously could be divided into four general categories:

1. Wide-field laryngectomies. In this operation, the lymph nodes along the anterior and lateral portions of the internal jugular vein as well as the nodes in the paratracheal area were removed. There was considerable variation in the extent to which the internal jugular vein was cleared of surrounding lymph-node-bearing tissue.

2. Bilateral upper neck dissections (supraomohyoid dissections). In this procedure, the nodes along the internal jugular vein to the level of the omohyoid were removed, as were the nodes in the submandibular and submental triangles. In most instances, the lymph nodes in the upper posterior triangle around the spinal accessory nerve were also removed.

3. Functional or modified neck dissections. Although this was a nonstandardized procedure and depended on the individual surgeon, a functional neck dissection done at UTMDAH generally consisted of removal of the nodes lateral, anterior, and medial to the internal jugular vein from the angle of the mandible to the clavicle. The nodes above the upper third of the spinal accessory nerve in the upper posterior triangle of the neck and the nodes above the cervical and brachial plexuses were included in the dissection. In cases in which the procedure was being performed for cancer of the larynx, pharyngeal wall, or base of the tongue, the nodes in the submandibular and submental triangles were frequently not removed unless the clinical conditions dictated it.

4. Radical neck dissections. All operations were considered radical neck dissections when the sternocleidomastoid muscle and internal jugular veins were removed, whether or not the spinal accessory nerve was preserved.

To avoid too many subclassifications, all the neck dissections were placed in one of three categories: (1) bilateral neck dissection, which included cases involving either a bilateral modified neck dissection, a bilateral radical neck dissection, or a modified neck dissection on one side and a radical neck dissection on the other (Table 13–1); (2) wide-field laryngectomy; or (3) bilateral upper-neck dissection.

These patients were not all "pure patients"; that is, some had been treated previously. In fact, all patients in the category of recurrent cancer of the laryngeal area had been treated by radiotherapy either at UTMDAH or elsewhere, and then had recurrences. In all the other categories, there were patients who had had some form of treatment prior to definitive treatment at UTMDAH. They were included in the analysis, though if they had been excluded the results would appear better. It was hoped that including all of the patients who had some form of bilateral neck dissection might eliminate bias in reporting and actually reflect better the fate of patients referred to

Table 13–1. Patients Having Synchronous Bilateral Neck Dissection

SITE OF PRIMARY TUMOR	*Number*	TREATMENT OF NECK *BMND**	*RMND**	NUMBER OF PATIENTS WITH NODES HISTOLOGICALLY POSITIVE FOR DISEASE *Unilaterally (%)*	*Bilaterally (%)*
Supraglottic larynx	92	43	49†	43 (47)	33 (36)
Pyriform sinus	69	24	45‡	40 (58)	22 (32)
Pharyngeal wall	38	23	15	18 (47)	15 (40)
Floor of mouth	48	32	16	10 (21)	16 (33)
Glottis	25	18	7	7 (28)	2 (8)
Base of tongue	19	13	6	11 (58)	6 (32)
Oral tongue	18	10	8	7 (39)	5 (28)
Cervical esophagus and postcricoid	21	19	2	2 (57)	3 (14)
Other parts of oral cavity	13	8	5	4 (31)	5 (38)
Unknown primary	1		1	0 (0)	1 (100)
Total	344			152 (44)	108 (30)

*BMND = bilateral modified neck dissection; RMND = radical neck dissection.
†Two patients had a bilateral radical neck dissection.
‡One patient had a bilateral radical neck dissection.

UTMDAH for treatment. Five-year survivals are absolute survivals, and the fate of other patients who did not reach the 5-year mark are reported in the analysis of each subgroup of patients.

There was a considerable disparity between clinical and pathologic staging of nodes, as seen in Table 13–2. Most of the false-positive clinical staging occurred in cancer of the floor of the mouth in which a submaxillary gland enlarged due to obstruction of the duct or direct extension of the cancer could be mistaken for a metastatic node.

Overall treatment results for this group of patients are given in Table 13–3. Although the mortality rate is higher than that previously reported by Ballantyne, it is lower than that reported by Sako (1985)—10 percent for synchronous bilateral neck dissections. Miscellaneous findings are reported in Table 13–4, which shows the frequency of the use of pre- and postoperative irradiation.

BILATERAL NECK DISSECTION

Cancer of Cervical Esophagus and Postcricoid Region

Two patients in this series of 21 cases had cancer that occurred in previously irradiated fields. In one, the irradiation was given postoperatively for breast cancer; in the second, the irradiation was given for treatment of a cancer of the tongue. Two patients had had previous radiation therapy to cure cancer of the cervical esophagus, and one patient had received 600 cGy in three fractions elsewhere prior to referral. One other patient had had an emergency tracheostomy. The postcricoid region was believed to be the site of origin of the cancer in two patients; it was the cervical esophagus in the remainder.

Staging. The primary tumor in one patient was classified T_2; in four patients, T_3; and in 14 patients, T_4. Two primary tumors were not classified because they were recurrent.

The nodes of 15 patients were classified N0; nine were positive for disease. One patient had nodes histologically positive for disease classified N1, one had nodes positive for disease classified N2a, and one had nodes positive for disease classified N2b. Three patients had nodes bilaterally positive for disease classified N3b. In addition to the spread to regional nodes, five specimens showed direct invasion of the thyroid gland, and one patient who had a large postcricoid carcinoma involving the pharyngeal wall was found to have a retropharyngeal node positive for disease. Evaluating paratracheal nodes as histologically positive for disease is probably inaccurate, since in the large cancers extending outside the esophageal wall, the paratracheal

Table 13–2. Differences in Clinical and Pathologic Staging In Patients Having Bilateral Neck Dissection

SITE	N0*	UNI†	BI‡	N1*	UNI†	BI‡	N2a*	UNI†	BI‡	N2b*	UNI†	BI‡	N3a*	UNI†	BI‡	N3b*	UNI†	BI‡
Supraglottic	30	13	6	25	17	3	7	5	2	12	7	5	0	0	0	18	1	17
Pyriform sinus	13	5	1	15	9	6	14	11	3	14	12	2	5	3	2	8	0	8
Pharyngeal wall	12	3	4	6	3	5	3	2	2	2	0	3	3	0	7	7	1	6
Floor of mouth	19	4	1	10	5	1	4	0	2	3	0	2	1	0	1	11	1	9
Glottis	19	4	0	2	1	0	1	1	0	1	1	0	1	0	1	1	0	1
Base of tongue	4	2	0	4	4	0	2	1	1	3	3	0	0	0	0	6	1	5
Oral tongue	7	1	2	5	3	0	0	0	0	2	1	1	2	2	0	2	0	2
Cervical esophagus and postcricoid	15	9	0	1	1	0	1	1	0	1	1	0	0	0	0	3	0	3
Other parts of oral cavity	4	0	1	2	2	0	1	0	0	2	1	1	2	0	2	2	1	1
Unknown primary	0	0	0	0	0	0	0	0	0	0	0	0	0	0	0	1	0	1
Total	123	41	15	73	48	13	35	22	10	40	28	11	14	8	6	59	5	53

*Classifications determined clinically.
†Unilateral positive nodes determined pathologically.
‡Bilateral positive nodes determined pathologically.

Table 13-3. Summary of Treatment Results in Patients Having Bilateral Neck Dissection

PRIMARY SITE	NO. OF PATIENTS	NO. OF BIL. POS. NODES	5-YR SURVIVAL WITH BIL. POS. NODES	POST-OP DEATHS	DEATHS FROM LOC.-REG. RECURRENCE	ABSOLUTE 5-YR SURVIVAL (%)
Cervical esophagus	21	3	1	6	2	4 (19)
Glottic	25	2	0	1	2	13 (52)
Oral tongue	18	5	2	0	5*	9 (50)
Base of tongue	19	6	3	1	3	10 (53)
Pyriform sinus	69	22	5	4	6	25 (36)
Pharyngeal wall	38	15	3	2	15	12 (32)
Floor of mouth	48	16	4	2	3	29 (60)
Supraglottic larynx	92	33	11	5	10	42 (46)
Other parts of oral cavity	13	5	1	0	3	4 (31)
Unknown primary	1	1	1	0	0	1 (100)
Total	344	108	31†	21	49	149 (44)

*3 occurred in patients previously treated.
†17 did not receive any radiation therapy; 14 did.
bil. pos. nodes = bilateral positive nodes determined by pathologic examination; loc.-reg. recurrence = local-regional recurrence.

nodes were probably engulfed by the primary neoplasm.

Treatment. All except one of the primary cancers were treated by laryngopharyngo-esophagectomy. One patient whose disease was classified T2N0 had a bilateral modified neck dissection and resection of the cancer of the posterior wall of the cervical esophagus, with repair by skin graft. One node positive for disease was found in the operative specimen. The patient received 5000 cGy postoperatively, and at 10 months was found to have a small-cell carcinoma of the lung, of which he died. Defects in the other patients were repaired with colon transfer in five instances, stomach pull-up in one case, and regional flap in 14.

Adjunctive Therapy. Radiation therapy was given postoperatively to two patients in the immediate postoperative period. Two other patients who developed metastatic tumor in the neck received postoperative therapy after a radical neck dissection with local control. One of the latter died at 3 years of distant metastasis, and the other at 6 years of other causes. Two patients received chemoimmunotherapy; one of them, who had cervical and paratracheal nodes positive for disease bilaterally, died of cancer of the prostate after 7 years.

Table 13-4. Patients with Bilateral Neck Dissection: Miscellaneous Results

SITE	NO. OF PATIENTS	OCCURRENCE IN PREVIOUSLY RADIATED FIELDS	NO. RECEIVING RADIATION	
			Pre-op	*Post-op*
Supraglottic	92	2	9	40
Pyriform sinus	69	1	1	47
Pharyngeal wall	38	1	2	15
Floor of mouth	48	0	1	7
Glottis	25	0	1*	4
Base of tongue	19	1	2	4
Oral tongue	18	0	1	3
Cervical esophagus and postcricoid	21	2	0	2
Other parts of oral cavity	13	0	1	3
Unknown primary	1	0	0	0
Total	344	7	18	125

*Pre-op therapy begun elsewhere.

Recurrences. Two neck recurrences were controlled by neck dissection and postoperative irradiation. Two local recurrences were not controlled, one occurring in a patient who developed the cancer in the radiation fields used to treat a cancer of the tongue. This patient also developed multiple myeloma.

Complications. Surgical complications were numerous and varied and included a chylothorax in a patient who had had previous radiation therapy to the supraclavicular area and mediastinum for a breast cancer. This proved to be lethal. Most of the complications were related to problems incidental to repair by flaps, and might have been avoided by immediate repair by gastric pull-up or free jejunal graft. There were six postoperative deaths.

Survival of Patients with Nodes Bilaterally Positive for Disease. One patient with nodes histologically positive bilaterally for disease in the neck and paratracheal area survived for 7 years. A second patient, found to have tumor in the thyroid and connective tissue as well as in 20 lymph nodes, died of other causes after 3 months and before he developed local recurrence or distant metastases. The third patient, who had received 600 cGy of radiation prior to referral, was found to have 12 nodes in the neck and seven paratracheal nodes positive for disease, as well as cancer in the paraesophageal connective tissue. He received chemotherapy postoperatively and died after 13 months from distant metastasis.

Other Primary Cancers. In one patient, a second primary cancer was located in the midesophagus; in two, it was located in the thyroid. A secondary primary cancer occurred in the tongue in one patient, and in the prostate in another. One patient had multiple myeloma in addition to cancer of the cervical esophagus. A second primary tumor was located in the lung in one patient. One patient was found to have a parathyroid adenoma as well as cancer of the cervical esophagus.

Survival. Only four of the 21 patients (19%) survived for 5 or more years. One survivor had lateral cervical and paratracheal nodes bilaterally positive for disease. One of the long-term survivors had received 5000 cGy as a curative dose for cancer of the cervical esophagus; had had a bilateral modified neck dissection in which one node was found to be positive; had had a laryngectomy and cervical esophagectomy with repair by colon interposition; and survives at 7 years.

Comment. Although the problems associated with cancer of the cervical esophagus and postcricoid regions are primarily local and concern the conflict between removing adequate amounts of trachea, esophagus, and paraesophageal tissues and leaving enough tissue to repair the defect, it is apparent that a significant number of patients do have cervical lymph-node metastases. Removal of neck nodes should be done at the time of removal of the primary cancer. If the neck nodes are not clinically positive for disease, a bilateral modified neck dissection is a reasonable procedure. If the nodes are of such size that a modified neck dissection is not feasible, a radical neck dissection may be done on the side of greatest involvement and a modified neck dissection on the other. Whether postoperative irradiation therapy is of value cannot be determined from this small series.

Glottic Cancer

Only three patients in the group of 25 who had glottic cancer had had any prior treatment. One had a previous emergency tracheostomy; a second a tracheostomy, thyrotomy, and removal of prelaryngeal nodes; and a third had received 1200 cGy of radiation, had become obstructed, and then had an emergency tracheostomy. The third patient had T4N1 disease, and had a radical neck dissection on one side and a modified neck dissection on the other; one node histologically positive for disease was recovered from the side of the radical neck dissection. Postoperatively, he developed a salivary fistula and carotid perforation, of which he died.

Staging. Eleven of the primary tumors were classified T_3; 14 were classified T_4. Nineteen patients had nodes classified N0 (four histologically positive for disease. Two patients had nodes classified N1 (one histologically positive for disease). One patient had nodes classified N2a (histologically positive for disease); one patient had nodes classified N2b (histologically positive for disease). One patient had nodes classified N3a (histologically positive for disease bilaterally), and one patient had nodes classified N3b (histologically positive for disease bilaterally).

Treatment. All patients had total laryngectomies. Seven had radical neck dissection on one side and modified neck dissection on the other, and 18 had bilateral modified neck dissections.

Subglottic Extension. Seventeen patients were found to have subglottic extension in the operative specimen, but there were no stomal recurrences. Ten of the 17 survived for more than 5 years, four received postoperative irradiation, and of these two died of other causes within less than 5 years, one died of either local or distant metastases in 13 months, and one died within 5 months with metastases to heart and liver, 3 months after the completion of radiation therapy. This last patient had an 8-cm mass in one side of the neck that was treated by radical neck dissection on that side and by modified neck dissection on the other, with one node histologically positive for disease found in the side of the modified neck dissection.

Recurrences. There was only one fully documented local recurrence in the group, which occurred in a patient whose disease was classified T3N0 and treated with a modified neck dissection on one side and a less-radical procedure on the other. In the operative specimen, there was found to be supraglottic and subglottic extension and one lymph node positive for disease. Recurrence that developed in the opposite side of the neck was detected and treated unsuccessfully elsewhere.

A probable local recurrence occurred in a patient whose disease was classified T4N3b and treated by a radical neck dissection on one side and a modified neck dissection on the other; multiple nodes were histologically positive for disease. Radiation therapy was started at 2.5 months, but the patient died at 13 months of either distant metastasis or distant metastasis and local recurrence.

Other Primary Cancers. Two second primary cancers occurred in the lung and one in the cervical esophagus. One patient had synchronous pyriform sinus cancer, one had incidental thyroid cancer, and one had cancer of the ovary in addition to glottic cancer.

Survival of Patients with Nodes Bilaterally Positive for Disease. Theree were only two patients with nodes bilaterally positive for disease, and both died of distant metastases, at 5 and 13 months.

Five-Year Survival. Thirteen of 25 patients in this group survived for 5 or more years, eight died of other causes or distant metastases, one died of a second primary cancer of the lung, and two were classified as having died of local recurrence. There was one postoperative death.

Comment. It is quite likely that a bilateral modified neck dissection is adequate treatment for subclinical metastases, and that the presence of subglottic extension is not necessarily an ominous sign if the trachea is transected low enough (two or three rings below tumor) and if a paratracheal node dissection is done. It is also apparent that if metastases are large and multiple, postoperative irradiation may reduce the risk of local recurrences but will probably not significantly prolong survival.

Cancer of the Oral Tongue

Patients with cancer of the oral tongue had an unfavorable prognosis, since five of the 18 patients had recurrent cancer after previous treatment—three following irradiation therapy, one after surgery, and one after irradiation and surgery. It was in this group of previously treated patients that most of the recurrences and deaths from cancer occurred, since only one of the five (the patient who had recurrence following both surgery and irradiation) survived for mor than 5 years.

Staging. Seven primary tumors were classified T_2, eight were classified T_3, and three were classified T_4.

Seven patients had nodes classified N0 (three histologically positive for disease, two bilaterally) and five had nodes classified N1 (two histologically negative for disease). All the patients with nodes classified N2b (two), N3a (two), and N3b (two) had clinical impressions confirmed histologically.

Treatment. Surgical treatment for the primary tumors consisted of partial glossectomy in 13 patients, partial glossectomy combined with marginal resection of mandible in two, and segmental resection with glossectomy in two. A total glossectomy with resection of the mandible was done in one patient. Treatment of the neck consisted of bilateral modified neck dissection for 10 patients. Eight patients had a radical neck dissection on one side and a modified neck dissection on the other.

Adjunctive Therapy. Of the 14 patients who had not had irradiation therapy prior to treatment at UTMDAH, one had preoperative irradiation here, and three had postoperative irradiation. Postoperative irradiation therapy was planned for one patient referred for treatment for cancer of the tongue recurrent after surgery, but the proposed treatment was refused by the patient. Local recurrence and distant metastases promptly occurred, and the patient died after 3.5 months. The tumor of the patient who received preoperative irradiation was initially classified T2N1; that patient was found to have metastatic papillary and follicular cancer of the thyroid. He died at 4 years, probably of local recurrence and cancer of the thyroid. Only one of the patients who received postoperative irradiation survived for more than 5 years. One patient with 33 nodes positive for disease received postoperative irradiation, was found to have distant metastases at the completion of irradiation, and died at 4 months.

Recurrences. Among the 13 previously untreated patients, there was one proven local recurrence that was not controlled, one possible local recurrence in the patient who received preoperative irradiation, and no recurrences in the neck. Recurrences in the neck and at local sites developed in three of the five patients previously treated. Another patient died at 2 months of infection probably secondary to chemotherapy.

Survival of Patients with Nodes Bilaterally Positive for Disease. Five patients in the group were found to have nodes bilaterally histologically positive for disease (one patient in the group previously treated). Two of the five patients survived for more than 5 years; one received postoperative irradiation and one had no adjunctive treatment. The latter patient's tumor was classified T3N3b, and that patient was found to have eight nodes histologically positive for disease on one side and one on the other. No further treatment was given and the patient is alive at 12 years.

Other Primary Cancer. A second primary adenocarcinoma of the lung was resected in one patient who survived 12 years; 2 patients were found to have incidental cancers of the thyroid (which may have contributed to the death of one of the patients); and one patient had multiple separate intraoral cancers.

Five-Year Survival. Eight of 13 previously untreated patients survived for 5 or more years, with one dying of proven local recurrence, one of possible local recurrence or recurrence in the tongue and thyroid, and the remainder of other causes or of distant metastases. Only one of the five previously treated patients survived for more than 5 years.

Comment. Synchronous bilateral neck dissection seems to be a satisfactory method of treatment of lymph nodes both clinically negative and positive for disease in the neck. Postoperative irradiation might have benefitted the patient who had developed uncontrolled local recurrence; when given to the patients with multiple nodes histologically positive for disease, it reduced the risk of local recurrence but did not alter their ultimate fate, since the majority of patients receiving this treatment died of distant metastases.

Base-of-Tongue Cancer

Of the 19 patients with cancer of the base of the tongue, three had had previous irradiation, two for attempted cure of a known primary cancer and one with metastatic nodes whose primary site was unknown. In one patient, the cancer developed in fields employed for irradiation of a lymphoma of the thyroid, and one patient had had a node removed prior to referral.

Staging. Three of the primary tumors were classified T_1, four were classified T_2, five were classified T_3, and six were classified T_4; one was unclassified because of prior treatment.

Four patients had nodes classified N0 (two histologically positive for disease); four had nodes classified N1 (all positive for disease). Two had nodes classified N2a (both positive, one positive bilaterally), three had nodes classified N2b (all histologically positive), and six had nodes classified N3b (five of six positive bilaterally). One cancer recurrent after radiation was unclassified.

Treatment. Three patients had resection of the base of the tongue only. Three patients had resection of the base of the tongue and partial pharyngectomy, and one had resection of the base of the tongue and partial laryngectomy. Seven patients had a total laryngectomy along with resection of the base of the tongue, and two had a total glossectomy and laryngectomy. Three patients had biopsies only. The intent in two of those cases was to remove the nodes following irradiation therapy, which was intended to be curative for the base-of-the-tongue lesion. In the third, the biopsy preceded removal of bilateral cervical masses, with the aim of curing the base-of-the-tongue primary and any residual disease in the neck with postoperative irradition.

Thirteen patients had bilateral modified neck dissections, and six had radical neck dissections on one side and modified neck dissections on the other.

Adjunctive Therapy. Of the previously untreated patients, four received postoperative radiation therapy and two received preoperative radiation. The diseases of the patients who received preoperative irradiation were both classified as T1N3b, with the radiation given to cure the primary, and the bilateral modified neck dissection done to control any residual cancer in the neck. One of the two survived for 10 years; the other died at 15 months of distant metastasis.

Survival of Patients with Nodes Bilaterally Positive for Disease. Six patients had nodes histologically positive for disease bilaterally, and three of them survived more than 5 years (one received preoperative irradiation, one received postoperative irradiation, and one received no adjunctive treatment). Two patients who received postoperative irradiation died of local and distant metastasis, and one who received preoperative irradiation died of distant metastasis. One of the patients who died of local recurrence had both lymphatic permeation and retropharyngeal nodes positive for disease.

Recurrences. There were two recurrences in the neck, both occurring in patients who had had nodes positive for disease bilaterally and received postoperative irradiation. There was one possible but undocumented local recurrence occurring in a nonirradiated patient at 4 years. Of the neck disease recurrences, one occurred in a patient who had had a radical neck dissection and the other in a patient who had had a bilateral modified neck dissection.

Five-Year Survival. Of these 19 patients, 10 lived 5 or more years without evidence of cancer; three died of distant metastases; three died of their cancers, either at the primary site or in the neck; one died of a new primary cancer of the lung; and one of other causes. There was one postoperative death.

Comment. The relatively good survival rate of 10 of 19 patients at 5 years, and the relatively low recurrence rate despite the fact that all except two patients had nodes histiologically positive for disease, indicates that the treatment selected was relatively effective in controlling both the primary cancer and the metastatic disease in the neck.

Cancer of the Pyriform Sinus

All 69 patients in this series were previously untreated for their pyriform sinus cancer, except for two patients who had had node biopsies. The patients with recurrent cancer are included in the text under recurrent cancer of the laryngeal region.

Staging. Six primary tumors were classified T_2, 29 were classified T_3, and 34 were classified T_4.

The nodes of 13 patients were classified N0 (five positive and one bilaterally positive for disease), the nodes of 15 patients were classified N1 (all positive for disease, with six positive bilaterally), and the nodes of 14 patients were classified N2a (all histologically positive for disease, with three positive bilaterally). The nodes of 14 patients were classified N2b (all histologically positive for disease, with two positive bilaterally); the nodes of five, N3a (all positive for disease with two positive bilaterally); and the nodes of eight, N3b (all positive for disease bilaterally). Sixty-two of the 69 patients had nodes histologically positive for disease, with 22 positive for disease bilaterally.

Treatment. All patients had a total laryngectomy as part of their treatment except for two. One, whose disease was classified T3N3a, had a radical neck dissection on one side and a modified neck dissection on the other, and a supraglottic laryngectomy with removal of pyriform sinus followed by postoperative irradiation. There was no apparent difficulty in swallowing, but the patient died at 28 months of distant metastasis. The second patient had disease classified T2N3B; preoperative irradiation was given with the aim of curing the primary tumor, which was followed by a bilateral modified neck dissection. The patient died at 6 years of other causes. Treatment of the neck consisted of bilateral modified neck dissection in 24 patients, a radical neck dissection on one side and a modified neck dissection on the other in 44, and a bilateral radical neck dissection in one.

Adjunctive Therapy. Forty-seven patients received postoperative irradiation therapy, 21 were not so treated immediately, and one patient received preoperative irradiation. Of the 21 patients who did not receive irradiation as part of the planned procedure, four died in the postoperative period. Irradiation therapy was not given to the others for a variety of reasons, such as the incidental finding of cancer of the prostate in the operative specimen from the neck, poor general condition, multiplicity of nodes, postoperative problems in wound healing, and the presence of known or suspected lung cancer. One patient did not receive postoperative irradiation because the cancer occurred in fields that had previously been irradiated for a cancer of the anterior tonsillar pillar.

Three patients received irradiation long after the original surgery, one for a new cancer of the base of the tongue, and another for recurrent cancer occurring in the submental area on the side of a radical neck dissection. The third received irradiation for local recurrence because immediate postoperative irradiation had been considered inadvisable because of previous irradiation therapy for a cancer of the tongue.

Recurrences. In addition to the last-mentioned patient in whom further irradiation was unsuccessful, there were six other patients who developed neck-disease recurrences. A stomal recurrence and neck-disease recurrence developed in spite of postoperative irradiation therapy in one patient who developed a pyriform sinus cancer with multiple nodes positive for disease while undergoing chemotherapy for metastatic melanoma. Of the five other neck disease recurrences, one developed in a patient who had previously had both sides of the neck included in the radiation treatment fields used for an anterior tonsillar pillar cancer and who could receive no more irradiation. Three recurrences in the neck developed within previously irradiated fields on the side of a modified neck dissection, and further treatment efforts were to no avail. There was one submental recurrence on the side of a radical neck dissection in a patient who did not receive postoperative irradiation. Although the recurrent cancer was apparently controlled by radiation therapy, the patient died within 15 months of distant metastases. All recurrences developed in necks in which nodes histologically positive for disease were found, except in the one patient who developed cancer within fields previously irradiated for another primary cancer.

Survival of Patients with Nodes Bilaterally Positive for Disease. Although only eight patients had disease clinically classified N3b, 22 were found to have nodes histologically positive for disease. Five of this group survived for more than 5 years: one received preoperative irradiation, two received postoperative irradiation, and two received no adjunctive treatment. One other patient with nodes histologically positive for disease bilaterally who received no postoperative irradiation survived for 3.5 years, then died of other causes. There were two postoperative deaths and one neck disease recurrence; the other patients died of either distant metastases, other causes, or, in one case, a second primary cancer of the esophagus.

Five-Year Survival. Twenty-five of the 69 (36%) survived for 5 or more years: 18 died within less than 5 years of distant metastases, 11 of other causes, 5 of other primaries, and 6 of local or regional recurrence. There were four postoperative deaths. Five patients were found to have more than 20 nodes positive for disease, and none survived more than 2 years; in fact, one died during the course of postoperative irradiation therapy.

Other Primary Cancers. Other cancers of the upper aerodigestive tract were fairly common, occurring prior to, at the time of, or subsequent to the treatment of the cancer of the pyriform sinus. The sites involved by other primaries were the pharyngeal wall (four), base of the tongue (one), oral tongue (one), floor of the mouth (two), and anterior tonsillar pillar (two). Two patients developed cancer of the lung. One patient died of cancer of the pancreas, one of cancer of the esophagus, and two of prostate cancer. Two were found to have incidental cancer of the thyroid.

Incidental Findings. Three patients had retropharyngeal nodes histologically positive for disease, and in another patient their presence was strongly suggested by the clinical course of the disease. In five cases, the thyroid gland was directly invaded by cancer. In one patient, a primary or metastatic cancer of the lung was treated by wedge resection at 1 year, and the patient died at 7 years of other causes.

Complications. There was one carotid perforation that required ligation but produced no neurological sequelae. Delayed wound healing or fistula formation occurred in seven patients.

Severe dysphagia occurred as a result of radiation therapy in five patients. In one of them, the strictured area had to be opened, with subsequent death probably resulting from aspiration. One patient died either of inability to take adequate food through the area of stricture, or local recurrence. Death occurred during the course of radiation therapy given postoperatively to a patient who was found to have 48 nodes positive for disease.

Comment. Synchronous bilateral neck dissection combined with adequate resection of the primary cancer seems to be a reasonable way to treat cancer of the pyriform sinus. Almost all the patients will have nodes histologically positive for disease, almost a third of those positive bilaterally.

The use of postoperative irradiation seems to reduce the risk of local recurrence, but many who receive such adjunctive therapy die of distant metastases even though the local cancer is controlled. The fact that there were as many 5-year survivors with histologically positive nodes bilaterally who did not receive postoperative irradiation as those who did suggests that not all patients with nodes histologically positive for disease need receive adjunctive treatment.

Cancer of the Pharyngeal Wall

There were 38 patients in this group, two of whom had extensive recurrent cancers after previous irradiation. One of the two had a carotid artery perforation, from which he died at 2 months. The other had ligation of the carotid during the postoperative period that caused hemiplegia, and he succumbed to recurrent cancer. Cancer developed within previously irradiated fields in one patient. Two patients had treatment prior to surgery—preoperative irradiation in one, and chemotherapy and preoperative irradiation in the other. Both died of local and regional recurrence.

Staging. Three patients had primary tumors classified T_2, 8 had primary tumors classified T_3, and 27 had tumors classified T_4.

A total of 12 patients had nodes classified N0; seven were histologically positive for disease, four of those bilaterally. Nine patients had nodes histologically positive for disease classified N1; three of those were positive bilaterally. Five patients had nodes positive for disease classified N2a; two of those were positive bilaterally. Two patients had nodes positive for disease classified N2b; three had nodes positive for disease classified N3a; and seven had nodes positive for disease classified N3b (six of those were bilaterally positive). The retropharyngeal nodes played a very significant role in the outcome of the cancer in these patients. In 14 they were found to be positive for disease on one or both sides; in three others, it was believed after reviewing their clinical courses that their nodes must have been positive for disease because all three patients developed the characteristic ipsilateral neck pain radiating over the ear to the supraorbital area.

Treatment. Surgery consisted of bilateral modified neck dissection in 23 patients, and radical neck dissection on one side and modified neck dissection on the other in 15. Laryngopharyngectomy was done in 27 patients, and in 11 patients, pharyngectomy was performed and the larynx was preserved.

Survival of Patients with Nodes Bilaterally Positive for Disease. Of the 15 patients with nodes histologically positive for disease bilaterally, only three survived more than 5 years. One received postoperative irradiation; the other two did not. One of those two had a total of 23 nodes positive for disease, including two retropharyngeal nodes on one side and three retropharyngeal nodes on the other.

Adjunctive Therapy. Two patients received irradiation preoperatively and 15 received irradiation therapy postoperatively. The patients receiving irradiation benefited very little from it, because the majority died of local and regional recurrence; only four patients survived for 5 years. In one of them, the postoperative irradiation was started 7 months postoperatively.

Recurrences. Fifteen patients developed local or regional recurrence. In only one of them was surgery apparently effective in achieving local tumor control, though the patient died of cancer of the esophagus within 6 months of the surgery for recurrences. One patient developed a recurrent node in the same side as a modified neck dissection while awaiting radiation therapy; the postoperative irradiation was not effective in subsequently controlling the cancer.

Cancers of the pharyngeal wall present challenging problems from the surgical standpoint because their location places them immediately adjacent to the carotid arteries. The internal carotid arteries in two patients in this series were surrounded by cancer and resected without neurologic sequelae. An additional problem is the occurrence of the cancer next to the prevertebral fascia. Ordinarily, the tumor is confined by the fascia of the posterior pharyngeal wall, but this fascia is incomplete in the nasopharynx, and extensive cancers that grow up to the nasopharynx may become attached to the prevertebral fascia in the nasopharyngeal area.

The retropharyngeal nodes also create a problem because if the cancers break outside the node capsules, they may extend along the internal carotid arteries or prevertebral fascia. This possibility could be assessed by preoperative computerized tomography (CT) scans.

Five-Year Survival. Twelve patients survived more than 5 years, six died of other causes in less than 5 years, one died of distant metastases, and two of other primary tumors. There were two postoperative deaths. Fifteen patients died of local or regional recurrence, or both, and one patient was lost to follow-up.

Comment. The local and regional recurrence rate of cancers of the pharyngeal wall exceeds the 5-year survival rate. It is conceivable that some patients with this type of cancer might have benefitted from postoperative irradiation as far as local control of cancer is concerned. It is unlikely that any combination of irradiation, chemotherapy, and surgery would have benefited many of the patients with advanced cancers. The only survivors were those who had complete removal of the primary cancer and adequate surgery for the lateral cervical and retropharyngeal lymph nodes.

Cancer of the Floor of the Mouth

Forty-eight patients were classified as having cancer of the floor of the mouth, and had a synchronous bilateral neck dissection as part of their treatment. Of the 48, two patients had recurrences after surgery, four had been treated previously by irradiation therapy, and one patient whose cancer was classified T3N3b was seen and treated, even though his initial chest x-ray showed probable pulmonary metastasis.

Staging. The primary tumors of two patients were classified T_X. The primary tumor of one patient was classified T_1. Thirteen patients had primary tumors classified T_2, 18 had primary tumors classified T_3, sand 14 had primary tumors classified T_4.

The nodes of 19 patients were classified N0; four of those were positive and one bilaterally positive for disease. Ten patients had nodes classified N1; 6 of those were histologically positive for disease. The nodes of four patients were classified N2a; two were negative and two were histologically positive bilaterally for disease. Of the three patients with nodes classified N2b, one was negative and two were histologically positive bilaterally for disease. One patient had nodes classified N3a that were histologically positive bilaterally for disease, and 11 had nodes classified N3b (one histologically negative, one positive on one side only, and nine positive bilaterally for disease). In one patient, a neck node clinically positive for disease was found to contain metastatic thyroid cancer, and the thyroid was removed at the time of the neck dissection.

Treatment. Treatment of the primary tumor consisted of the following procedures: wide excision only in 15 patients; wide excision with partial glossectomy in one patient; wide excision of the floor of the mouth plus marginal resection of the mandible in 14 patients; wide excision of the floor of the mouth and the tongue plus segmental resection of the mandible in five patients; resection of the floor of the mouth plus segmental resection of the mandible in 11 patients; resection of the mandible, total glossectomy, and partial maxillary resection in one patient; and resection of the floor of the mouth plus synchronous resection of the soft palate in one patient.

Sixteen patients were treated with radical neck dissection on one side and modified neck dissection on the other, and 32 patients were treated with bilateral modified neck dissection.

Adjunctive Treatment. Seven patients received postoperative irradiation. Of those patients, two survived for more than 5 years, one died 26 days after the completion of the postoperative irradiation, three died of distant metastases within 2 years, and one died of cancer of the lung at 3 years. One patient had had preoperative irradiation elsewhere and had a bilateral neck dissection and resection of the floor of the mouth, with no tumor found in the operative specimen. Death occurred at 52 months from other causes. Preoperative irradiation was given at UTMDAH to one patient whose disease was classified T3N1 and who had had a left radical and right modified neck dissection, with segmental resection of the mandible and no tumor found in the operative specimen. Local recurrence in the skin of the chin and tongue led to death at 22 months.

Survival of Patients with Positive Nodes Bilaterally for Disease. Of the 16 patients with nodes histologically positive for disease bilaterally, two died in the postoperative period. Five of the patients completed a course of postoperative irradiation, and one could not tolerate the treatment. No patient who received postoperative irradiation survived 5 years. Four of the eight patients who received no postoperative irradiation survived more than 5 years. One of these had 10 nodes positive for disease plus tumor in the connective tissue.

Recurrences. Two patients had local recurrences in the skin of the chin, one of which was controlled by further surgery. Two patients developed recurrences in the neck and primary tumor area; both recurrences were controlled by further surgery, with the addition of postoperative irradiation in one case. One patient who could not tolerate postoperative irradiation developed recurrence in the neck and tongue that was apparently controlled by further surgery, though the patient died at 7 months of distant metastasis following the surgery for neck recurrence. Retropharyngeal node metastases caused regional recurrence in a patient who had simultaneous cancers of the soft palate and floor of the mouth. Only three patients died of locally uncontrolled cancer.

Five-Year Survival. Twenty-nine of the 48 survived 5 or more years, 14 died in less than 5 years of distant metastases or other causes, and three died of uncontrolled local cancer. There were two postoperative deaths.

Other Primary Cancers. Twelve of the patients (25%) had second primary cancers. Four occurred in the lung and three in the pharyngeal wall. There were single cases of second primary tumors in the base of the tongue, oral tongue, gum, epiglottis, pyriform sinus, larynx, soft palate, and breast. More than one second primary tumor occurred in several patients.

Comment. The relatively low recurrence rate in the neck and primary tumor area indicates that surgery and bilateral neck dissection is an effective means of treating cancer of the floor of the mouth and cervical lymph nodes occultly or clinically positive for disease. Postoperative irradiation was infrequently used, so it is difficult to assess the impact the use of this modality might have in the treatment scheme.

Cancer of the Supraglottic Larynx

Ninety-two patients are included in this group, but a considerable number had had prior therapy of some sort in the region of the larynx, which influenced the selection of treatment. In two patients, the cancer occurred within fields that had previously been irradiated for another primary cancer. Three had had emergency tracheostomies; in one, a cervical mass had been removed and a thyroidectomy had been done, and in another the tracheostomy was followed by cryosurgery. Two had had open biopsies of cervical masses, and one of them had had a radon seed implant throughout the laryngeal area. The problem of treatment was complicated in one patient by the simultaneous presence of chronic leukemia; a recurrent cancer of the upper lip that had produced a metastatic mass that was directly attached to the mandible; and a laryngeal cancer classified T_3. One other patient had a simultaneous gum and laryngeal cancer.

Staging. Seven patients had primary tumors classified T_2. Fifty patients had tumors classified T_3. Thirty-five patients had tumors classified T_4.

Thirty patients had nodes classified N0; 18 of those were histologically positive for disease, six bilaterally. Twenty-five patients had nodes classified N1; 20 of those were positive for disease, three bilaterally. Seven patients had nodes positive for disease classified N2a; two were bilaterally positive. Twelve patients had nodes positive for disease classified N2b; five were positive bilaterally. Eighteen patients had nodes positive for disease classified N3b; 17 were positively bilaterally.

Treatment. Supraglottic laryngectomy was performed in six patients, and followed by postoperative radiation therapy in one of them. One patient required a laryngectomy at 2.5 months because of continued aspiration, and died at 2 years of other causes. Four of the five patients not receiving postoperative irradiation and the one patient who did survived more than 5 years. In three patients whose disease was classified T2N3b, preoperative irradiation was given to cure the primary cancer followed by surgery to remove the nodes, but in only one case was this successful. In an additional patient whose disease was classified T2N3b, the nodes were removed first, and radiation therapy given to cure the primary and any residual metastases in the neck. Biopsy of the larynx at 6 months showed only radiation necrosis, but the patient died 1 month later of gunshot wounds to the head and chest. In all other patients in the series, a total laryngectomy was done.

Forty-three patients had bilateral modified neck dissections; 47 had radical neck dissections on one side and modified neck dissections on the other; and in two patients, bilateral radical neck dissection was performed.

Adjunctive Therapy. Nine patients received preoperative irradiation and 40 received postoperative irradiation. In several patients, postoperative irradiation had been planned but could not be accomplished either because of problems in wound healing or patient refusal. One of the patients for whom postoperative irradiation had been planned had multiple problems during the postoperative period and x-ray therapy could not be given, but the patient survived more than 10 years despite having eight nodes histologically positive for disease in the neck dissection specimen.

Recurrences. There were nine documented cases of recurrence in the neck or primary tumor area. In two other patients, recurrence was highly probable but not proven. One of the neck recurrences occurred in a patient who had had a bilateral modified neck dissection, and the recurrence was treated satisfactorily by further surgery. In another instance, recurrence appeared within the neck on the side of the modified neck dissection while the patient was awaiting therapy, but it was not controlled by radiation therapy. Recurrence developed in the neck of one patient who had had a bilateral radical neck dissection; it was not controlled. In another patient for whom postoperative irradiation therapy had been planned, recurrence that was not controlled developed in the side of the radical neck dissection. The other recurrences developed in patients who had received either pre- or postoperative irradiation, and the recurrences developed in the side of the radical neck dissection. Ten of the 11 patients died of locally recurrent cancer.

Survival of Patients with Nodes Bilaterally Positive for Disease. Thirty-three patients had nodes histologically positive for disease bilaterally; four of them died during the postoperative period. Eleven survived more than 5 years, five had no postoperative irradiation, and five received irradiation postoperatively. In one patient, the irradiation was given preoperatively. There were seven neck disease recurrences in this group.

Five-Year Survival. Forty-two of the 92 patients survived 5 or more years. Sixteen died of distant metastases, 13 of other causes, 10 of local recurrence, and three of second primaries. Three died either during or immediately after irradiation therapy, and there were five postoperative deaths.

Complications of Surgery. Of the five postoperative deaths, one occurred in a patient whose cancer developed within previously irradiated fields. A radical neck dissection was done on one side and a modified neck dissection on the other; there was poor wound healing with carotid perforation requiring ligation, which resulted in neurologic sequelae and death. One patient who died had chronic leukemia and separate primary tumors of the upper lip and larynx. This patient had poor wound healing, with death resulting from multiple organ failure. The other three deaths were unexpected and largely unexplained. A total of seven patients had poor wound healing (including those previously mentioned); among them, one patient developed a chyle fistula. Six patients developed salivary fistulas. One additional patient required carotid ligation that did not result in neurologic sequelae, and in one case the carotid artery was removed without incident.

Complications of Radiation Therapy. Two patients died during the course of postoperative irradiation, and a third died of severe dysphagia shortly after completion of radiation therapy. Four other patients developed strictures. One patient developed radiation myelopathy with paraplegia, but is surviving with difficulty at 6 years.

Second Primary Cancer. Seven second primary cancers occurred in the lung—two in the pharyngeal wall, and one each in the gum, upper lip, esophagus, floor of the mouth, and the bladder. Two patients were found to have an incidental cancer of the thyroid that was of no significance during the course of the disease. Two patients underwent segmental resection of either a second primary lung cancer or metastasis, and one survives at 7 years.

Comment. This is a difficult group of patients to analyze because of the previous treatment given, and the multiplicity of variables in the surgical procedures, extent of disease, and employment of adjunctive therapy. As could be expected, the outcome of the disease was largely dependent on the extent of the nodal disease and extranodal spread, with postoperative irradiation being of benefit in reducing the risk of local recurrence. The same number of patients with nodes bilaterally positive for disease who did not receive postoperative irradiation survived as those who did.

Cancer of Other Parts of the Oral Cavity

Of the 13 patients in this group, nine had cancers of the lower gum, one of the upper gum, two of the palate, and one of the lower lip. In several, the cancers were so extensive that more than one site was involved—e.g., lower lip and gum, or gum and floor of the mouth. Only 1 patient had had prior treatment—surgery to the lower gum as part of the treatment for multiple intraoral primary tumors.

Staging. Three patients had primary tumors classified T_2, two had primary tumors classified T_3, and eight had primary tumors classified T_4.

Four patients had nodes classified N0, one of them histologically positive for disease bilaterally. Two patients had nodes histologically positive for disease classified N1. One patient had nodes histologically negative for disease classified N2a (mass was direct extension). Two patients had nodes histologically positive for disease (one of them bilaterally) classified N2b. Two patients had nodes bilaterally histologically positive for disease classified N3a. Two patients had nodes classified N3b; one was histologically positive for disease bilaterally. The other was said to be negative for disease, but the patient had received preoperative irradiation. In one patient with surgically treated upper gum cancer initially classified N0, the classification of the neck disease were changed to N3b at 3 months.

Treatment. Surgery was the primary tumor treatment in 12 patients. In the remaining case of a soft-palate cancer, preoperative irradiation was given for a lesion classified as T2N3b with the aim of curing the palate lesion by irradiation and perform surgery for the neck disease. A bilateral modified neck dissection was done after the irradiation therapy, and no nodes histologically positive for disease were found, but the patient developed recurrence in the retropharyngeal area and neck, of which she died. In the cases of cancer of the lower gum, a segmental resection of the mandible was done in six patients, and a marginal resection in three.

In one case, in which nodes bilaterally positive for disease developed after treatment of a cancer of the upper gum, a bilateral modified dissection was done, with tumor found at the base of the skull. Of the other patients, seven had a bilateral modified neck dissection, and five had a radical neck dissection on one side and a modified neck dissection on the other.

Adjunctive Therapy. Preoperative irradiation therapy was given to one patient with a palate lesion, and postoperative irradiation was given to three others. In one patient, the irradiation treatment was not started until 6 months after the surgery; in the patient with cancer of the upper gum, the irradiation was given only to the face region, with the nodes bilaterally positive for disease becoming apparent after completion of the radiation therapy.

Recurrences. Both patients with cancers of the palate developed recurrent cancer in the retropharyngeal nodes despite the use of irradiation therapy, preoperatively in one and postoperatively in the other. The patient who received preoperative irradiation also developed neck disease recurrences despite the absence of nodes histologically positive for disease at the time of the bilateral modified neck dissection. One other patient developed uncontrolled neck disease recurrence after treatment for an extensive cancer of the lower lip, with nodes histologically positive for disease bilaterally. He could conceivably have benefited from postoperative irradiation.

Survival of Patients with Nodes Bilaterally Positive for Disease. Only two of the five patients with nodes bilaterally histologically positive for disease survived more than 3 years. One, with cancer of the lower gum classified T4N2b, had a radical neck dissection on one side and a modified neck dissection on the other, with nodes histologically positive for disease in both sides of the neck. He did not receive postoperative irradiation, and died at 4 years of other causes. The other patient, who had cancer of the lower gum classified T4N0, was treated by bilateral modified neck dissection, with nodes histologically positive for disease found in both sides of the neck. Postoperative irradiation was started at 6 months, and the patient died at 6 years of cancer of the lung.

Five-Year Survival. Only four of the 13 patients survived 5 or more years. Three of the 10 who did not survive died of local or regional recurrence, and six died of other causes or distant metastases.

Comment. The only conclusion that can be drawn from this small series is that cancers of the palate can spread to the retropharyngeal nodes.

Metastatic Cancer from an Unknown Primary

Only 1 patient had synchronous bilateral neck dissection for metastatic cancer from an unknown primary tumor. He previously had had nodes removed from the right side of the neck that were positive for squamous cell carcinoma. No primary cancer was found. Since there were nodes clinically positive for disease in the left upper neck, right radical and left modified neck dissections were done, with no tumor found in the right side of the neck and three nodes histologically positive for disease found in the left side. No additional treatment was given. At 13.5 years there has been no evidence of recurrence, and a primary cancer has not been found.

Recurrent Cancer in the Laryngeal Region

One hundred and three patients who had received radiation therapy as a curative measure for cancer in the laryngeal region underwent a surgical attempt to cure the recurrent cancer. Patients were almost evenly divided between those who had had their initial treatment at UTMDAH and those who had had their initial radiation therapy elsewhere. Although most presented with nodes clinically negative for disease, some patients either gave a history of having masses in the neck prior to treatment, or were treated at UTMDAH, so the initial nodal status was known. Because several sites were involved and a variety of approaches were used to remove apparent or possible involved nodes, each site was analyzed separately.

Cancer of the Supraglottic Larynx Recurrent After Irradiation Therapy. There were 19 patients in this group, 11 of whom had had their irradiation therapy at UTMDAH and eight who had had it elsewhere. Results were not significantly different between the two groups, so they were analyzed together.

Treatment. A total laryngectomy was done in each case, and tumor was present in all except for one, in whom only radiation necrosis was present.

In 15 instances, a wide-field laryngectomy alone was done. Three patients had a bilateral modified neck dissection, and one patient had a radical neck dissection on one side and a modified neck dissection on the other. In only four patients were nodes histologically positive for disease; they were bilaterally positive in one of these patients, who had had an emergency tracheostomy prior to arrival at the hospital. Treatment was bilateral modified neck dissection, laryngectomy, and partial pharyngectomy. Four nodes positive for disease were found on one side and one positive for disease on the other. A neck dissection 6 months later showed metastatic tumor in one node and in connective tissue. The patient died at 2.5 years of distant metastasis.

Recurrence. Nine patients developed neck disease recurrence, which was controlled by further surgery in four cases; in three patients, surgery was employed, and the fourth received chemotherapy and radiation therapy. In the fourth, recurrence developed in the side of the neck that had been initially found to have 12 nodes histologically positive for disease. The patient is well at 6 years after treatment, with no further recurrences. Another patient had successful control of cancer recurring in the opposite side of the neck as well as in both retropharyngeal areas. One local recurrence in the pharyngeal mucosa was controlled by further surgery.

Complications. Most patients were left with controlled fistulas, and though there were some problems in closing some of them, exposure of the carotid artery was reduced. There was one carotid perforation requiring ligation, but no neurologic sequelae resulted.

Five-Year Survival. Nine patients survived more than 5 years. Three died of other causes or distant metastases, two of other primaries, and five of neck recurrence.

Recurrent Cancer of the Pyriform Sinus. Only one patient of the seven in this group was initially treated at UTMDAH. This patient presented with a cancer classified T2N1 and was treated for cure by radiation therapy. The treatment failed, and the patient had a wide-field laryngectomy, which showed no positive nodes. A retropharyngeal node developed disease that was proved to be cancer by aspiration biopsy. Death occurred secondary to hemorrhage from the retropharyngeal node.

Treatment. Four patients had radical neck dissections on one side and modified neck dissections on the other, two had bilateral modified neck dissections, and one had only a wide-field laryngectomy. Nodes histologically positive for disease were found in four patients; in one, the nodes were bilaterally positive. All patients with nodes histologically positive for disease died, three of local or regional recurrence and one of other causes.

Complications. All patients were left with controlled fistulas, and there was considerable difficulty in closing some of them. One carotid perforation occurred with no immediate sequelae, but the patient died after an additional attempt to cover the stump of the carotid artery.

Recurrences. There were four recurrences in the neck, none of which were controlled. There was one proven metastasis to a retropharyngeal node and one possible metastasis to the lung.

Five-Year Survival. No patient survived 5 years. Of the few who did not develop local or regional recurrence, one died postoperatively after an attempt to cover the carotid artery, and one died of other causes. This dismal story reflects the difficulty in dealing with patients whose treatment fails following radiation therapy for cancer of the pyriform sinus. The physician is limited by the constraints imposed on dealing with tissues following radiation therapy to the entire neck.

There is an obvious reluctance to do a retropharyngeal node dissection in these patients, even though it is recognized that cancers of the pyriform sinus that involve the pharyngeal wall have a significant incidence of metastasis to the retropharyngeal nodes.

Recurrent Cancer of the Glottis. Seventy-seven patients with recurrent cancer in the glottic region were seen for an attempt at surgical salvage treatment. Thirty-seven of these patients had their initial treatment at UTMDAH; 40 received their treatment elsewhere. There was very little difference between the two patient groups, so they were analyzed together. Of the total group, two patients died in the postoperative period, 54 did not develop any recurrence following the initial salvage surgery, and 21 developed further recurrence, for an initial failure rate of 30 percent (including the patients who died postoperatively).

Patients Not Having Further Recurrence. Thirty-eight of the 54 patients not developing further recurrence were treated with wide-field laryngectomy and 16 with bilateral modified neck dissection. Only one patient was found to have a node histologically positive for disease.

FIVE-YEAR SURVIVAL. Of the 54 patients not having further recurrence, 40 survived more than 5 years, 10 died of other causes, two died of distant metastasis, and two were lost to follow-up.

Patients with Further Recurrence. Nineteen of the 21 patients in this group had total laryngectomy initially. One patient who had a partial laryngectomy at first, then a total laryngectomy to treat the recurrence, is an 8-year survivor. The second patient originally had a partial laryngectomy, but then required a total laryngectomy for recurrence, and at that time was found to have nodes bilaterally positive for disease. He died of recurrence in his neck.

TREATMENT. Sixteen patients had a wide-field laryngectomy; six, a bilateral modified neck dissection; and one, a radical neck dissection on one side and a modified neck dissection on the other. Lymph nodes positive for disease were found at the time of initial surgery in five patients; two were bilaterally positive for disease, and there was direct invasion of the thyroid gland in three cases.

One of the patients with nodes bilaterally positive for disease may have had a second primary causing the metastases. He was initially seen with a cancer of the glottic region, and treated by radiation therapy. When recurrence was found, he had a bilateral modified neck dissection and total laryngectomy. The tumor was believed to involve the pyriform sinus; 15 of 16 nodes on one side and 10 of 12 nodes on the other were histologically positive for disease. Recurrence and distant metastases developed while the patient was still in the hospital.

Of the 10 patients initially treated at UTMDAH, one had a local recurrence following partial laryngectomy that was not controlled, and seven had neck recurrences, two of which were controlled, one by chemotherapy only, one by surgery plus chemotherapy.

Of the 13 patients initially treated elsewhere, there were two postoperative deaths and six uncontrolled local or stomal recurrences. One stomal recurrence did not become apparent until 6.5 years after the salvage surgery. Two patients developed neck recurrences that were controlled by additional surgery, and three developed neck-disease recurrences and did not respond to further treatment. There was one serious surgical complication in this group of patients: a perforation of the carotid artery, which required ligation but did not result in nuerological sequelae.

FIVE-YEAR SURVIVAL. Six of this group of patients lived 5 or more years. One interesting patient had recurrent cancer in the neck controlled by additional surgery and had asynchronous resection of bilateral pulmonary metastases, but no further evidence of cancer for 8 years.

Comment. The relatively high rate of treatment failure in the neck in the absence of nodes clinically positive for disease initially suggests that these patients might have benefited from a more extensive bilateral modified neck dissection. The local-treatment failure rate could possibly have been improved by a more extensive paratracheal node dissection and a lower resection of the trachea. In two instances, however, the cancer grew rapidly and invaded deeply along the tracheoesophageal groove to the great vessels, and no treatment could conceivably have altered the outcome.

Treatment results for this group of patients with recurrent cancer in the laryngeal region are summarized in Table 13–5. The relatively high risk (22%) of local or regional failure could probably be reduced by doing more than a wide-field laryngectomy, particularly in patients with a history of nodal involvement in the neck prior to treatment, or in cancers occurring in a site known to have a high incidence of regional lymphatic spread.

CANCER OF THE LARYNGEAL REGION TREATED BY WIDE-FIELD LARYNGECTOMY

It was difficult to neatly categorize all patients with cancer of the laryngeal area according to both site of primary origin and treatment of the neck nodes. Classification according to site of origin was based on the clinical evaluation and the pathologic findings, with the recognition that the two did not always agree. In the case of the extensive tumors involving several sites, the apparent center of the lesion was used to classify the site. Similarly, it was not always easy to decide whether wide-field laryngectomy or laryngectomy plus modified neck dissection had been done because the description of the number and location of the nodes removed sometimes seemed to be inadequately stated on the pathology report. Nonetheless, it appeared that a resection of the primary and an apparent wide-field laryngectomy was done on 88 patients with glottic cancers, 68 with supraglottic cancers, and 21 with pyriform sinus cancers.

Because each site differed as to frequency of nodal metastasis and other factors, the sites were analyzed separately. Because some patients received radiation as an adjunct to the surgical treatment and some did not, those who did receive radiation therapy as a planned part of the procedure were analyzed separately from those who did not.

Treatment results are summarized for this group of patients in Table 13–6. This group by and large represented patients with earlier disease than those reported under bilateral neck dissection. The operative mortality of 2.3 percent is lower than that reported for the patients having bilateral neck dissection, but this series did not include any patients with cancers of the cervical esophagus or postcricoid region, which had the highest surgical mortality rate in the group of patients having synchronous bilateral neck dissections.

Table 13–5. Summary of Treatment Results in Patients with Recurrent Cancer in Laryngeal Area

PRIMARY SITE	NO. OF PATIENTS	BILATERALLY POS. NODE		POST-OP DEATHS	DEAD OF LOC.-REG. RECURRENCE	ABSOLUTE 5-YR SURVIVAL (%)
		No.	*5-yr survivors*			
Supraglottic larynx	19	1	0	0	5	9 (47)
Pyriform sinus	7	1	0	0	5	0 (0)
Glottis	77	0	0	2	12	46 (60)
Total	103	2	0	2	22	55 (53)

Table 13–6. Summary of Treatment Results in Cancers of Laryngeal Region Treated by Wide Field Laryngectomy

PRIMARY SITE	NO. OF PATIENTS	NO. OF PATIENTS WITH HIST. POS. NODES. BIL.		POST-OP DEATHS	DEAD OF LOC.-REG. RECURRENCE	ABSOLUTE 5-YR SURVIVAL (%)
		No.	*5-yr survivors*			
Glottis						
no radiation planned	51*	0	0	1	3	34 (67)
radiation planned	37	1	0	0	7	19 (51)
Supraglottic						
no radiation planned	20	0	0	1	1	11 (55)
radiation planned	47	5	2	1	3	30 (64)
Pyriform sinus						
no radiation planned	4	0	0	1†	0	3 (75)
radiation planned	17	0	0	0	2	9 (53)
Total	176	6	2	4	16	106 (60)

*One patient had 1 week of therapy elsewhere, followed by emergency tracheotomy; wide-field laryngectomy here, then staged bilateral neck dissection and therapy for retropharyngeal metastasis. The patient died from radiation myelopathy.
†From carotid perforation in a patient whose cancer occured in field irradiated for other primary.

Cancer of the Glottic Region

Cancer of the Glottic Region Treated by Wide-Field Laryngectomy Without Postoperative Irradiation. There were 51 patients in this group. Four had had emergency tracheostomies prior to referral, and one of the four also had had 1 week of radiation therapy. Another patient had an emergency tracheostomy on arrival at the hospital because the treatment of his gastric obstruction seemed more pressing than the treatment of the laryngeal cancer. None of these five patients survived five years, although only one died of a stomal recurrence. In addition to these five patients, one patient had had a previous cord stripping, and another a cordectomy. Cancer developed within irradiated fields in one patient who had had radiation therapy 16 years previously for metastasis from a unknown primary.

Staging. The primary tumors of 41 patients were classified T_3; the primary tumors of 10 were classified T_4.

The nodes of 49 patients were classified N0 (four were histologically positive for disease), and the nodes of the other two were classified N1 (none was positive for disease). Subglottic extension was reported in 26 patients, and of them, 19 survived 5 or more years.

Recurrences. Two patients developed stomal recurrences, one of them at 4 years. Neither recurrence occurred in patients whose operative specimen was reported to show subglottic extension, but one did occur in a patient who had an emergency tracheostomy prior to relief of gastric obstruction.

There were five recurrences in the neck, one developing in a patient who had previously had irradiation therapy to both sides of the neck for an unknown primary. In four patients, surgery was followed by postoperative irradiation; two of the four survived 5 or more years, and the third died of distant metastasis at 20 months. The fourth patient had had 1 week of irradiation therapy and an emergency tracheostomy prior to referral. A wide-field laryngectomy was done, and three nodes positive for disease were found. Subsequently, a dissection of the left side of the neck was done, followed by a dissection of the right side of the neck. When an aspiration biopsy of a retropharyngeal node showed squamous cell carcinoma, the patient received irradiation to a dosage of 4617 cGy. The patient developed transverse myelitis, to which he succumbed.

Five-Year Survival. Thirty-four of the 51 patients survived more than 5 years. Two died of distant metastases, 11 of other causes, and three of local or regional recurrence. There was one postoperative death from a perforated viscus, and one patient was lost to follow-up.

Cancer of the Glottic Region Treated by Wide-Field Laryngectomy with Postoperative Irradiation. Thirty-seven patients underwent wide-field laryngectomy and postoperative irradiation. It was not always clear whether the addition of the postoperative irradiation was planned or dictated by the operative findings. Four patients in this group had had some previous surgery for their laryngeal carcinoma, and four had had an emergency tracheostomy.

Staging. Twenty-two primary tumors were classified as T_3, and 15 as T_4. Disease in 35 necks was classified as N0, with eight being histologically positive; one as N1 in which no positive nodes were found; and one as N3b in a patient who had previously had a laryngofissure and a synchronous cancer of the lung.

All but 2 patients completed their postoperative irradiation. One was found to have three positive nodes in his neck, which was clinically negative for disease. He stopped his radiation after 1800 cGy and developed a neck recurrence, from which he died. The other, whose disease was classified N3b and who had synchronous lung cancer, stopped treatment after 2050 cGy, and also developed recurrent cancer in the neck.

Recurrences. Twelve patients were found to have subglottic extension in the operative specimen; one of them developed a stomal recurrence. There were six recurrences, five developing in necks in which nodes histologically positive for disease had been found, and one in a neck histologically negative for disease. Two of the neck-disease recurrences occurred in the patients who stopped irradiation therapy. None of the six patients with neck-disease recurrences nor the one with the stomal recurrence lived.

Complications of Radiation Therapy. There was one serious complication occurring at 8 months consisting of intrathoracic ligation of the carotid artery without neurologic sequelae. One patient developed a stricture and died at 10 months of either the stricture or recurrent cancer; another patient developed a stricture and fistula at 2.5 years.

Other Primary Cancers. Five patients had synchronous or subsequent lung cancer, and three developed new primary cancers within the irradiated fields—one in the pharynx, one in the base of the tongue, and one in the palate.

Five-Year Survival. Of the 37 patients, 19 (51%) survived without evidence of cancer for 5 or more years. Nine died of other causes or distant metastasis, two died of other primary cancers, and seven of recurrent cancer within the neck or stoma.

Comparing the two groups—those who received postoperative irradiation and those who did not—it is apparent that there were more patients with disease classified T_4 and more with nodes histologically positive for disease in the group receiving postoperative irradiation. It is also apparent that in those patients who were found to have nodes histologically positive for disease, postoperative irradiation therapy was not always effective in controlling the occult cancer within the neck.

Cancer of the Supraglottic Larynx

Sixty-seven patients were included in this group. Twenty did not receive radiation therapy postoperatively; 47 did.

Cancer of the Supraglottic Larynx Treated by Wide-Field Laryngectomy Without Postoperative Irradiation. One of the 20 patients treated by wide-field laryngectomy but not postoperative irradiation had had a supraglottic laryngectomy elsewhere, and was referred to UTMDAH for problems with aspiration; laryngectomy was completed and no tumor was found. The other 19 were untreated beforehand for their laryngeal cancer.

Staging. One patient's tumor was classified T_X, 12 patients had tumors classified T_3, and seven had tumors classified T_4.

Seventeen patients had nodes classified N0 (three were histologically positive for disease), two patients had nodes classified N1 (both histologically negative), and one patient had nodes classified N2a (four nodes histologically positive for disease).

Recurrence. One patient who had previously had an emergency tracheostomy developed a stomal recurrence that was not controlled by further surgery and irradiation. A patient who was found to have one node histologically positive for disease on the right side subsequently developed metastases on the left side of the neck that were treated by radical neck dissection. It was believed by the surgeon that all of the tumor had not been removed. The patient was treated by radiation therapy twice daily, and had had no recurrence at 12 years. The patient whose disease was classified N2a and who was found to have four positive nodes on one side underwent a radical neck dissection on the opposite side. No nodes histologically positive for disease were found; the patient was placed on chemoimmunotherapy and survives at 8 years.

Five-Year Survival. Although none of these patients received postoperative irradiation in a planned manner, postoperative irradiation was advised for one patient, who refused, and died of other causes at 8 years. Of the other 19 patients, 10 survived more than 5 years. Three died of other primary tumors in less than 5 years. Four died of other causes, there was one postoperative death by stroke at 2 days. One patient died of recurrent cancer.

Other Primary Cancers. One patient had previously been treated for Hodgkin's disease and also had lung cancer. One patient had three separate synchronous primary cancers in the tongue, the larynx, and the lung. One patient had synchronous lung and larynx cancers and had his lung cancer treated before his larynx cancer. Another patient died of cancer of the ovary.

Cancer of the Supraglottic Larynx Treated by Radiation Therapy and Wide-Field Laryngectomy. For some of the patients in this group of 47, irradiation was planned because of the initial clinical findings, and some received radiation therapy because of the operative findings. Two patients had emergency tracheostomies prior to referral. One patient had started irradiation elsewhere and had received 800 cGy. He had a wide-field laryngectomy at UTMDAH, with one lymph node positive for disease found, received postoperative radiation to a dose of 4998 cGy, developed Lehrmitte's syndrome and recurrence in the side of the original positive node, and died at 16 months.

Preoperative irradiation therapy was started on one patient whose disease was classified T3N2b, but had to be stopped because of bleeding. A wide-field laryngectomy was performed, with one node positive for disease found in the operative specimen. Multiple problems ensued, leading to gastrostomy and, finally, death from sepsis and aspiration pneumonia.

Staging. Six patients had primary tumors classified T_2 and 30 had primary tumors classified T_3. Eleven patients had primary tumors classified T_4.

Thirty-three patients had nodes classified N0; eight were positive, with one bilaterally positive for disease. Seven patients had nodes classified N1, of which six were positive, two of them bilaterally positive for disease. One patient had nodes positive for disease classified N2a, and seven had nodes classified N2b (five were positive, of which two were bilaterally positive for disease). Twenty-one of the 47 patients (44%) had nodes histologically positive for disease, with five (10%) positive for disease bilaterally.

Treatment. In nine patients, a supraglottic laryngectomy was done, followed by postoperative irradiation. Seven of the nine survived more than 5 years, although one was never able to speak or swallow well. One died of aspiration pneumonia 3 months after completion of radiation therapy. One of the patients who had a supraglottic laryngectomy was found to have seven positive nodes, received only 2000 cGy of radiation therapy postoperatively, and survives at 6 years.

Recurrences. Three patients developed recurrent cancer within the neck that was untreatable. In one case, the patient had two synchronous primaries, one in the larynx and one in the soft palate. All the recurrences developed in necks that had been histologically positive for disease.

Deaths After Radiation Therapy. One patient died 6 days after completion of radiation therapy; another died at 39 days. One patient died at three months of aspiration pneumonia, and one died at 7 months with possible myxedema.

Five-Year Survival. Thirty patients (64%) survived 5 or more years. Seven patients died of other causes within 5 years, four of distant metastases, three of other primaries, and three of local recurrence. There was one postoperative death.

Other Primary Cancers. Five second primary cancers occurred in the lung and two in the bladder. Two second primary cancers developed in the floor of the mouth, one in the pharyngeal wall, one in the lip, and one in the palate. One incidental thyroid cancer was found.

Survival of Patients With Nodes Bilaterally Positive for Disease. Of the five patients with nodes bilaterally positive for disease, two survived 5 or more years, and one died of regional recurrence. The remaining two died of distant metastasis.

Comment. It is readily apparent that the patients who had postoperative irradiation in addition to the surgical procedure had more advanced primary cancer than those who received no adjunctive treatment. Since there was only one neck-disease failure in the patients who received no postoperative irradiation, an operative procedure alone seemed to be satisfactory for that group. The addition of postoperative irradiation seems to reduce, but does not eliminate, the risk of recurrence in the neck that has presumably been rendered free of metastatic tumor by a surgical procedure. It is quite likely that the small metastases found in necks that are clinically negative for disease may have different significance than the nodes found in necks clinically positive for disease, in which the nodes are more likely to be larger and have extracapsular extension.

Cancer of the Pyriform Sinus

Of the 21 patients with cancer of the pyriform sinus, four did not receive postoperative irradiation. The other 17 had postoperative irradiation, either planned or deemed necessary by the histologic findings.

Cancer of the Pyriform Sinus Treated by Wide-Field Laryngectomy and No Postoperative Irradiation. There were only four patients in this group, all with disease classified T3N0. In none of the specimens were the nodes histologically positive for disease. In one patient, the cancer occurred within fields irradiated 10 years earlier to treat Hodgkin's disease. There was poor healing and a carotid perforation requiring ligation. The patient died 27 days postoperatively. The remaining three patients all survived 5 or more years.

Cancer of the Pyriform Sinus Treated by Wide-Field Laryngectomy with Postoperative Irradiation. None of the 17 patients who received postoperative irradiation had been previously treated.

Staging. Two patients had primary tumors classified T_2, 14 had primary tumors classified T_3, and one had a primary tumor classified T_4.

Thirteen patients had nodes classified N0; seven were histologically positive for disease. Three patients had nodes histologically positive for disease classified N1, and one had nodes histologically positive for disease classified N2b. Sixty-five percent of the patients had nodes histologically positive for disease, none bilaterally positive.

Treatment. All except one patient had a total laryngectomy. A supraglottic laryngectomy was performed in a patient whose disease was initially classified T2N0, but the pathology report showed metastatic cancer in one node and in the connective tissue. Postoperative irradiation was given, but the patient developed neck-disease recurrence and distant metastases and died at 11 months.

Recurrences. Four patients developed apparent recurrent cancer in the neck. In two patients, disease appeared in the nodes before radiation therapy was begun. In one patient, histologic proof of recurrence was not obtained, but the patient received postoperative irradiation and survives at 11 years. It is quite possible that the nodes, which developed during the postoperative period, were not histologically positive for disease because the examination of the operative specimen showed no positive node. A second patient whose neck disease was classified N1 was found to have four nodes positive for disease in the neck; an additional node was removed at 1 month and found to contain metastatic cancer. Postoperative irradiation was given, with apparent control of the cancer in the neck, but the patient died of distant metastases at 8 months. There were two additional recurrences in the neck in the same sides as nodes positive for disease; neither patient lived.

Complications. One patient died during postoperative irradiation therapy 1.5 months after a dose of 2025 cGy. Three patients developed fistulas, one of which was closed with a tube pedicle in multiple stages; the others were not closed. A pharyngeal stoma was left at the time of surgery in one patient; postoperative irradiation was given, a feeding gastrostomy was needed, and multiple surgical stages over a 7-month period were required to close the stoma. Swallowing was never entirely satisfactory. One patient developed a stricture and had to be tube-fed. One patient developed radiation myelopathy, which may have contributed to his death.

Five-Year Survival. Nine patients survived 5 or more years. Two died of regional recurrence, and the remainder died either of other causes or of distant metastases within less than 5 years.

Comment. Even though patients with cancer of the pyriform sinus treated by wide-field laryngectomy plus postoperative irradiation have the most favorable prognoses of any patients with cancer of the pyriform sinus, there are problems associated with treatment. The percentages of nodes histologically positive for disease in the neck clinically negative for disease is high. Postoperative irradiation is not innocuous, even though it may seem to be the logical treatment.

SYNCHRONOUS BILATERAL UPPER NECK DISSECTION

The 81 cases included in this group were difficult to analyze because of the multiplicity of sites involved and variations in the extent of nodal dissection. Rather than separating the neck dissections into a number of subgroups, we considered patients in this series to have a bilateral upper neck dissection if the dissection did not go below the omohyoid. There were considerable differences in the extent to which the lymph nodes about the upper third of the spinal accessory nerve were removed.

To further confuse the issue, some patients received irradiation therapy preoperatively, whereas others received it postoperatively; some received no irradiation therapy. Prior treatment had failed to cure some patients, and they presented with uncontrolled primary tumors and regional metastases. Others presented with presumably controlled primary tumors, but with regional metastases. To make some sense of the confusing array of variables, cases were analyzed according to whether or not radiation therapy was employed; in each category, each primary site was analyzed separately.

Treatment results for patients with bilateral upper neck dissection are summarized in Table 13–7. The dismal results and high risk of local or regional recurrence probably reflect more the difficulty in achieving satisfactory results in previously treated patients than a failure of surgical selection or use of adjunctive treatment. It can be seen in the text that a number of recurrences in the neck were in patients not selected for immediate postoperative irradiation. Although many of these were controlled by further surgery, there is the suggestion that a more extensive surgical procedure done ini-

Table 13–7. Summary of Treatment Results with Bilateral Upper Neck Dissection

PRIMARY SITE	NO. OF PATIENTS	BIL. POS. NODES		POST-OP DEATHS	DEAD OF LOC.-REG. RECURRENCES	ABSOLUTE 5-YR SURVIVAL (%)
		No.	*5-yr survival*			
No planned radiation						
Floor of mouth	26	0	0	2	4	14 (54)
Lower lip	7	1	1	1	1	5 (71)
Skin	3	1	1	0	0	3 (100)
Oral tongue	1	0	0	0	1	0 (0)
Subtotal	37	2	2	3	5	22 (61)
Radiation pre- or post-op						
Floor of mouth	24	12	2	0	7	6 (25)
Lip	9	1	0	0	5	3 (33)
Nose	7	4	0	0	5	2 (29)
Miscellaneous	4	4	0	0	4	0 (0)
Subtotal	44	21	2	0	21	11 (25)

tially might have resulted in fewer of these recurrences.

Bilateral Upper Neck Dissection with No Planned Postoperative Irradiation Therapy

There were 37 patients in this category. Twenty-six had cancer of the floor of the mouth, seven had cancer of the lower lip, three had skin cancers, and one had cancer of the oral tongue.

Cancer of the Floor of the Mouth. Two patients had had prior irradiation therapy. One patients who had been treated elsewhere was treated with resection of the recurrent cancer, marginal resection of the mandible, and bilateral upper-neck dissection. No tumor was found in the nodes, but at 5.5 years local recurrence became evident and tumor was found in the hypoglossal nerve. One patient treated at UTMDAH required resection of the anterior arch and bilateral upper-neck dissection. No tumor was found in the nodes. The patient died at 81 months of primary or metastatic cancer of the lung.

Staging. Two patients had primary tumors classified T_1, 18 had primary tumors classified T_2, three had primary tumors classified T_4, and two were unclassified.

Twenty patients had nodes classified N0 (two were histologically positive for disease), and six had nodes classified N1 (two were positive for disease).

Recurrences. Although only four of the patients were found to have nodes histologically positive for disease, seven patients developed recurrences in the neck, which were controlled by further surgery and radiation in five, and not controlled in two. Of the recurrences, four occurred in necks histologically negative for disease, two occurred in the side of the neck opposite the side from which nodes histologically positive for disease had been recovered, and one developed lower in the neck, from which a node histologically positive for disease was recovered. It is apparent from this small number of cases that bilateral upper-neck dissection is not successful in controlling occult metastases, though subsequent control was achieved in five of the seven patients. Four patients developed recurrent cancer at the primary site, and in two cases it was controlled.

Five-Year Survival. Fourteen patients survived 5 or more years. Five died of other causes, one of distant metastasis, and four of local or regional recurrence. There were two postoperative deaths.

Cancer of the Lower Lip. Seven patients were seen, four of whom had had prior treatment. One patient presented with recurrent cancer of the skin of the nose and lower lip, with regional metastases. Tumor grew up the inferior alveolar nerve, which led to death in 8 months. In three patients, the cancer of the lip was controlled and the patient was referred for metastatic disease in the neck, though in one case a submental metastasis had been previously removed and no tumor was found in the operative specimen. One patient, whose previously treated lip cancer was classified N2a, was found to have nine positive nodes in the neck-dissection specimen, and died during the postoperative period of peritonitis from a perforated appendix.

Staging. Three patients had T_1 disease, one primary tumor was classified T_2, one was classified T_3, and two were classified T_4. One patient had nodes histologically positive for disease classified N0, five had nodes classified N1 (four were histologically positive and one of them was bilaterally positive for disease), and one had nodes classified N2a (nine nodes positive for disease.)

Recurrences. There was only one local recurrence—in the patient whose cancer grew up the inferior alveolar nerve.

Five-Year Survival. Five patients survived 5 or more years, including one patient who was found to have bilateral nodal metastases, with five positive nodes on one side and three on the other. There was one postoperative death.

Skin Cancers. Three patients with previously treated skin cancers were treated with bilateral upper neck dissection. All patients had nodes positive for disease, with one having bilaterally positive nodes and connective tissue extension. There were no recurrences, and all patients survived 5 or more years.

Cancer of the Oral Tongue. There was only one patient with cancer of the oral tongue, which was classified T4N0. No tumor was found in the nodes, but tumor was found in the lingual and inferior alveolar nerves. Death occurred because of intracranial extension.

Bilateral Upper-Neck Dissection with Pre- or Postoperative Irradiation

There were 44 patients in this group, 24 with cancer of the floor of the mouth, nine with cancer of the lip, seven with cancer of the tip of the nose, and four with cancers in miscellaneous sites.

Cancer of the Floor of the Mouth. Of the 24 patients with cancer of the floor of the mouth, 18 were previously untreated when seen at UTMDAH, one had disease recurrent after elective radiation therapy given at UTMDAH, two had disease recurrent after surgery, and three presented with the primary cancer controlled but with metastases in the neck. Six patients were chosen to receive preoperative irradiation.

Staging. Three patients had primary tumors classified T_X and three had primary tumors classified T_1. Six primary tumors were classified T_2, seven were classified T_3, and five were classified T_4.

Eleven patients had nodes classified N0; five of those were histologically positive for disease. Two patients had nodes classified N1; one was histologically positive for disease. Two patients had nodes positive for disease classified N2a, and one had nodes positive for disease classified N2b; seven had nodes classified N3b (six were histologically positive for disease). Fifteen of the 24 (62%) had nodes histologically positive for disease, and of these, 12 (50%) were positive bilaterally.

Recurrences. Disease appeared in the neck nodes during or immediately prior to radiation therapy in two patients. In one of them, there was apparent local control, though the patient died at 8 months of distant metastasis. Recurrence in the neck of 1 patient was controlled by further surgery. In seven patients, local or regional recurrence, sometimes both, developed but was not controlled.

Five-Year Survival. Of the 12 patients with bilateral cervical metastasis, 10 died within 2 years of local or regional recurrence of distant metastasis, and two survived more than 5 years.

Six patients in the entire group survived 5 or more years. Four died of other causes, six died of distant metastasis, one died of a second primary cancer of the esophagus, and seven died of local recurrence, regional recurrence, or both.

Cancer of the Lip. There were nine patients in this group, three with cancer of the upper lip and six with cancer of the lower lip. Only four of these patients were previously untreated, and of these, two had preoperative irradiation at UTMDAH. Of the total group, one patient had synchronous recurrent primary cancers of the upper lip and gum, one had disease that recurred after surgery, two had controlled primary tumors but metastatic cancer in the neck, and one had a lower-lip cancer recurrent after irradiation.

Five patients developed recurrent cancer within the neck or at the primary site, none of which was controlled. One patient had histologically proven bilateral metastasis and underwent a bilateral dissection more extensive on one side than on the other. He received postoperative radiation and developed a mass in the side of the lesser dissection, but also developed distant metastases, from which he died before anything could be done about the diseased node in the neck.

Five-Year Survival. Three patients survived more than 5 years, one died of distant metastasis, and five died of local or regional recurrence. Two of the survivors had received preoperative irradiation, and one had no nodes histologically positive for disease in the operative specimen.

Patients with Cancer of the Skin of the Nasal Vestibule and Tip of the Nose. There were seven patients in this group, only one of whom had not been previously treated. All underwent resection of the nose and bilateral upper neck dissection. The patients who had been previously treated had recurrent disease after irradiation or surgery; in one case, the presence of a lymphoma was a complicating factor. This patient had a rapidly growing cancer that was treated by preoperative irradiation, then surgery, with nodes bilaterally positive for disease found in the operative specimen. He developed local recurrence and died.

Recurrences. All of the patients had nodes histologically positive for disease, with four positive bilaterally. None of the patients with nodes bilaterally positive for disease survived for any length of time. Five of the seven patients developed local or regional recurrence that caused their deaths. In two instances, the use of a complete bilateral radical neck dissection would not have been effective because the recurrent tumor developed within the parotid area. In one instance, the patient developed a neck recurrence in the side of the neck that had previously had less-than-optimal treatment, but also developed a recurrence in the parotid region. This patient was treated, with favorable results, by neck dissection and parotidectomy, followed by additional radiation therapy.

Five-Year Survival. Only two patients survived more than 5 years, the others dying of neck or local recurrence. Cancers of the nose that metastasize are difficult to control by surgery, since the nodes involved may be in the preauricular area or along the facial vessels, as well as in the tail of the parotid and neck. If radiation therapy is employed, it should be used in the "moustache" technique to cover the nose, the upper lip, the nodes along the facial vessels, and the tail of the parotid as well as the neck. Cancer may metastasize to the regional nodes, but it also may spread up the infraorbital nerve (the route of spread that caused the death of one of the patients in this series).

Cancer of Miscellaneous Sites. One patient had a cancer of the maxillary sinus. This patient underwent a maxillary resection and postoperative radiation therapy to the maxillary sinus and left side of the neck, followed by a bilateral upper-neck dissection that showed nodes histologically positive for disease bilaterally. Postoperative radiation therapy was given to the right side of the neck, but within 2 months recurrent cancer was found throughout the face and back of the neck.

A second patient had synchronous primary cancers of the base of the tongue and the anterior floor of the mouth and was treated by resection of the base of the tongue and epiglottis, with bilateral upper-neck dissection. A single node histologically positive for disease was found in each side of the neck. The patient had postoperative radiation therapy, then had to have a laryngectomy. He apparently did not develop local or regional recurrence, but did develop recurrence in the chest wall at the site of a deltopectoral flap.

A third patient had had prior surgery and radiation for a cancer of the oral tongue that was classified T4N1 when seen. Total glossectomy and bilateral upper-neck dissection was done, and nodes positive for disease were found in both sides of the neck. Postoperative irradiation therapy was started, but was discontinued because of rapid recurrence of tumor.

The fourth patient had cancer of the upper gum and palate classified T4N3b. After a course of preoperative irradiation, a bilateral upper-neck dissection was done, which showed nodes histologically positive for disease bilaterally. Postoperative radiation was started, but was terminated when the tumor was found extending up into the cranium.

Treatment of these four cases was probably doomed to failure from the beginning, except in the patient with synchronous cancers of the base of the tongue and the floor of the mouth. In that case, a bilateral modified neck dissection, resection of the base of the tongue and laryngectomy, and resection of the cancer of the floor of the mouth might have been a preferable form of treatment.

DISCUSSION

Most of the treatment results occasioned very little surprise, although the rate of local and regional failure in cancer of the pharyngeal walls was distressing, and probably reflects more an unwise attempt to treat all patients presenting with this problem rather than inadequate surgery or failure to combine treatment modalities. The risk of regional recurrence in patients treated for glottic cancer by wide-field laryngectomy and postoperative irradiation was unexpectedly high, and remains unexplained. Patients treated for cancer of the glottic area by radiation therapy who developed recurrence and then had an attempt at surgical salvage, showed a higher-than-expected risk of local and regional recurrence, which suggests that something more than a wide-field laryngectomy might have been more effective.

Two incidental findings are interesting. Sixty of the 703 patients had either positive retropharyngeal nodes at the time of the initial treatment or developed them during the progress of their cancer. The incidence was highest in cancers of the pharyngeal wall, but was also significant in cancers of the pyriform sinus and soft palate, and could occur whenever routes of lymphatic spread to the lateral cervical nodes were disrupted by surgery or radiation. The retropharyngeal nodes then became a primary drainage site. An incidental finding was the presence in the neck-dissection specimens or thyroid gland of thyroid cancer in 22 instances (all papillary and follicular). In only one instance was this of any possible clinical significance.

The addition of radiation therapy to the surgical procedure seemed to reduce the risk of local recurrence. Such multimodality therapy exacted a price in that several patients died during the course of radiation therapy or immediately afterwards. The number of patients having dysphagia and strictures of the esophagus was significantly increased over those who did not have adjunctive treatment, and radiation myelopathy contributed to the problems in several patients. Cancer occurred in seven patients within the radiated fields used to treat prior cancers, and the treatment problems in those patients were markedly increased. Cancer also occurred subsequently in the irradiated fields among patients surviving combined treatment.

It was not possible to determine the value of adjunctive irradiation in increasing survival. The fact that of the 5-year survivors among those patients with nodes histologically positive bilaterally having bilateral neck dissection, 17 received no irradiation and 14 did, indicates that postoperative irradiation is not always necessary. A better means to determine the necessity of adjunctive treatment is required.

CONCLUSIONS

1. Bilateral neck dissection performed synchronously can be done with a reasonable mortality and morbidity. The mortality rate for wide-field laryngectomy is less than that for bilateral neck dissection.
2. There is a considerable discrepancy between clinical and pathologic staging of the status of cervical lymph nodes. Elective neck dissection seems to be a reasonable approach to the problem of clinically occult cervical lymph-node metastasis, and it does not seem to add to the morbidity.
3. Adjunctive irradiation seems to reduce the risk of local recurrence, though it may not add much to the 5-year survival rate. More patients in this series with histologically positive nodes bilaterally survived without radiation than did those receiving radiation.
4. Postoperative irradiation cannot be given without side effects, some of which can be lethal. A better means of determining the necessity for adjunctive therapy must be found. The mere presence of histologically positive nodes, unilaterally or bilaterally, is not an absolute indication for the use of adjunctive treatment.
5. Few successes are achieved in the treatment of patients with cancer after radiation therapy if both the nodes and the primary site contain residual cancer. This is particularly true for cancers of the pharyngeal wall and pyriform sinus.
6. When cancers occur in fields previously treated by irradiation for another primary cancer, the surgical problems are compounded and treatment results are poor.
7. Recurrent cancers of the nose and upper lip with cervical-node metastases are difficult surgical problems with a poor salvage rate.

REFERENCES

Ballantyne, A. J., and Jackson, G. L.: Synchronous bilateral neck dissection. *Am. J. Surg.*, 144:452–55, 1982.

Crile, G., Sr.: Excision of cancer of the head and neck with special reference to the plan of dissection based upon one hundred thirty two operations. *J.A.M.A.*, 47:1780–86, 1906.

Martin, H. E., del Valle, B., Ehrlich, H., and Cahan, W. G.: Neck dissection. *Cancer*, 4:441–99, 1951.

Sako, K.: Simultaneous bilateral neck dissection. In Chretien, P. B., Johns, M. E., Shedd, D. P., Strong, E. W., Ward, P. H. (eds.): *Head and Neck Cancer*, Vol. 1, pp. 166–68, B.C. Decker, Philadelphia, 1985.

CHAPTER 14

Squamous Cell Carcinoma Metastatic to the Neck from an Unknown Primary Site

Robert C. Wang, Helmuth Goepfert, Annabel Barber, and Patricia F. Wolf

EDITORS' COMMENT

As its name implies, the unknown primary tumor metastatic to the neck is a perplexing entity, one that begins with the initial visit of the patient. Questions are always raised about the thoroughness of the evaluation, the type and aggressiveness of treatment, and the adequacy of follow-up. This is one area of head and neck cancer treatment where surgeons are forced to use all their clinical acumen to tailor the correct treatment for a given patient because each patient is unique in presentation and clinical findings. Dr. Wang and Dr. Goepfert have provided us with a valuable tool to accomplish this—an exhaustive literature review, coupled with a 30-year review of the disease entity at the University of Texas M.D. Anderson Hospital and Tumor Institute at Houston.

As expected, the authors confirm the work of others in identifying significant factors in the determination of survival: neck-disease stage, residual disease after surgery, connective-tissue disease, recurrence in the neck, and distant metastasis. There are also a number of unexpected findings in this review that do not appear to determine survival: discovery of the primary, histologic differentiation, pretreatment biopsy of the neck (confirming the findings of Million in Chapter 8), type of neck dissection performed, or the presence of low neck nodes in combination with other areas of nodal disease.

The authors use these and other facts to reach logical conclusions about the treatment of the patient with an unknown squamous carcinoma metastatic to the neck. The N1 and N2a neck can be treated with radiation or surgery with equal effectiveness. Modifications of the neck dissection should be liberally used in surgical treatment of the neck. Patients with poorly differentiated tumors should have definitive radiation to Waldeyer's ring as well as to the neck. Finally, observation only, following excisional biopsy of minimal disease, cannot be recommended.

INTRODUCTION

In his review of 3800 consecutive head and neck cancer patients, Martin (1944) found only 55 in which no primary lesions were ever discovered. Metastatic carcinoma to cervical lymph nodes with a primary tumor remaining unknown even after exhaustive investigation is rare and intriguing. It poses questions of tumor origin and biology, as well as what optimal therapy should be. Because of the limited number of cases usually encountered, past series have tended to combine different histologic types, or stages of neck disease or both, with notable exception (Spiro, 1983). This chapter will focus on squamous cell carcinomas metastatic to the neck from unknown primary lesions.

MATERIALS AND METHODS

We reviewed 218 records of patients treated at The University of Texas M.D. Anderson Hospital and Tumor Institute at Houston (UTMDAH) from 1953 to 1983 listing squamous cell carcinoma metastatic to the neck, with unknown primaries. Seventy-eight patients were excluded because of previous treatment, subsequent definitive treatment elsewhere, lack of pathologic confirmation, lack of follow-up, and finding the primary site on initial evaluation at UTMDAH or discoveries at postmortem examination, leaving only 140 cases suitable for this study.

The mean age was 59 years; the median, 60 years; with 78 percent of patients between 50 and 79 years. Males outnumbered females four to one. Sixty patient records were reviewed from the first half of the study period, the remaining 80 from the last 15 years. Follow-up was unlimited, lasting up to 23 years; median follow-up interval was 53.5 months. Tobacco was used by 64 percent of the patients and not used by 16 percent; 20 percent of the records failed to show tobacco use. Because of the high frequency of cutaneous squamous cell carcinomas in our patient population, skin cancer histories were noted in 90 percent of the records, with cancer being present in 24 percent and absent in 66 percent.

After initial clinical examination failed to reveal a primary lesion, patients underwent direct inspection of the laryngopharynx and directed (on the basis of node location) biopsies of the nasopharynx, as well as of the tonsil, base of the tongue, the hypopharynx, and any suspicious mucosal or skin areas. Bronchoscopy, esophagoscopy, and such studies as chest x-ray, nasopharyngeal and laryngeal tomograms, barium swallow, sputum cytology, thyroid scan, and roentgenographic examination of the gastrointestinal and genitourinary tracts were performed when the treating physician deemed it necessary.

Pretreatment histologic diagnosis was made by needle aspiration in 13 percent of the patients, incisional biopsy in 38.5 percent (performed elsewhere before referral), and excisional biopsy in 38.5 percent. In the remaining 10 percent, diagnosis was confirmed by frozen section at the time of neck dissection. All slides from biopsies performed elsewhere were reviewed at UTMDAH before definitive therapy, which was initiated in all cases within 4 weeks of biopsy.

Neck staging was in accordance with the American Joint Committee, 1980 classification, and is shown in Table 14–1. NX refers to unclassifiable neck disease because of previous biopsy and subsequent diffuse induration or, much more commonly, lack of palpable disease. Of the NX cases, 54 percent underwent excisional biopsy that left no residual palpable disease.

TREATMENT

The treatment modalities are listed in Table 14–2. In addition, one patient underwent surgery followed by chemotherapy, and one underwent surgery followed by radiation and chemotherapy. The no-treatment group consisted of 13 cases with no definitive palpable disease after biopsy was performed elsewhere (close observation was elected in lieu of treatment), and one patient with metastatic colon adenocarcinoma who had a neck-node biopsy

Table 14–1. Neck Staging, According to the American Joint Committee 1980 Classification

STAGE	NO. OF PATIENTS (%)
NX	42
N1	14
N2a	13
N2b	8
N3a	12
N3b	11

Table 14–2. Treatment Modalities (UTMDAH)

MODALITY	NO	(%)
Surgery only	51	(37)
XRT only	47	(34)
Combined:		
Pre-op XRT	10	(7)
Post-op XRT	16	(12)
None	14	(10)
Total	138	(100)

of squamous carcinoma died shortly thereafter of colon cancer.

Classic radical neck dissections, with or without 11th nerve preservation, were performed in 50 cases; the procedure was unilateral in 49 cases. Modified radical neck dissections, preserving the 11th nerve, sternocleidomastoid muscle, and internal jugular vein, was performed in 14 cases; in 13 it was unilateral. Unilateral limited upper-neck, submandibular, or submental dissections and parotidectomy with upper neck dissections were performed in 19 cases. In one patient, an upper-neck dissection was performed on one side and submandibular area dissection on the other.

Megavoltage radiation has been used at UTMDAH since 1954. In general, a 5000-cGy minimum midline dose is delivered to the upper neck and nasopharyngeal areas via parallel opposed lateral portals, and 5000 cGy to the lower neck area via an anterior field. Portals were moved off the spinal cord after 4500 cGy, and a midline block was used to protect the larynx. An additional 1000-cGy boost by the electron beam was administered to any palpable nodes that remained after megavoltage therapy. Postoperative radiation was usually given if there was multiple positive nodes or nodal areas, connective-tissue invasion, or suspicion of residual microscopic disease. Postoperative radiotherapy was delivered within 6 weeks of surgery.

In the radiation-only group, 83 percent received more than 5000 cGy compared with 75 percent and 50 percent of the post- and preoperative radiation groups, respectively. The remainder received 4500 to 5000 cGy, except for one patient in the radiation-only group and four patients in the preoperative radiation group, who were given less than 4500 cGy.

Follow-up visits were generally made every 2 to 4 months for the first 2 years, 4 to 6 months until 5 years, and yearly thereafter.

Computer analysis was aided by procedures contained in the Statistical Package for the Social Sciences, version 9(Nie et al., 1975). This included frequency distributions, cross-tabulations with chi-square analysis, and the actuarial method of calculating survival functions. Survival curves were plotted on the basis of deaths attributable to head and neck cancer and deaths from all causes.

RESULTS

Disease status at last evaluation is shown in Table 14–3. Of those with no evidence of disease, 83 percent had at least 2 years of follow-up, and 69 percent had more than 5 years' follow-up. Actuarial survival for the entire group regardless of cause of death was 70 percent at 2 years and 55 percent at 5 years; the rates were 82 percent and 79 percent at 2 and 5 years, respectively, if analysis was limited to deaths from head and neck cancer.

Survival according to type of treatment is shown in Table 14–4. Surgery produced significantly better results than radiation alone (87% vs. 69% 5-year actuarial survival limited to death from head and neck cancer), but this difference reflects, at least in part, a bias because patients with stage N3a neck disease were believed to be inoperable and were thus selected for curative radiotherapy. If patients with residual disease after therapy were omitted, there appears to be no difference in effectiveness between surgery or radiation therapy alone (89% vs. 87% 5-year actuarial survival, with analysis limited to death from head and

Table 14–3. Disease Status on Last Evaluation

	NO. OF PATIENTS (%)
Free of cancer	75
Dead of:	
Neck failure	14
Distant metastasis	4
Primary cancer	2
Neck failure and distant metastasis	3
Combination of above	1
Unknown	1

Table 14–4. Actuarial Survival by Treatment Modality

MODALITY	2 YR (%)	5 YR (%)
Surgery	92	87*
Radiation	69	69*
Combined:		
Pre-op	60	60
Post-op	79	70
No treatment	91 (10/11)	71 (5/7)

*$p = < 0.05$.

neck cancer). Nevertheless, it is interesting that surgery alone was able to control disease in all six patients with neck disease of stage N3a and both with N2b disease (one with connective-tissue invasion), whereas in the radiation-only group, five of seven with stage N3a neck disease and four of 13 with N2b neck disease had residual cancer after treatment. The two remaining patients with N2b neck disease suffered from recurrence. The no-treatment group did well by comparison, with a 70 percent 5-year actuarial survival when based on deaths from cancer. This high rate reflects the initial presence of minimal disease. There were no significant differences in survival other than that between the surgery- and radiation-only groups.

Survival by nodal stage is shown in Table 14–5. Patients with NX, N1, or N2a disease had significantly better survival at 5 years than those with N2b or N3a disease ($p = < 0.05$). The N3b group was intermediate in survival. In this group, survival was probably a function of the proportion of the particular stages.

Residual disease after therapy had a dismal prognosis. All patients were dead within 2 years, except for one, who had N2b disease and was given curative radiotherapy. Surgical salvage consisted of radical neck dissection, and the patient was free of cancer at last contact more than 8 years after presentation. Residual disease was more common in the radiation-only group (11 of 47, or 23%) than in the surgery-only group (1 of 51, or 2%). It is difficult to determine the role of selection bias, especially in patients with N2b and N3a stage disease for radiotherapy.

Table 14–5. Actuarial Survival by Stage

STAGE	NO. OF PATIENTS	2 YR (%)	5 YR (%)
NX	59	93	88
N1	19	89	89
N2a	18	100	92
N2b	11	55	55
N3a	17	36	36
N3b	16	65	65

The recurrence rate for neck disease was similar among those at risk in the surgery- and radiation-only groups (12% and 8%, respectively). The small number of patients in the other treatment categories precludes meaningful analysis, with three of nine patients in the preoperative group and four of 16 patients in the postoperative radiation group developing recurrence. It should be mentioned that the recurrence rate in the no-treatment group was significantly higher (six of 13, or 46%, $p = < 0.005$). Of all the recurrences, 64 percent occurred within 2 years, 86 percent within 5 years, and 100 percent within 10 years. Recurrences outside of surgical or radiation fields happened in 37.5 percent of patients, with no significant differences among the treatment groups.

Five-year survival as a function of recurrence was 48 percent, compared with 95 percent if no recurrence or residual disease was manifest ($p = < 0.05$). Of the 16 who developed recurrences in the treated groups, 12 died of disease and three died of other causes, all within 5 years. Only one survived more than 5 years free of recurrence.

Salvage was successful in three of six surgery-only patients, and futile in all three patients in the radiation-only and combined-therapy groups in which salvage was attempted. Among the three successful cases, one patient died within a year and another within 4 years, both of unrelated causes. The third was followed for 14 years with no recurrence, at which time he died of either primary lung cancer or distant metastasis from an unknown primary.

In the no-treatment group, all six patients who had recurrences underwent successful salvage therapy, with neck disease being controlled for at least 2 years. One developed distant metastasis and died of disease; the remaining five were free of disease recurrence for from 2 to 15 years of follow-up.

Primary lesions were eventually discovered in 23 patients, or 16 percent of the total. Of these 23, only 10 (43%) were manifest within the first 2 years, 16 (70%) by 5 years, and all by 10 years (Table 14–6). One lung and one esophagus primary were found. There were significantly more primaries (14 of 51, or 27%; $p = < 0.05$) developing in the surgery-only group than in the radiation-only (3 of 47, or 6%) or combined-therapy groups (4 of 26, or 15%). Of seven radiated patients, three developed a primary within radiated fields (two oral cavity, one nasopharynx). The fact that a primary lesion was discovered did not affect survival at 5 and 10 years, nor were recurrences in the neck more common after primary lesions were found than before in those who ultimately developed primaries.

Distant metastases occurred in 14 of 140 patients, or 10 percent. All except two had distant metastases within a year of treatment, and had persistent or recurrent neck cancer. The two exceptions developed pulmonary nodules at 12 and 22 years; these metastases are unlikely to be related to their original disease. Lung was the most common site of distant metastases (10), followed by liver (two), bone (one), and a combination of lung and bone (one). All patients with distant metastases died of disease.

Connective tissue invasion in the 77 operative cases was found in 36% of them, as shown in Table 14–7. The individual percentages refer to the respective node stages. Recurrence in the neck was found in 29 percent of those with connective-tissue disease versus 10 percent in those without ($p = < 0.05$). The rate of distant metastases was increased, but not significantly (11% vs. 4%), in those with connective-tissue disease. Survival was definitely affected adversely by the presence of connective-tissue disease, as seen in Table 14–8. The differences may be even greater, because early extracapsular spread of tumor has not been investigated routinely at UTMDAH until the last 5 years. Postoperative radiation was not found to be more effective in controlling connective-tissue disease in the neck, but the small numbers and selection bias in this series do not allow further conclusions.

A significant difference ($p = < 0.05$) in 5-year survival based on deaths from head and neck cancer was present between those patients with up to two nodal areas involved pathologically (90%) compared with those with more than two areas involved (63%).

The following factors had no significant influence on recurrence in the neck distant metastases or survival: histologic differentiation, pretreatment biopsy, history of skin cancer, age, type of neck dissection, detection of putative primary cancer on follow-up, and the presence of supraclavicular or low posterior cervical-node involvement, singly or in combination with other areas.

Table 14–6. Sites of Primary Squamous Cell Cancer Discovered on Follow-Up

SITES	2 YR	5 YR	10 YR
Skin	4	2	1
Oral cavity	1	1	3
Oropharynx	3	2	0
Nasopharynx	1	0	0
Larynx	0	0	2
Other	1	1	1
Cumulative total	10	16	23

Table 14–7. Connective-Tissue Invasion by Nodal Stage

STAGE	NO. OF PATIENTS
NX	34 (21)
N1	9 (0)
N2a	15 (60)
N2b	6 (50)
N3a	9 (78)
N3b	4 (50)
Total	77 (36)

DISCUSSION

Less than 3 percent of head and neck cancers present as unknown primary lesions metastatic to the neck (Martin, 1944; Marchetta,

Table 14–8. Influence of Connective-Tissue Disease on Determinate Survival

	2 YR	5 YR
Present	71	66*
Absent	95	90

*$p = < 0.05$

1963; Fried, 1975). Comess reported, in 1957, that of 1189 cases of metastatic carcinoma of the cervical lymph nodes, 103 (8.7%) had unknown primaries. Of those patients with a neck mass as the presenting symptom in Martin's series (1944), 33 percent had no primary lesion found within 1 month of presentation. The proportion of squamous cell carcinoma in neck metastases from unknown primaries ranges from 14.5 to 86 percent in the different series reported (Acquarelli, 1961; Barrie, 1970; Coker, 1977; Didolkar, 1977; Fitzpatrick, 1974; Fried, 1975; Jesse, 1966; Jesse, 1973; Leipzig, 1981; Nordstrom, 1979; Pacini, 1981; Pico, 1971; Shaw, 1970; Spiro, 1983; Yang, 1983). Primary lesions remained occult in 84 percent of the patients in our series. Seventy-one of these 117 patients, however, were followed for less than 5 years—mainly because of death from disease or other causes—leaving 46 patients followed for more than 5 years who did not manifest primary lesions. Similarly, omitting seven primaries found more than 5 years after presentation leaves 16 primaries found within 5 years. This is a 74 percent incidence of occult primaries.

A compilation from several authors (Acquarelli, 1961; Coker, 1977; Comess, 1957; France, 1963; Fried, 1975; Martin, 1944; Smith, 1967; Spiro, 1983) of the proportion of primaries eventually isolated in squamous cell carcinoma neck metastases of occult origin is displayed in Table 14–9. The primary lesion was discovered in 11–54 percent of patients, discoveries that appeared to worsen the prognosis when all histologies are considered (Coker, 1977; Jesse, 1966; Jesse, 1973; Marchetta, 1963; Smith, 1967). In Commes' series (1957), 16 survivors (14 with squamous cell carcinoma) did not have their primaries found. In Spiro's study (1983), there was no difference in outcome as a result of primary lesion identification. In this study, the finding of the primary tumor did not affect survival, but did occur more in those treated surgically only. The previous report from UTMDAH by Jesse in 1973 aluded to a relative paucity of eventually found primaries in the irradiated-only cases (6% vs. 20% in the surgery-alone group).

The nasopharynx, base of tongue, and lung have been the most frequently reported sites of primary location, followed by tonsil, hypopharynx, and supraglottic larynx in those with originally occult primary lesions of the squamous cell type (Acquarelli, 1961; Barrie, 1970; Coker, 1977; Comess, 1957; Didolkar, 1977; France, 1963; Fried, 1975; Greenberg, 1966; Jesse, 1966; Jesse, 1973; Leipzig, 1981; Marchetta, 1963; Martin, 1944; Nordstrom, 1979; Pacini, 1981; Pico, 1971; Robinson, 1959; Shaw, 1970; Smith, 1967; Spiro, 1983). As Martin suggested in 1944, it is reasonable to allow a 5-year period for the appearance of primaries, distant metastases, or recurrence in the neck related to the original neck disease. As a recent report by Vikram (1984) shows, however, there can be a second primary development rate of 5 percent a year in head and neck cancer patients, especially in the lung and esophagus. It may be impossible to distinguish second primary lesions from occult primaries finally surfacing or from solitary lung metastases, but recurrences and primary tu-

Table 14–9. Survival Results for Patients with Unknown Primary Tumors Metastatic to the Neck of Squamous Cell Carcinoma

AUTHOR	NO. OF CASES	FOLLOW-UP (ANALYSIS)	SURVIVAL (%)
Spiro (1983)	79	5 yr (absolute)	50
Pacini (1981)	42	5 yr (absolute)	23
Leipzig (1981)	32	3 yr (absolute)	40
Didolkar (1977)	37	5 yr (life table)	14
Coker (1977)	39	5 yr (life table)	54
Fried (1975)	28	3 yr (absolute)	28
Barrie (1970)	104	5 yr (determinate)	31
Greenberg (1966)	16	5 yr (absolute)	0
France (1963)	19	Unlimited (absolute)	11
Robinson (1959)	9	Unlimited (absolute)	33
Comess (1957)	42	Unlimited (absolute)	33

mor appearances after a 5-year disease-free interval should be suspected as representing a second disease process.

It cannot be reiterated or stressed enough that a patient with a neck mass suspicious for cancer, whether already biopsied or not, must be extensively evaluated for an inapparent primary lesion. Directed biopsies based upon known patterns of cervical nodal metastases (Johnson, 1981; Lindberg, 1972; Molnari, 1977) should be performed if no gross lesions are demonstrable. Anti-Epstein-Barr virus antibody titers may be beneficial in defining occult nasopharyngeal carcinoma, especially IgA antiviral capsid antigen (Pearson, 1983). The skin should not be overlooked as a potential source of metastatic squamous cell carcinoma.

Only after exhaustive investigation has failed to reveal a primary lesion should material be removed from the neck mass for pathologic identification, preferably by fine-needle aspiration or wide excision of a discrete lesion. Incisional biopsy should be avoided. McGuirt (1978) suggested in his retrospective case-controlled study that pretreatment biopsy significantly increases the rate of distant metastases, as well as seeming to increase regional recurrence and wound complications. A recent study by Robbins (1985) offers evidence to the contrary, provided patients get prompt adequate treatment. The same was shown by Razack in 1977 who, using historical controls, found no difference in neck-disease recurrence or survival if prior biopsy had been performed. Distant metastases were not examined separately. In this study, no adverse effect of pretreatment biopsy was unequivocally demonstrated.

Survival results in several series on squamous cell carcinoma only concerning unknown primaries metastatic to the neck are presented in Table 14–10. Five-year survival ranged from 0 to 54%, and our results compare favorably with 55% 5-year actuarial survival when analysis was based on all deaths.

Reports of outcome by treatment for all histologies vary. In 1973, Jesse found no difference in 5-year actuarial survival between surgery and radiation alone. Some workers (Comess, 1957; France, 1963), however, have shown better results with definitive radiotherapy; others (Coker, 1977); Nordstrom, 1979) have shown better results with surgical extirpation. Nodal stage has correlated with outcome in all large series (Coker, 1977; Jesse, 1973; Nordstrom, 1979; Pacini, 1981; Spiro, 1983) in which this parameter has been studied. The N3b stage represents a heterogeneous group, and the results are probably determined by treatment for the side of the neck with the highest disease stage.

Table 14–10. Percentage of Primary Tumors Found (Squamous Cell Carcinoma Only)

AUTHOR	PERCENTAGE
Spiro (1983)	15
Coker (1977)	29*
Fried (1975)	39
Smith (1967)	54
France (1963)	11
Aquarelli (1961)	40†
Comes (1957)	40
Martin (1944)	23

*Including anaplastic Cancer.
†Six of 10 by autopsy.

Extracapsular tumor extension, an important histologic factor that adversely affects survival (Johnson, 1981), was more frequent in higher-staged neck disease in Spiro's series (1983). In our report, connective-tissue invasion was linked with both poorer prognosis and advanced stage of neck disease. Postoperative radiotherapy can reduce the recurrence rate associated with extracapsular extension, and certainly should be considered for these patients (Vikram, 1984).

Multiple level or nodal-area involvement has been associated with poorer prognosis (Pacini, 1981; Strong, 1969), and our data support this. Postoperative radiation may be able to eliminate the added risk incurred by multiple-level disease (Vikram, 1984). Supraclavicular nodal metastases yielded poor survival according to some reports (Jesse, 1973; Fitzpatrick, 1974; Yang, 1983), but this may be related to a higher relative proportion of supraclavicular disease in the adenocarcinoma patients (Fitzpatrick, 1974; Spiro, 1983). Didolkar (1977) and Spiro (1983) found much poorer 5-year survival rates for patients with adenocarcinoma (5% and 0%, respectively) than with squamous cell carcinoma (14% and 50%, respectively).

In our opinion, recommendations regarding treatment of squamous cell carcinoma metastatic to the neck with an unknown primary can be made based on the results of the present and other series. Patients with N1 and N2a stage disease can be treated effectively with either surgery or radiation alone. Surgery should be in the form of modified neck dissection, with judicious preservation of the sternocleidomastoid muscle, internal jugular vein, and accessory nerve. Patients with N2b and N3a neck disease that are operable should have a neck dissection, modified when possible. Postoperative radiation is indicated in patients with connective-tissue disease, more than two nodal areas involved pathologically, or likely residual microscopic disease.

Patients with lymphoepithelioma of the neck without a primary site should receive definitive radiation to fields including the nasopharynx and tonsillar areas, with surgery reserved for the few with persistent cancer. It is intriguing to note that no primary was ever found in the seven cases of lymphoepithelioma in this series, even though two patients were treated by surgery alone. Patients with advanced neck disease thought to be inoperable should receive radiotherapy, chemotherapy, or both, to reduce size and fixation and provide respectability. Curative radiation alone after complete response to chemotherapy may also be considered.

We must speculate about the tumor biology in patients whose primary lesions are never discovered, especially the 25 patients followed for more than 5 years who underwent only surgical extirpation of neck disease. The simplest explanation is that these secondary lesions arose in branchial-cleft remnants. This subject has been extensively reviewed by Batsakis (1979, 1981), who believed that most, if not all, reports of such branchial cleft lesions cannot fulfill the criteria for them set by Martin in 1950—namely: (1) The cervical tumor must occur along a line extending just anterior to the tragus, downward along the anterior border of the sternocleidomastoid muscle to the clavicle. (2) The histologic appearance of the neoplasm must be consistent with origin from tissue known to be present in branchial vestiges. (3) No primary lesion should be discovered for at least 5 years. (4) The best criterion is the histologic demonstration of carcinoma arising in the wall of a structure consistent with a branchial cyst. Certainly, the literature is devoid of series of branchial-cleft cysts that had microscopic foci of squamous cell carcinoma. The existence of branchiogenic squamous cell carcinoma has not been disproved, but it must be accepted only after it meets strict criteria.

Another theory to be entertained is the spontaneous regression of cancer at the primary site. The "seed and soil" theory of tumor cell biology (Fidler, 1982) could account for different antigenic subpopulations of tumor cells in the primary areas versus the metastatic areas, to allow for selective immunologic elimination of cancer at the primary location.

A review of spontaneous regression of squamous cell carcinoma (Everson, 1966) showed one case each of larynx, lung, and oral tongue. The laryngeal tumor reported was a true vocal-cord tumor, and "regression" could be explained by total excision of the tumor at the time of vocal-cord stripping biopsy. The right-lung squamous cell carcinoma regression was documented histologically and radiographically. Follow-up continued for more than 5 years, and clinical examinations and radiographs showed no recurrence. New lesions, however, were observed on radiographs in the left lung 5 years after initial biopsy. The third case—that of an elderly woman with a large ulcerated oral tongue lesion and bilateral cervical adenopathy—was presented as a letter to the editor (Roxburg, 1935). A biopsy was performed and read as "cancer," with no further specification of histology. After the patient refused operative treatment and the use of potassium permanganate mouthwash, the primary and regional disease disappeared "in a short time." The patient died 7 years later of pneumonia. There was no mention of an autopsy or the duration of continued head and neck examinations. Thus, only one satisfactorily documented case of spontaneous regression of squamous cell carcinoma is present in the literature.

Based on the many reported series of metastatic squamous cell carcinoma to the neck with never-discovered primaries, including the present study, we can hypothesize that there is a capacity for subclinical, small, perhaps microscopic foci of squamous cell carcinoma from upper aerodigestive tract mucosa or skin to regress spontaneously, and for subpopulations of cells with special metastatic potential to escape immunologic surveillance and manifest as regional nodal disease.

REFERENCES

Acquarelli, M. J., Matsimga, R. S., and Cruze, K.: Metastatic carcinoma of the neck of unknown primary origin. *Laryngoscope*, 71:962–74, 1961.

American Joint Committee on Cancer: Staging of Cancer of Head and Neck Sites, 1980.

Barrie, J. R., Knapper, W. H., and Strong, E. W.: Cervical nodal metastases of unknown origin. *Am. J. Surg.*, 120:466–70, 1970.

Batsakis, J. G.: *Tumors of the Head and Neck*, 2nd ed., Williams and Wilkins, Baltimore, 1979.

Batsakis, J. G.: The pathology of head and neck tumors: The occult primary and metastases to the head and neck, Part 10. *Head Neck Surg.*, 3:409–23, 1981.

Coker, D. D., Casterline, P. F., Chambers, R. G., and Jacques, D. A.: Metastases to lymph nodes of the head and neck from an unknown primary site. *Am. J. Surg.*, 134:517–22, 1977.

Comess, M. D., Beahrs, O. H., and Dockerty, M. B.: Cervical metastasis from occult carcinoma. *Surg. Gynecol. Obstet.*, 104:607–17, 1957.

Davis, R. S., Flynn, M. D., and Moore, C.: An unusual presentation of carcinoma of the lung: 26 patients with cervical node metastases. *J. Surg. Oncol.*, 9:503–7, 1977.

Didolkar, M. D., Fanous, N., Elias, E. G., and Moore, R. H.: Metastatic carcinoma from occult primary tumors. A study of 254 patients. *Ann. Surg.*, 186:625–30, 1977.

Everson, T. C., and Cole, W. H.: *Spontaneous Regression of Cancer*. Philadelphia, W.B. Saunders, 1966.

Fidler, I. J., and Hart, L. I.: Biological diversity in metastatic neoplams. Origins and implications. *Science*, 47:998–1003, 1982.

Fitzpatrick, P. J., and Kotalik, J. F.: Cervical metastases from an unknown primary tumor. *Therapeutic Radiology*, 110:659–63, 1974.

France, C. J., and Lucas, R.: The management and prognosis of metastatic neoplasm of the neck with an unknown primary. *Am. J. Surg.*, 106:835–59, 1963.

Fried, M. P., Diehl, Jr., W. H., Brownson, R. J., Sessions, D. G., and Ogura, J. H.: Cervical metastasis from an unknown primary. *Ann. Otol. Rhinol. Laryngol.*, 84:152–57, 1975.

Greenberg, B. E.: Cervical lymph node metastasis from unknown primary sites. An unresolved problem in management. *Cancer*, 19:1091–95, 1966.

Jesse, R. H., and Neff, L. E.: Metastatic carcinoma in cervical nodes with an unknown primary lesion. *Am. J. Surg.*, 112:547–53, 1966.

Jesse, R. H., Perez, C. A., and Fletcher, G. H.: Cervical lymph node metastasis: Unknown primary cancer. *Cancer*, 31:854–59, 1973.

Johnson, J. T., and Newman, R. K.: The anatomic locations of neck metastasis from occult squamous cell carcinoma. *Otolaryngol. Head Neck Surg.*, 89:54–58, 1981.

Johnson, J. T., Barnes, E. L., Myers, E. N., Schramm, V. L., Jr., Borochovitz, D., and Sigler, B. A.: The extracapsular spread of tumors in cervical-node metastasis. *Arch. Otolaryngol.*, 107:725–29, 1981.

Leipzig, B., Winter, M. L., and Hokanson, J. A.: Cervical nodal metastases of unknown origin. *Laryngoscope*, 91:593–98, 1981.

Lindberg, R.: Distribution of cervical node metastasis from squamous cell carcinoma of the upper respiratory and digestive tracts. *Cancer*, 29:1446–49, 1972.

Marchetta, F. C., Murphy, W. T., and Kovaric, J. J.: Carcinoma of the neck. *Am. J. Surg.*, 106:974–79, 1963.

Martin, H., and Morfit, H. M.: Cervical lymph node metastasis as the first symptom of cancer. *Surg. Gynecol. Obstet.*, 78:133–59, 1944.

Martin, H., Morfit, H. M., and Ehrlich, H.: The case for branchiogenic cancer (malignant branchioma). *Ann. Surg.*, 132:867–87, 1950.

McGuirt, W. F., and McCabe, D. F.: Significance of node biopsy before definitive treatment of cervical metastatic carcinoma. *Laryngoscope*, 88:594–97, 1978.

Molnari, R., Cantu, G., Chesa, F., Podrecca, S., Milani, F., and Del Vecchio, M.: A statistical approach to detection of the primary cancer based on the site of neck lymph node metastases. *Tumori*, 63:267–82, 1977.

Nie, N. H., Hull, C. H., Jenkins, J. G., Steinbrenner, K., and Bent, D. H.: *SPSS—Statistical Package for the Social Sciences*, McGraw-Hill, New York, 1975.

Nordstrom, D. G., Tewfik, H. H., and Latourette, H. B.: Cervical lymph node metastases from an unknown primary. *Int. J. Radiat. Oncol. Biol. Phys.*, 5:73–76, 1979.

Pacini, P., Olmi, P., Cellai, E., and Chavacci, A.: Cervical lymph node metastases from an unknown primary tumour. *Acta Radiol. Oncol.*, 20:311–14, 1981.

Pearson, G. R., Weiland, L. H., Neel, H. B., Taylor, W., Earle, J., Mulroney, S. E., Goepfert, H., Lanier, A., Talvot, M. L., Pilch, B., Goodman, M., Huang, A., Levine, P. H., Hyams, V., Moran, E., Henle, G., and Henle, W.: Application of Esptein-Barr virus (EBV) serology to the diagnosis of North American nasopharyngeal carcinoma. *Cancer*, 51:260–68, 1983.

Pico, J., Frias, Z., and Bosch, A.: Cervical lymph node metastases from carcinoma of undetermined origin. *Am. J. Roentgenol.*, 111:95–102, 1971.

Razack, M. S., Sako, K., and Marchetta, F. C.: Influence of initial neck node biopsy on the incidence of recurrence in the neck and survival in patients who subsequently undergo curative resectional surgery. *J. Surg. Oncol.*, 9:347–52, 1977.

Robinson, D. W.: The management of metastases in

lymph nodes when the primary tumor cannot be found. *Plas. Reconstr. Surg.*, 23:27–35, 1959.

Roxburg, D.: Spontaneous regression of cancer. *Br. Med. J.*, 1:39, 1935.

Shaw, H. J.: Metastatic carcinoma in cervical lymph nodes with occult primary tumor—diagnosis and treatment. *J. Laryngol. Otol.,* 84:249–65, 1970.

Smith, P. E., Krementz, E. T., and Chapman, W.: Metastatic cancer without a detectable primary site. *Am. J. Surg.*, 113:633–37, 1967.

Spiro, R. H., DeRose, G., and Strong, E. W.: Cervical metastasis of occult origin. *Am. J. Surg.*, 146:441–46, 1983.

Strong, E. W.: Preoperative radiation and neck dissection. *Surg. Clin. North. Am.*, 49:271–76, 1969.

Vikram, B., Strong, E. W., Shah, J. P., and Spiro, R.: Failure at the primary site following multimodality treatment in advanced head and neck cancer. *Head Neck Surg.*, 6:720–23, 1984.

Vikram, B.: Changing patterns of failure in advanced head and neck cancer. *Arch. Otolaryngol.*, 110:564–65, 1984.

Yang, Z. Y., Hu, Y. H., Yan, J. H., Cai, W. M., Qin, D. X., Xu, G. Z., and Wu, X. L.: Lymph node metastases in the neck from an unknown primary. *Acta Radiol. Oncol.*, 22:17–22, 1983.

PART FIVE:

CHEMOTHERAPEUTIC CONSIDERATIONS

CHAPTER 15

Adjuvant Chemotherapy in Head and Neck Cancer:

Critical Review and Prospects

Waun K. Hong and Isaiah W. Dimery

EDITORS' COMMENT

In the next two chapters, Dr. Hong and Dr. Dimery, members of the Section of Head and Neck Medical Oncology, Department of Medicine, University of Texas M.D. Anderson Hospital and Tumor Institute at Houston, identify the literature and report on both their own and others' experiences in the use of chemotherapeutic agents as applied to cancer of the head and neck.

Most of us will agree that this is the most confusing aspect of head and neck cancer—what is the appropriate role of chemotherapy in the treatment of head and neck cancer? We have all seen the patient with a dramatic response to chemotherapy: we know that it is an effective tool in some patients; we just don't know which patients. We all agree that the patient with N+ disease has a high risk of developing systemic disease, which in turn must be treated by a systemic therapy—chemotherapy. But there appears to be little agreement on when, what, how much, and how long drugs should be used.

At times, there seem to be as many permutations of treatment as there are patients. This is compounded by the fact that this treatment modality has an additional twist. Unlike surgery or radiation, which are almost always carried to completion by the physician, patient compliance is essential in order to obtain meaningful data from any study of chemotherapy.

In these chapters, the authors have attempted to make some order out of the wealth of literature on the subject. They have perhaps the most difficult task of any author in this book. Dr. Hong and Dr. Dimery note the historical data of single and combined agent trials when used as an induction adjuvant. They identify the fact that there have been few randomized, adjuvant studies large enough to account for the numerous variables, such as performance status, primary site, and stage of disease. In order to accrue enough patients, multiinstitutional studies must be used. The problems with initiation, bias, and uniform reporting inherent in these studies is known by all investigators.

Finally, any study involving an experimental treatment modality must ask the critical question—what is the effect on distant metastases and eventually patient survival? To this point, *no* studies have demonstrated a significant, reproducible effect on either factor. We await the answer that should come from work such as that presented by Dr. Hong and Dr. Dimery.

INTRODUCTION

The choice of treatment for head and neck cancer depends on the size and location of the primary tumor, the status of regional lymph nodes, and metastases to distant organs (Carter, 1977; Hong and Bromer, 1983). The effectiveness of surgery and/or radiotherapy in curing patients with relatively early stages of squamous carcinomas of the head and neck is well established (Carter, 1977). These treatment methods, however, have not provided adequate tumor control in patients who present with advanced local and regional diseases (Goldsmith and Carter, 1975).

Two-year survival rates in patients with stages III and IV resectable carcinoma range from 40 to 60 percent. Local tumor control remains a major problem because local recurrences occur in up to 40 to 60 percent of the patients and are the caues of death in approximately 20 to 30 percent of cases. Distant metastases occur in 20 to 30 percent of cases, and second primary malignancies also develop in approximately 20 percent of patients with head and neck cancer (Wolf, 1984). Multiple concurrently existing medical problems of patients with head and neck cancer may cause death in up to 20 percent (Wolf, 1984).

These unfavorable statistics, coupled with the functional and cosmetic deformities associated with treatment and tumor recurrence, have led to the clinical investigation of adjuvant chemotherapy for patients at high risk for local and distant recurrence (Tarpley et al., 1975; Wolf, 1984).

Until recently, chemotherapy was reserved for patients with recurrence of disease following surgery and/or radiotherapy (Bertino et al., 1975; Carter, 1977). Extensive prior treatment and poor performance and nutritional status of these patients predictably led to a poor response with chemotherapy (Bertino et al., 1975; Mead and Jacobs, 1982; Carter, 1977). Many studies have shown little survival benefit or symptomatic palliation for those receiving chemotherapy (Hong and Bromer, 1983).

Recently, several clinical trials have indicated higher response rates and longer response duration in previously untreated patients than in patients previously treated with recurrent tumors (Hong and Bromer, 1983). These observations are substantiated by the efficacy of chemotherapy prior to surgery in several animal tumor models (Burchenel, 1976; Forbes, 1984).

The rationale for theoretical advantages of chemotherapy prior to surgery and/or radiotherapy is: (1) increased tolerance of chemotherapy with better nutritional and performance statuses; (2) intact vascularity to the tumor beds; (3) increased killing of tumor cells in rapidly growing tumors and the potential eradication of subclinical metastastic disease; and (4) possible enhanced efficacy of local treatment by cytoreduction from chemotherapy (Tarpley et al., 1975; Wolf, 1984).

The possible adverse effects of induction chemotherapy prior to definitive treatment are: (1) delay of surgery from complications of chemotherapy; (2) inaccurate tumor margin because of dramatic tumor response; and (3) increased immunosuppression and potential increased risks from postoperative radiotherapy (Tarpley et al., 1975; Hong et al., 1979).

The large number of chemotherapeutic drugs active against head and neck squamous cell carcinoma, and the encouraging results of adjuvant chemotherapeutic trials in other types of solid tumors, have encouraged the design of adjuvant chemotherapy programs for head and neck cancer.

ADJUVANT CHEMOTHERAPY TRIALS

The selection of chemotherapeutic agents for induction regimens has evolved from experience in the single-agent or combination-regimen treatment of patients with advanced recurrent tumors.

Single-Agent Trials

Methotrexate (MTX) is considered to be one of the most active drugs in the treatment of squamous cell cancer of the head and neck. Recently, MTX has been used in moderate and high doses with leucovorin rescue to enhance the therapeutic index and to rescue normal

Table 15-1. Induction Adjuvant Single-Agent Chemotherapy

DRUG REGIMEN	INVESTIGATOR	NO. OF PATIENTS	CR* (%)	PR (%)	OR (%)
Methotrexate-leucovorin	Tarpley et al., 1975	30	0	77	77
Methotrexate-leucovorin	Kirkwood et al., 1981	23	0	52	52
Methotrexate-leucovorin	Taylor et al., 1978	32	3	37	40
Bleomycin infusion	Popkin et al., 1984	21	5	28	33
Cisplatin	Wittes et al., 1984	22	3	37	40
Cisplatin	Jacobs et al., 1978	18	6	34	39

*CR = complete response; PR = partial response; OR = overall response.

cells. Three nonrandomized pilot studies of preoperative adjuvant high or intermediate doses of MTX with leucovorin rescue have been published (Tarpley et al., 1975; Kirkwood et al., 1981; Taylor et al., 1978).

Bleomycin is an agent very extensively studied in head and neck cancer. The initial use of bleomycin was as an intermittent intravenous bolus push. Recently, an *in vitro* study has suggested the improved therapeutic index of continuous infusion of bleomycin. Therefore, bleomycin has been used as a continuous 24-hour infusion for 7 days in head and neck cancer (Popkin et al., 1984).

Cisplatin has substantial activity in squamous cell cancer of the head and neck. The nature of the dose-response curve for cisplatin in head and neck cancer has not been well defined, but intravenous doses of 80 to 120 mg/m^2 every 3 to 4 weeks are probably most appropriate (Wittes et al., 1979; Jacobs et al., 1978).

Methotrexate, bleomycin, and cisplatin have produced response rates of 40 percent, mostly partial responses. Few, if any, complete response have resulted from single-agent treatment; therefore, the role of single agents in induction adjuvant trials seems limited, although there have been at least six such nonrandomized trials reported, as summarized in Table 15-1.

Combination Trials

The experience with combination chemotherapy in the treatment of recurrent head and neck cancer has not been encouraging. Therefore, there has been a recent emphasis on the use of combination chemotherapy as the initial treatment prior to surgery and/or radiotherapy in advanced head and neck cancer. Cisplatin in conjunction with bleomycin infusion was perhaps the first combination induction regimen for head and neck cancer (Table 15-2).

Randolph et al. (1978) used cisplatin at 120 mg/m^2 on days 1 and 22, plus continuous bleomycin infusion for 7 days, days 3 to 10. A

Table 15-2. Combination Induction Regimens in Advanced Head and Neck Cancer

DRUG REGIMEN	INVESTIGATOR	NO. OF PATIENTS	*CR (%)	PR (%)	OR (%)
Cisplatin + bleomycin	Randolph et al., 1978	21	19	52	71
Cisplatin + bleomycin	Hong and Bromer, 1983	58	20	52	72
Cisplatin + bleomycin	Glick et al., 1980	29	0	48	48
Cisplatin + bleomycin	Israel et al., 1983	57	18	60	78
Cisplatin + bleomycin + methotrexate	Ervin et al., 1984	93	24	64	88
Cisplatin + bleomycin + methotrexate	Tannock et al., 1982	33	10	50	60
Cisplatin + bleomycin + vincristine	Al-Sarraf et al., 1981	77	29	51	80
Cisplatin + bleomycin + vincristine	Spaulding et al., 1980	46	23	65	88
Cisplatin + bleomycin + vincristine	Amrein et al., 1982	37	5	62	67
Cisplatin + bleomycin + velban	Perry et al., 1982	64	22	43	65
Cisplatin + bleomycin + vincristine + methotrexate	Schuller et al., 1983	58	28	38	66
Cisplatin + bleomycin + mitomycin-C	Israel et al., 1983	53	25	75	90
Cisplatin + bleomycin + velban + methotrexate + 5-fluorouracil	Krasnow et al., 1984	25	36	32	68

*CR = complete response; PR = partial response; OR = overall response.

71 percent overall response rate—with a 19 percent complete response rate—was noted in 21 patients with advanced head and neck cancer (Randolph et al., 1978). Since then, at least four nonrandomized studies have been reported (Hong et al., 1979; Hong and Bromer, 1983; Glick et al., 1980; Israel et al., 1983).

To improve the overall response rate, other agents have been added to the cisplatin and bleomycin regimen (Table 15-2). Mostly, methotrexate or a Vinca alkaloid has been added to form combination induction regimens. There have been observed response rates of 60 to 80%, 20 percent with clinical complete responses, which is clearly superior to results from single-agent trials (Ervin et al., 1984; Tannock et al., 1982; Amrein et al., 1983; Perry et al., 1982; Schuller et al., 1983; Al-Sarraf et al., 1981; Israel et al., 1983; Krasnow et al., 1984).

Recently, investigators at Wayne State University used a continuous infusion of 5-fluorouracil (5-FU) instead of bleomycin in patients with poor pulmonary function. The 5-FU, 1000 mg/m^2/day for 5 days, was added to cisplatin, 100 mg/m^2 intravenously, every 3 weeks for three courses. The initial report was very impressive, with clinical complete response attained in 54 percent of patients. Since that report, there have been reports of at least four studies of cisplatin with 5-FU; they are summarized in Table 15-3. Most studies conclude that this cisplatin and 5-FU regimen is an effective one, with fewer toxic effects than bleomycin in patients with head and neck cancer (Kish et al., 1981; Decker et al., 1983; National Cancer Institute pilot study, 1983; Krueger et al., 1985).

Table 15-3. Induction Cisplatin + 5-Fluorouracil Regimen in Advanced Head and Neck Cancer

INVESTIGATOR	NO. OF PATIENTS	CR* (%)	PR (%)	OR (%)
Kish et al., 1984	85	54	39	93
National Cancer Institute Pilot Study, 1984	20	35	50	85
Kies et al., 1984b	51	41	51	92
Krueger et al., 1985	17	35	35	70

*CR = complete response; PR = partial response; OR = overall response.

Other Combination Trials Without Cisplatin

Price and Hill (1983) at Royal Marsden Hospital in London have explored the use of a nonplatinum-containing regimen as the initial treatment for patients with advanced head and neck cancer. The regimen consisted of vincristine, bleomycin, methotrexate, 5-FU, and hydrocortisone given over 24 hours as induction therapy on days 1 and 14 and prior to definitive local treatment. Of 200 patients, 195 were assessed for response to chemotherapy on day 28; the overall objective response rate was 67 percent (131 patients), with mostly partial responses and only a few complete responses. The complete local control rate following local therapy was significantly higher in responders than in nonresponders to chemotherapy. Price and Hill have concluded that responders to chemotherapy live significantly longer than nonresponders, for all patients.

Randomized Adjuvant Chemotherapy Trials

Few adjuvant studies have been designed as controlled randomized trials, or have been large enough to account for important differences in patient prognostic variables such as performance status, tumor site, and stage of disease. In 1978, to determine the efficacy of the preoperative use of adjuvant chemotherapy in patients with potentially curable head and neck cancer, the National Cancer Institute initiated a multiinstutitional prospective randomized trial. A single course of combination chemotherapy using cisplatin and bleomycin was used as the preoperative regimen. Monthly courses of cisplatin alone were used as the maintenance regimen following surgery and radiotherapy. The overall tumor response rate was 50 percent, including a low complete response rate of 8 percent, which is no higher than complete response rates obtained in single-agent trials. During the design of this trial, a single course of chemotherapy was selected because of uncertainty about toxic effects that might delay or prevent subsequent treatment with surgery and radiotherapy. Overall survival at 2 years was 59 percent in the standard arm and 56 percent and 58 percent in the adjuvant chemotherapy groups (Wolf et al., 1984).

Taylor et al. (1984) also found that adjuvant methotrexate as a single agent given prior to definitive treatment yielded no survival benefit in head and neck cancer.

Holoye et al. (1984) at the Medical College of Wisconsin have reported that their prospective trial of induction chemotherapy using bleomycin with cytoxan, methotrexate, and 5-FU prior to radiotherapy and surgery did not improve overall survival at 2 years. Results of three randomized studies of adjuvant induction chemotherapy are summarized in Table 15-4.

SEQUENTIAL ADJUVANT CHEMOTHERAPY AND RADIOTHERAPY WITHOUT SURGERY IN ADVANCED HEAD AND NECK CANCER

Radiation therapy has excellent cure rates for patients in early stages of head and neck cancer. The results in patients with advanced, inoperable cancers, however, are very poor with radiotherapy alone. In an attempt to improve this poor outcome, adjuvant chemotherapy is currently being evaluated as part of a combined modality approach for advanced head and neck cancer.

Adjuvant chemotherapy has been given prior to radiotherapy to decrease tumor bulk and therefore to decrease the number of hypoxic cells. The sequential use of adjuvant chemotherapy and radiotherapy has permitted the monitoring and correlation of the sequential response patterns produced by each modality of treatment. Many investigators have observed that responders to chemotherapy can be predicted to have further response to subsequent radiotherapy. Conversely, patients who fail to respond to chemotherapy can be predicted to fail to respond to radiotherapy (Ensley et al., 1984; Price and Hill, 1983; Sheetz et al., 1984). Ervin et al. (1984) reported that patients achieving total or nearly total regression of tumor following chemotherapy alone achieve complete local control with radiotherapy alone without surgery. At least eight studies of such sequential induction therapy have been reported, and are summarized in Table 15-5.

Most investigators have identified subgroups that are more likely to benefit from adjuvant sequential chemotherapy and radiotherapy. That sequential chemotherapy and radiotherapy are capable of achieving a higher complete response rate than radiotherapy alone may have some impact on the management of advanced head and neck cancer.

TOLERANCE AND COMPLICATIONS OF SURGERY AND/OR RADIOTHERAPY AFTER INDUCTION CHEMOTHERAPY

In general, the toxic effects of induction chemotherapy regimens have been mild, or at least moderate and tolerable. Chemotherapy used prior to radiotherapy may result in increased normal tissue damage, leading to less

Table 15-4. Randomized Trial of Adjuvant Induction Chemotherapy

INSTITUTION	DRUGS	NO. OF PATIENTS	CR + PR* (%) (%)	METHOD	2-YR SURVIVAL RATE (%)
National Cancer Institute Trial	Cisplatin + bleomycin	411	8 + 40	S + R*	59
				C + S + R	56
				C + S + R + C	58
Northwestern University	Methotrexate	90	6 + 34	S and/or R	39
				C + S and/or R + C	37
Med. College of Wisconsin	Bleomycin + cytoxan, methotrexate, 5-fluorouracil	83	4 + 62	R + S	42
				C + R + S	28

*CR = complete response; PR = partial response; C = chemotherapy; S = surgery; R = radiotherapy.

Table 15–5. Local Control Rate of Sequential Induction Chemotherapy and Radiotherapy in Advanced Head and Neck Cancer

DRUGS	INVESTIGATOR	cGy	LOCAL CONTROL RATE (%)
Cisplatin	Schaefer et al., 1983	6500	(11/28) 39
Cisplatin + bleomycin	Hong et al., 1979	6–7000	(24/39) 61
Cisplatin + bleomycin	Glick et al., 1980	6–7000	(9/29) 31
Vincristine + 5-fluorouracil + methotrexate + bleomycin + hydrocortisone	Price and Hill, 1983	6–6500	(150/218) 69
Cisplatin + bleomycin	Coughlin et al., 1984	6–6800	(18/21) 84
Cisplatin + bleomycin + vincristine	Kukla et al., 1984	6–7000	(11/26) 42
Cisplatin + bleomycin + methotrexate	Tannock et al., 1981	5–6000	(13/33) 40
Bleomycin + methotrexate + vincristine	Figuero-Valles et al., 1982	6–7000	(16/38) 41

effective radiation-dose delivery. Pretreatment chemotherapy does not appear to intensify serious toxic effects of subsequent irradiation, other than in some degree of acceleration of mucositis and skin changes (Glick et al., 1980; Weichselbaum et al. 1981; Ensley et al., 1984; Tannock et al., 1982; Hong et al., 1979; Coughlin et al., 1984). The long-term toxic effects of chemotherapy and radiotherapy, however, need to be evaluated.

Surgery after induction chemotherapy has been accomplished without difficulty. Recent National Cancer Institute trials demonstrate no delays in surgery because of toxicity and no increase in surgical complications (Wolf et al., 1984).

IMPACT OF ACHIEVING COMPLETE RESPONSE WITH EFFECTIVE REGIMENS

High rates of complete response have traditionally been hallmarks of progress in cancer chemotherapy. Previous studies have frequently demonstrated persistent histologic evidence of tumor, at least in half the clinically complete responders, at the time of surgery, which indicates the need to have surgery and/or radiotherapy as the definitive treatment (Kies et al., 1984; Schuller et al., 1983; Decker et al., 1983). Several studies have also demonstrated an improvement in survival for patients achieving a complete response to chemotherapy prior to local therapy, compared with patients with partial or no response (Kies et al., 1984; Decker et al., 1983; Ervin et al., 1984). Whether the attainment of a complete response only identifies patients whose tumor biologically favors improvement, or whether the treatment actually contributes to the favorable outcome, is controversial.

CONCLUSIONS OF PREVIOUS ADJUVANT CHEMOTHERAPY TRIALS

1. Randomized or nonrandomized studies confirm the feasibility of preoperative chemotherapy without surgical complications and with a tolerable level of toxicity in relation to radiotherapy.

2. Primary tumor and regional node responses to chemotherapy were mostly correlated. Tumor response has been significantly related to T and N stages.

3. Substantial local control rates without increasing radiotherapeutic toxic effects have been achieved in advanced cancer with sequential chemotherapy and radiotherapy. The response to chemotherapy predicts further response to local radiotherapy.

4. Clinical complete responses in single-agent trials and in randomized combination-regimen trials have been less than 5 percent because of the use of ineffective regimens or suboptimal doses of drugs.

5. An increased complete response rate has been produced with more effective regimens, in particular a complete response rate of 35 to 50 percent with cisplatin and 5-FU regimens.

6. Achieving a complete response with chemotherapy improves overall survival, and is crucial because no tumor cells can be found in surgical specimens in half of these complete responses.

7. So far, several nonrandomized studies have demonstrated that, compared with conventional treatment, induction chemotherapy

as adjuvant treatment has not seemed to affect distant recurrence rate.

ONGOING CLINICAL TRIALS

There are currently several clinical trials of adjuvant chemotherapy in head and neck cancer.

1. The Head and Neck Intergroup Study. This randomized trial is investigating the value of postoperative adjuvant chemotherapy to surgery and radiotherapy in operable stage III or IV head and neck cancer. The chemotherapy regimen used is 100 mg/m^2 of cisplatin and 1000 mg/m^2 of 5-FU per day, continuously infused for 5 days every 3 weeks for three courses. Chemotherapy is being given following surgery and prior to radiotherapy.

2. The Veterans Administration Cooperative Laryngeal Cancer Study. This is a randomized clinical trial to determine whether induction chemotherapy followed by radiotherapy is an alternative to or improvement on laryngectomy and postoperative radiotherapy. The control group is receiving surgery and postoperative radiotherapy. The experimental group is receiving induction chemotherapy with cisplatin and 5-FU for a minimum of two cycles, after which tumor response is assessed. Patients showing no response receive surgery, followed by radiotherapy, and patients who show a response receive one additional cycle of chemotherapy, then radiotherapy. Patients who show persistent disease have a salvage laryngectomy.

The aim of the study is to investigate the value of sequential chemotherapy and radiotherapy in head and neck cancer. Any progress from this study would be a great contribution to the treatment of laryngeal cancer because the larynx would be preserved and the quality of life improved, even if the overall survival rate remained unchanged.

3. Adjuvant trials at UTMDAH. The first study is investigating the value of postoperative adjuvant chemotherapy in patients who are at risk for distant metastases. Any patients presenting with N2b, N3a, N3b, or N3c tumors are candidates for the study. After surgery and radiotherapy, patients will be randomized to either undergo or not undergo chemotherapy. The chemotherapy regimen is a combination of cisplatin and 5-FU for three courses.

The second study is investigating the value of 13-*cis*-retinoic acid to surgery and/or radiotherapy in patients who are at risk for local recurrence and second primary neoplasm. This study is a double-blind randomization trial. The dose of 13-*cis*-retinoic acid is 100 mg/m^2 orally, with treatment lasting 12 months.

FUTURE DIRECTIONS

The high rate of clinical complete response with effective regimens in previous trials suggests that chemotherapy will play an important role in designing future studies.

It is well established that patients who achieve a complete response to chemotherapy have overall improved survival rates. Therefore, the question is how to attain a higher complete response rate with new strategies. The previously established feasibility of induction chemotherapy indicates that intensive multicourse or noncross-resistant drugs could be given to improve overall complete response rates (DeVita, 1983; Goldie and Coldman, 1979).

Another possible new approach is the use of combined intensive regional chemotherapy and systemic chemotherapy to increase local control and to reduce distant metastases. Many questions regarding the selection of drugs, and the intensity, methods, duration, timing, and sequence of chemotherapy with respect to surgery and radiotherapy have yet to be addressed. Experimental treatment regimens must be rationally designed and rigidly controlled so that the analysis of accurate data will improve patient care.

REFERENCES

Al-Sarraf, N., Drelichman, A., Jacobs, J., et al. Adjuvant chemotherapy with cisplatinum, oncovin, bleomycin followed by surgery and/or radiotherapy in patients with advanced previously untreated head and neck cancer: final report. In Salmon, S., and Jones, S. (eds.): *Adjuvant Therapy of Cancer III*, pp. 145–52. Grune and Stratton, New York, 1981.

Amrein, P. C., Fingert, H., and Weitzman, S. A.: Cisplatin, vincristine, bleomycin therapy in squamous cell carcinoma of the head and neck. *J. Clin. Oncol.*, 1:421–27, 1983.

Bertino, J. R., Boston, B., and Capizzi, R. L.: The role of chemotherapy in the management of head and neck cancer: a review. *Cancer*, 36:752–58, 1975.

Burchenel, J. H.: Adjuvant therapy—theory, practice, and potential. *Cancer*, 317:46–57, 1976.

Carter, S. K.: The chemotherapy of head and neck cancer. *Semin. Oncol.*, 4:413–24, 1977.

Coughlin, C. T., Grace, M., O'Donnell, J., LeMarbre, P. J., Morain, W. D., Geurkink, N. A., and McIntyre, O. R.: Combined modality approach in the management of locally advanced head and neck cancer. *Cancer Treat. Rep.*, 68:591–97, 1984.

Decker, D. A., Drelichman, A., Jacobs, J., Hoschner, J., Kinzie, J., Loh, J., Weaver, A., and Al-Sarraf, M.: Adjuvant chemotherapy with cis-diaminedichloroplatinum II and 120-hour infusion 5-fluorouracil in stage III and IV squamous cell carcinoma of the head and neck. *Cancer*, 51:1353–55, 1983.

DeVita, V. T.: The relationship between tumor mass and resistance to chemotherapy. *Cancer*, 51:1209–20, 1983.

Elias, E. G., Chretien, P. B., Monnard, E., Kahn, T., Bouchelle, W. H., Wiernik, P. H., Lipson, S. D., Hande, K. R., and Zentai, T.: Chemotherapy prior to local therapy in advanced squamous cell carcinoma of the head and neck. Preliminary assessment of an intensive drug regimen. *Cancer*, 43:1025–31, 1979.

Ensley, J. F., Jacobs, J. R., Weaver, A., Kinzie, J., Crissman, J., Kish, J. A., Cummings, G., and Al-Sarraf, M.: Correlation between response cisplatin-combination chemotherapy and subsequent radiotherapy in previously untreated patients with advanced squamous cell cancer of the head and neck. *Cancer*, 54:811–14, 1984.

Ervin, T. J., Weichsalbaum, R., Fabian, R. L., Miller, D., Norris; C. M., Posner, M. R., Rose, C., Lockhart, P., Tuttle, S. A., MacIntyre, J. M, and Frei, E.: Advanced squamous carcinoma of the head and neck. A preliminary report of neoadjuvant chemotherapy with cisplatin; bleomycin; and methotrexate. *Arch. Otolaryngol.*; 110:241–54, 1984.

Figuero-Valles, N. R., Marcial, V. A., Velez-Garcia, E., Cintron, J., and Vallecillo, L. A.: Multidrug chemotherapy (vincristine-bleomycin-methotrexate) followed by radiotherapy in inoperable carcinomas of the head and neck. *Am. J. Clin. Oncol.*, (CCT) 5:399–404, 1982.

Forbes, J. F.: The biology of surgery and adjuvant therapy. In Salmon, S., and Jones, S. (eds.): *Adjuvant Therapy of Cancer IV*, pp. 47–54. Grune and Stratton, New York, 1984.

Glick, J. H., Marcial, V., Richter, M., and Velez-Garcia, E.: The adjuvant treatment of inoperable stage III and IV epidermoid carcinoma of the head and neck with platinum and bleomycin infusions prior to definitive radiotherapy: An RTOG study. *Cancer*, 46:1919–24, 1980.

Goldie, J. H., and Coldman, A. J.: A mathematical model for relating the drug sensitivity of tumors to their spontaneous mutation rate. *Cancer Treat. Rep.*, 63:172, 1979.

Goldsmith, M. A., and Carter, S. K.: The integration of chemotherapy into a combined modality approach to cancer therapy versus squamous cell cancer of the head and neck cancer. *Cancer Treat. Rev.*, 2:137–58, 1975.

Holoye, P., Kun, L., Toohill, R., Byhardt, J., Duncavage, P., Ritch, T., Grossman, T., Cox, J., Hoffmann, R., and Malin, T.: Prospective randomized trial of adjuvant chemotherapy in head and neck cancer. *Proc. Am. Soc. Clin. Oncol.*, C-712, 1984.

Hong,, W. K., and Bromer, R.: Chemotherapy in head and neck cancer. *N. Engl. J. Med.*, 308:75–79, 1983.

Hong, W. K., Shapshay, S. M., Bhutani, R., Craft, M. L., Ucmakli, A., Yamaguchi, K. T., Vaughan, C. W., and Strong, M. S.: Induction chemotherapy in advanced squamous head and neck carcinoma with high-dose cisplatinum and bleomycin infusion. *Cancer*, 44:19–25, 1979.

Israel, L., Aquilar, J., Soudant, J., Penot, J. C., Breau, J. L., and Morere, J. F.: Bleomycin and cisplatinum with or without mitomycin-C in 110 previously untreated patients with head and neck cancer. *Am. J. Clin. Oncol.*, 5:305–11, 1983.

Jacobs, C., Bertino, J. R., Goffinet, D. R., Fee, W. E., and Goode, R. L.: 24-hour infusion of cisplatinum in head and neck cancer. *Cancer*, 42:2135–40, 1978.

Kies, M. S., Gordon, L. I., Hauck, W. W., et al.: Analysis of complete responders after initial treatment with chemotherapy in head and neck cancer. *Otolaryngol. Head Neck Surg.*, 92:(in press), 1984a.

Kies, M. S., Percaro, B. C., Gordon, L. I., et al.: Preoperative combination for advance-stage head and neck cancer: Promising early results. *Am. J. Surg.*, 148: 367–71, 1984b.

Kirkwood, J. M., Canellos, G. P., Ervin, T. J., Pitman, S. W., Weichselbaum, R., and Miller, D.: Increased therapeutic index using moderate-dose methotrexate and leucovorin in patients with advanced squamous carcinoma of the head and neck: a safe new effective regimen. *Cancer*, 47:2414–21, 1981.

Kish, J. A., Ensley, J., Weaver, A., Jacobs, J. R., Kinzie, J., Cummings, G., and Al-Sarraf, M. (eds.): Improvement of complete response rate to induction chemotherapy for advanced squamous cell carcinoma. *Adjuvant Therapy IV*, pp. 145–52. Grune and Stratton, New York, 1981.

Krasnow, S. H., Cohen, M. H., Johnston-Early, A., Citron, M. L., Fossieck, B. E., Mauk, C. M., Yenson, A., Banda, F. P., Lunzer, S., and deFries, H. O.: Combined therapy for stage III and IV head and neck cancer. *J. Clin. Oncol.*, 2:804–10, 1984.

Krueger, S., Sheetz, S., Levitan, N., Yang, H., Karp, D., et al.: Cisplatin and 5-FU infusion as an induction regimen in advanced squamous cell carcinoma of the head and neck. *Cancer Treat. Rep.*, in press.

Kukla, L. J., Rao, V. P., Mantravadi, P., Applebaum, E. L., and McGuire, W. P.: Preirradiation chemotherapy for advanced head and neck carcinomas. *Arch. Otolaryngol.*, 110:78–81, 1984.

Mead, G. M., and Jacobs, C.: Changing role of chemotherapy in treatment of head and neck cancer. *Am. J. Med.*, 73:582–95, 1982.

National Cancer Institute pilot study, personal communication, 1984.

Perry, D. J., Davis, R. K., and Weiss, R. B.: Combined modality treatment with combination chemotherapy for advanced carcinoma of the head and neck. *Proc. Am. Soc. Clin. Oncol.*, 1:193, 1982.

Popkin, J., Hong, W. K., Bromer, R., Hoffer, S. M., Doos, W. G., Willett, B. L., Katz, A. E., Vaughan, C. W., and Strong, M. S.: Induction bleomycin infusion in head and neck cancer. *Am. J. Clin. Oncol.*, 7:199–204, 1984.

Price, L. A.; and Hill; B. T.: Integration of safe initial combination chemotherapy with a high response rate and local therapy for untreated stage III and IV epidermoid cancer of the head and neck. *Cancer Treat. Rep.*, 67:535–39, 1983.

Randolph V. L., Vallejo, A., Spiro, R. H., Shah, J., Strong, E. W., Huvos, A. G., and Wittes, R. E.: Combination therapy of advanced head and neck cancer. *Cancer*, 41:460–67, 1978.

Schaefer, S. D., Middleton, R., Reisch, J., and Frenkel, G. P.: Cisplatinum induction chemotherapy in the multimodality initial treatment of advanced stage IV carcinoma of the head and neck. *Cancer*, 51:2168–74, 1983.

Schuller, D. E., Wilson, H. E., Smith, R. E., Batley, F., and James, A. D.: Preoperative reduction chemotherapy for locally advanced carcinoma of the oral cavity, oropharynx, and hypopharynx. *Cancer*, 51:15–19, 1983.

Sheetz, S., O'Donohue, J., Bromer, R., Vaughan, C., and Hong, W. K.: Response to initial chemotherapy predicts complete response to subsequent radiotherapy in advanced squamous cell carcinoma of the head and neck. *Proc. Am. Soc. Clin. Oncol.*, 3:183, 1984.

Spaulding, M. B., Klotch, D., Grille, J., and Lore, J. M.: Adjuvant chemotherapy in the treatment of advanced tumors of the head and neck. *Am. J. Surg.*, 140:538–42, 1980.

Tannock, I., Cummings, B., Sorrenti, V., and the ENT Group: Combination chemotherapy used prior to radiation therapy for locally advanced squamous cell carcinoma of the head and neck. *Cancer Treat. Rep.*, 66: 1421–24, 1982.

Tarpley, J. L., Chretien, P. B., Alexander A. S., et al.: High dose methotrexate as a preoperative adjuvant in the treatment of epidermoid carcinoma of the head and neck. *Am. J. Surg.*, 130:481–86, 1975.

Taylor, S. G., Bytell, D. G., DeWys, W. D., et al.: Adjuvant methotrexate and leucovorin in head and neck squamous cancer. *Arch. Otolaryngol.*, 104:647–51, 1978.

Taylor, S., Caldarelli, D. D., Norusis, M., Showel, J. L., Hutchinson, J. C., Holinger, L. D., Murthy, A. K., and Applebaum, E.: A randomized trial of adjuvant chemotherapy in head and neck squamous cancer. In Salmon, S., and Jones, S. (eds.): *Adjuvant Therapy of Cancer IV*, pp. 89–95. Grune and Stratton, New York, 1984.

Weishselbaum, B. R., Posner, M. R., Ervin, T. J., Fabian, R. L., and Miller, D.: Toxicity of aggressive multimodality therapy including cisplatinum, bleomycin, and methotrexate with radiation and/or surgery for advanced head and neck cancer. *Int. J. Radiat. Oncol. Biol. Phys.*, 8:909–13, 1981.

Wittes, R. G., Heller, K., Randolph, V., et al.: Cis-dichlorodiamineplatinum (II)-based chemotherapy as initial treatment of advanced head and neck cancer. *Cancer Treat. Rep.*, 63:1533–38, 1979.

Wolf, G.: An overview of preoperative chemotherapy: Where do we go from here? *Am. J. Otolaryngol.*, 5:77–79, 1984.

Wolf, G., Jacob, C., Makuch, R. W., and Vikram, B.: Adjuvant chemotherapy for head and neck squamous carcinomas. *Proc. Am. Soc. Clin. Oncol.*, 3:182, 1984.

CHAPTER 16

Chemotherapy of Recurrent Head and Neck Cancer

Isaiah W. Dimery, Sewa S. Legha, and Waun K. Hong

EDITORS' COMMENT

Recurrence of tumor, whether at the primary or regional site, is a grim harbinger of systemic disease. Appropriately used, conventional therapy (surgery, radiotherapy, or both) can control most tumor above the clavicles. The very nature of recurrence following this standard therapy makes a statement about the virulence of this new, recurrent tumor, whether at the primary site or in the neck.

It is this difficult clinical setting that Dr. Dimery, Dr. Legha, and Dr. Hong address. By noting the patient, tumor, and prior treatment factors that must be considered when objectively evaluating the choice of drug therapy, the authors add more pieces to the puzzle of the role of chemotherapy and head and neck cancer. By way of a literature review, Dr. Dimery cites the use of the four standard drugs and combination thereof; through this, we can all have a glimpse of the magnitude of the problem. It is only by knowledge of the strengths and weaknesses of prior studies that we will be able to find the place of chemotherapy in the definitive treatment of cancer in the neck.

INTRODUCTION

Patients with relapse at the primary head and neck site, in regional nodes, or in distant sites after initial surgery and/or radiation therapy with curative intent are defined as having recurrent tumors. Advanced-stage squamous cell carcinoma of the head and neck is associated with a high recurrence rate of up to 60 percent despite aggressive surgery, radiotherapy, or both. Despite control of the primary lesion, distant metastases are noted in 20 to 30 percent of cases within the first 2 years after initial treatment. As reported from The University of Texas M.D. Anderson Hospital and Tumor Institute at Houston (UTMDAH), despite local control rates as high as 80 to 90 percent in advanced primary and nodal sites, distant metastasis eventually developed in 47 to 50 percent of these patients (Byers et al., 1979; Mesic et al., 1981). The most frequent sites involved were lung, liver, and bone.

There is an air of uncertainty about whether a "standard treatment" for recurrent disease exists and whether that treatment involves single-drug therapy or a multiagent chemotherapeutic approach. Chemotherapy has historically been regarded as only a palliative measure for end-stage disease not amenable to retreatment with surgery or radiotherapy, and therefore not regarded as potentially curative. The majority of patients live on average of 6 months once the tumor has recurred. Given this circumstance, the final evaluable goal of successful treatment is a substantial prolongation of disease-free survival with a minimum of toxicity. This goal has not yet been reached: we are not able to halt the natural and inexorable course of the disease with the drugs presently available.

A number of important factors determine the response achieved in this group of patients. Patient-related factors (performance status, nutrition, and immune status) as well as tumor-related factors (site of the primary, site of recurrence, previous treatment modalities, and tumor differentiation) interact and affect how the treatment is tolerated and what the outcome is.

A number of drugs have been identified as active in head and neck cancer. These agents are methotrexate (MTX), bleomycin, 5-fluorouracil (5-FU), and cisplatin.

Methotrexate is considered the "standard drug" by which responses to all other chemotherapeutic treatments are measured, both in degree and duration of response. A logical point of reference for our discussion would be the evaluation of MTX and MTX-containing combinations and the therapeutic value of these combinations in the treatment of recurrent head and neck tumors. A comparison of the activity of MTX with that of other agents should also be considered, with emphasis on the duration of response and survival. New concepts concerning the sequential use of methotrexate and 5-FU and of 5-FU and cisplatin in combination have been formulated. New chemotherapeutic agents continue to come into clinical use, and the impact of their clinical trials will be discussed.

Methotrexate

Methotrexate is an inhibitor of the enzyme dihydrofolate reductase. As a result, DNA and RNA synthesis is impaired. The drug can be administered either orally or intravenously. Absorption of the drug via the oral route is almost complete when doses up to 30 mg/m^2 are administered, but less well-absorbed at higher doses (Henderson et al., 1965).

A report was published in 1963 on the use of amethopterin administered orally or intravenously on a monthly schedule for recurrent head and neck tumors (Papac et al., 1963). Responses were minor (17%) and duration of response fleeting (1 month). When the frequency of administration was increased from monthly to weekly doses, modest increases in both response and survival were seen (Lane et al., 1968). Further refinement of the schedule to 60 mg/m^2 weekly led to an increase in the overall response to 60 percent, with 26 percent being complete responses (CR) (Leone et al., 1968). Despite this improved response rate, the median duration of response was not improved (2-4 months).

The use of high-dose MTX was made possible by rescue of normal tissues with leucovorin factor. Numerous trials have been performed with varying doses combined with leucovorin (Levitt et al., 1973; Capizzi et al., 1970; Frei et al., 1980), but few studies have demonstrated CR, and the 50 to 60 percent partial response (PR) rates again generally lasted 2 to 4 months. When conventional dose administration was compared with high-dose administration in randomized prospective trials, no therapeutic advantage was gained by increasing the dose of MTX to 7.5 g/m^2 weekly (DeConti et al., 1973; Kirkwood et al., 1981; Woods et al., 1981). Recently, it was shown that patients with a good performance status and without hematogenous dissemination could benefit from this type of aggressive therapy with high-dose MTX in terms of an improved duration of disease control (Taylor et al., 1984).

Comparisons of oral and I.V. MTX therapy demonstrated no difference in response (Vogler et al., 1979). There were, however, CRs to I.V. therapy but no proven benefit in survival. Systemic toxicity was somewhat higher when this drug was given orally (Papac et al., 1963; Vogler et al., 1979). Both mucosal and bone-marrow toxicity were greater, and drug-related deaths were more frequent.

In summary (Table 16–1), MTX delivered

Table 16–1. Methotrexate Therapy in Head and Neck Cancer

METHOTREXATE SCHEDULE (REFERENCE)	EVALUABLE PATIENTS	RESPONSE (%) (CR + PR)
Low-dose schedule		
(Pitman, 1984)	566	165 (29)
All-dose schedules		
(Al-Sarraf, 1984)	942	291 (31)
Moderate dose + leucovorin		
(Mead, 1982)	129	64 (49.6)
Methotrexate vs. Methotrexate + leucovorin		
(Levitt, 1973)	41	44 vs. 60
(Vogler, 1979)	154	22 vs. 27 vs. 33*
(DeConti, 1981)	151	27 vs. 25
(Woods, 1976)	72	26 vs. 26 vs. 45†
(Kirkwood, 1981)	49	60 vs. 50
(Taylor, 1984)	37	22 vs. 32

*Two-dose schedules of methotrexate vs. methotrexate + leucovorin.
†Three-dose schedules of methotrexate + leucovorin.

by various routes (oral vs. intravenous), schedules (daily × 5, weekly, monthly), and doses (conventional, moderate, and high with leucovorin rescue) results in few complete responses. The overall response rate averages 30 to 40 percent, with the response lasting only 2 to 4 months. Oral therapy, although convenient and inexpensive, is associated with increased toxicity. High-dose MTX involving a very complex protocol for its safe administration has not been proved worth the potential problems. Weekly administration of conventional dose MTX (40–60 mg/m^2) until the development of toxicity (mild mucositis or myelosuppression), then biweekly administration, seems to be the schedule that offers optimal response with minimum side effects. The brief duration of the response, however, remains a severe limitation on the overall usefulness of this drug in the palliation of the patient with recurrent disease.

Bleomycin

The bleomycins are a group of antibiotics isolated from *Streptomyces verticillus* and consist of 13 different species. Next to MTX, they are the most-studied agents in head and neck cancer (Table 16–2), and are approved for the specific treatment of head and neck cancer. The primary cytotoxic action of the drugs is scission of free bases in the DNA molecule, resulting in strand breaks. Cells in the G2 phase of the cell cycle are most sensitive to its cytotoxic effects (Evans et al., 1981). Its single-agent activity is in the 15 to 20% range, and can be given by the I.M. or I.V. routes and by bolus or continuous infusion (Bertino et al., 1973; 1975).

Because of its lack of myelosuppressive toxicity, bleomycin gained popularity in combinations with MTX and cisplatin. Its pulmonary toxicity, however, is a major limitation, and the cumulative dose must be limited to 300 units.

Cis-diamminedichloroplatinum (Cisplatin)

Cisplatin is a platinum coordination complex that has antineoplastic activity against a variety of tumors. Its activity in head and neck carcinomas has made it one of the most widely used agents in combination chemotherapy regimens. The exact mechanism of action of cisplatin is unknown, though it has been shown

Table 16–2. Use of Single-Agent Bleomycin in Head and Neck Cancer

REFERENCE	NO. OF PATIENTS	NO. OF RESPONSES (%)
Bonnadonna et al. (1972)		
Halnan et al. (1972)		
Haas (1976)		
EORTC (1970)	360	84 (23.3)
Durkin (1976)		
Yagoda (1972)		

to inhibit DNA synthesis, possibly by forming inter- and intrastrand cross-links in DNA, thus functioning like an alkylating agent (Zwelling et al., 1979).

In 1975, cisplatin was introduced and proved to have activity in epidermoid carcinoma of the head and neck (Hill et al., 1975; Wittes et al., 1977). As with MTX, there were many variations in the dose schedule and length of administration of cisplatin (Table 16–3). In the early study, 0.5 to 2.5 mg/kg I.V. daily for 5 to 10 days repeated after a few days resulted in a 23 percent response rate (Hill et al., 1975). Using two dose schedules of 40 mg/m^2 I.V. every 3 weeks and 20 mg/m^2 I.V. daily × 5 days on a 4-week cycle produced response rates of 33 percent and 27 percent, respectively (Randolf et al., 1978).

Monthly or bimonthly dose schedules in two Southwest Oncology Group studies yielded similar response rates (Stephens et al., 1979; Panettiere et al., 1980). Two studies by Wittes and coworkers (1977, 1979), in one of which the cisplatin dose was 120 mg/m^2, a 30 percent response rate was reported. Results of daily low-dose administration of cisplatin (20 mg/m^2 × 5 days) compared in a randomized fashion with a high-dose regimen (120 mg/m^2 × 1 day) given every 3 weeks were not significantly different, with overall response rates of 26 percent and 33 percent, respectively (Sako et al., 1978). These results were comparable with results obtained in other studies (Wittes et al., 1979). The variations in dose scheduling were attempts to modify and possibly prevent the usual gastrointestinal and renal toxicity, while maintaining the antineoplastic activity of cisplatin.

Table 16–3. Single-Agent Cisplatin Therapy

REFERENCE	NO. OF PATIENTS	RESPONSE (%) (CR + PR)	
Randolf (1978)	13	8	23
Hill (1979)	31	23	
Wittes (1977)	26	8	23
Hong (1983)	21	5	24
Panettiere (1980)	65	8	17
Sako (1978)	15*	6.7	20
	15†	13.3	20
Jacobs (1978)	40‡	8	10
Creagan (1983)	33	12	
Overall Response	242	24	

*Low dose
†High dose
‡Infusion

Further attempts at this goal resulted in trials of prolonged drug infusion: A 24-hour infusion schedule used in 18 patients resulted in a response rate of 39 percent and some reduction in gastrointestinal and renal toxicity; when only the patients with recurrent disease were considered, there was a 50 percent response rate, with minimal toxicity (Jacobs et al., 1978). Another trial with continuous-infusion cisplatin demonstrated a considerably lower response rate (13%) despite the fact that these patients, unlike some of those in the previous study, had not received prior chemotherapy (Creagen et al., 1983).

Response duration in all these studies averaged 4 months for partial response and 8 months for complete responses. The accepted dose of 100 to 120 mg/m^2 I.V. every 3 to 4 weeks with vigorous hydration or mannitol diuresis appears to be the most appropriate schedule to date. No clear dose-response effect has been demonstrated for cisplatin in head and neck cancer.

METHOTREXATE VERSUS OTHER SINGLE AGENTS

How single agents compare with one another is difficult to determine from the literature because few randomized trials exist (Table 16–4). In a recent study, weekly MTX was compared with cisplatin given on days 1 and 8 on a 4-week cycle, in an attempt to identify the best form of palliative therapy (Hong et al., 1983). Although response rates (23.5% vs. 26%), durations of response (84 vs. 92 days), and median survival (6.1 vs. 6.3 months) were similar, the toxicity associated with MTX was less, and the treatment was better tolerated.

COMBINATION CHEMOTHERAPY

With the antitumor activity of single-agent chemotherapy established, combinations of

Table 16–4. Methotrexate and Cisplatin in Head and Neck Cancer

REFERENCE (DRUG)	NO. OF PATIENTS	RESPONSES		
		CR (%)	*PR (%)*	*Total (%)*
Hong (1983)				
(methotrexate)	21			23.5
(cisplatin)	23	4.3	21.7	26
Jacobs (1981)				
(methotrexate-cisplatin)	39	15	18	33
(cisplatin)	41	8	10	18
Drelichman (1983)				
(methotrexate)	24	8.3	25.0	33.3
(cisplatin-vincristine-bleomycin)	27	11.1	29.6	40.7
Davis (1979)				
(cisplatin)	30	3.3	10.0	13.3
(cisplatin-methotrexate-bleomycin)	27			11.1

these agents were expected to produce superior responses. Small, nonrandomized studies were performed, but the data from these studies were difficult to interpret for two reasons: patient populations were variable in terms of the primary and recurrent tumor site, and prior therapies were variable including any combination of the following: surgery, radiotherapy, chemotherapy. The studies involved such a heterogeneous group of patients that the information obtained was rarely reproducible, thus, no "standard combination" has been established.

Methotrexate and cisplatin, as the two most active agents, have frequently been combined (Table 16–4). In a small randomized trial, high-dose MTX and cisplatin were given to 22 patients (data not shown): 12 received MTX-cisplatin; 10 received cisplatin alone (Jacobs, 1981). A 25 percent response rate (three PRs) was obtained in the MTX-cisplatin group, compared with a 10 percent response rate (one CR) in the cisplatin group. This trial was expanded, and for the 80 patients randomized between the two arms, 18 percent achieved a response with cisplatin alone, compared with 33 percent with MTX-cisplatin ($p = 0.11$), but without improvement in overall survival (Jacobs, 1983).

A comparison was made of cisplatin versus cisplatin, MTX, and bleomycin in 57 patients with recurrent disease (Davis et al., 1979). Again, no response or survival advantage could be demonstrated with the combination treatment. Other studies have also shown higher response rates without survival advantage (Baher et al., 1979; Kaplan et al., 1981).

A randomized trial comparing weekly MTX with a combination of cisplatin, oncovin, and bleomycin did not result in a statistically significant response to the combinations (40.7%) compared with MTX alone (33.3%) (Drelichman et al., 1983). Gastrointestinal toxicity was a major side-effect of the cisplatin-containing combination, whereas myelosuppression was more frequent and severe with MTX. Cost containment may be a consideration too: in the same study, single-agent therapy cost one-fourth that of the combination (Drelichman et al., 1983).

Early studies combining cisplatin and bleomycin for previously treated (chemotherapy) patients yielded only an 11 percent response rate (Caradonna et al., 1979). The addition of MTX in several trials (Table 16–5) produced some of the first significant CR rates—16 to 23 percent—with high overall response rates of 60 to 75 percent (Caradonna et al., 1979; Vogl et al., 1979). Those patients achieving CR instead of PR did have a significantly higher overall survival of 21 months. These response factors seem to be the major indicators of prognosis. A 50 percent overall response rate (12.5% CR, 37.5% PR) was obtained with a combination of cisplatin, MTX, bleomycin, and vincristine (Rozencweig et al., 1984). Response occurred within two courses of therapy, with CR occurring after a median

Table 16-5. Cisplatin Combination Chemotherapy

REFERENCE	DRUGS	NO. OF PATIENTS	RESPONSES	
			CR(%)	*PR(%)*
Randolf (1978)	Cisplatin Bleomycin	12	33*	
Perry (1982)	Cisplatin Bleomycin Velban	42	14	31
Williams, (1982)	Cisplatin Bleomycin Velban	66	2	18
Vogl (1979)	Cisplatin Bleomycin Methotrexate	31	23	39
Von Hoff (1981)	Cisplatin Bleomycin Methotrexate	22	27*	
Caradonna (1979)	Cisplatin Bleomycin Methotrexate	19	16	58

*CR + PR

of 13 weeks. The average duration of CR (28 weeks) was superior to that of PR (16 weeks). No data were given in this particular evaluation to substantiate any survival benefit.

Cisplatin Combination Therapy Without Methotrexate

Other cisplatin-containing combinations without MTX do not differ in response results from those containing this agent. Activity was identified for the cisplatin and bleomycin induction combination (Peppard et al., 1980; Spaulding et al., 1980). When used in patients who have relapsed or were previously treated, only a 30 percent response rate (10/33) was achieved with cisplatin 80 mg/m^2 by continuous infusion over 24 hours, bleomycin 15 units/day continuous infusion for 4 days, and vincristine 1 mg/m^2 I.V. bolus (Amrein et al., 1983). The median response duration was 4 months, and the median survival, 12 months.

Cisplatin, vinblastine, and bleomycin has not been proved to be distinctly superior to MTX, but it is just as effective (Perry et al., 1982). In a randomized clinical trial, patients responded equally well to MTX alone (16.2%), compared with the cisplatin combination (20.0%) (Williams et al., 1982). Patients with distant metastases responded significantly better than those with local and regional disease to the combination (43.5%) compared with MTX alone (9.5%).

It is generally believed that the site of disease may determine the response. Most studies do not address the question of differences in response in local or regional versus distant metastatic sites. This may not be possible because of the small total number of patients in the report or because of the higher incidence of local and regional failure. Several reports, however, do address this issue. In patients treated with MTX alone, there was a response advantage in local or regional (52%) versus visceral (6%) involvement (Deconti et al., 1981; Taylor et al., 1984). This higher response rate, however, did not translate into a survival benefit. For patients given combination therapy, metastatic disease was a poor prognostic sign, with 73 percent of the patients failing to respond to chemotherapy. A marked difference of both response to 5-FU and cisplatin (36% vs. 89%) and survival (24 weeks vs. 32 weeks) was described for patients with or without disseminated disease, respectively (Kish et al., 1984). In most studies, however, there does not seem to be a statistically significant difference in response. By comparison, other authors have reported that responses in diseases at metastatic sites were higher than those achieved at local regional sites (Williams et al., 1982).

METHOTREXATE COMBINATION CHEMOTHERAPY WITHOUT CISPLATIN

Using the principles of stem-cell kinetics and cell-cycle specificity, several combinations of chemotherapy were designed. A five-drug regimen consisting of MTX with leucovorin, bleomycin, 5-FU, vincristine, and hydrocortisone, with (schedule B) or without (schedule A) Adriamycin, was administered over a 36-hour period in sequence so that cells in all phases of the cell cycle were killed by at least one of the drugs in the combination (Price et al., 1978). This very intensive combination was given to 27 patients who had received prior radiotherapy; a 56 percent response rate resulted. This kinetically based approach was thought to be advantageous over the traditional multiday regimens in terms of bone marrow toxicity and the convenience of being given in a short period of time. The Adriamycin-containing regimen was associated with greater side effects without improving the response rate, and it was discontinued.

The most recent analysis of this regimen in 61 patients with recurrent or metastatic tumors using schedule A resulted in a 41 percent objective response rate (Hill et al., 1984). Ten of the 25 responding patients became operable, and were candidates for salvage surgery. Only eight of 30 patients with metastatic disease responded to chemotherapy, and none achieved CR. Those patients achieving CR had a median survival of 24.5 months, but they were only a small subset of the patients treated. The regimen was of no value in previously irradiated patients because 92 percent of all such patients treated were dead at 2 years (Hill et al., 1984).

There are other permutations of drug combinations that add little information. One study, however, compared the effectiveness of each drug in the combination of bleomycin (B), Cytoxan (C), vincristine (O), methotrexate (M), and 5-FU (F) by withdrawing each, one at a time (Holoye et al., 1978). There was a 48 percent response with B-COMF, a 59 percent response with B-CMF, and a 31 percent response with B-CM. The median survival for complete and partial responders were 42 and 35 weeks, respectively, in this nonrandomized but consecutively treated group of patients.

Toxicity was severe with B-COMF, but acceptable with B-CMF. It was reported that response was optimal and toxicity minimal with the B-CMF regimen, and the remissions attained were superior to those resulting from single agents. In an abbreviated version of this regimen, also based on the cell-cycle synchrony principle, bleomycin by continuous infusion was administered over days 1 to 3, with Cytoxan, MTX, and 5-FU all given on day 5 (Cortes et al., 1981). The overall response rate was 54 percent, and the mediam duration of CR was 11 months; that of PR was 7 months. The median duration of survival was 15 for the CR group and 10 months for the PR group.

This experience was comparable to that of Holoye et al. (1978), and seemed to confirm the effectiveness and relative lack of toxicity of a noncisplatin-containing regimen. Survival benefits were three to four times those obtained with single-agent therapy.

5-Fluorouracil

5-Fluorocracil is less active against head and neck cancer than the other agents mentioned. In order to exert its activity, 5-FU must first be converted to the nucleotide 5-fluorodeoxyuridylate (F-dUMP), which inhibits thymidylate synthetase and thus blocks DNA synthesis, or converted to fluorouridine triphosphate (F-UTP), which is incorporated into RNA and so interferes with its function (Heidelberger et al., 1974).

5-Fluorouracil has definite activity, albeit limited, in advanced head and neck cancer (Glick et al., 1980). A single-agent response rate of 15 to 30 percent in patients with recurrent diseases has encouraged the use of this drug in combinations where it appeared to be therapeutically synergistic and lacked overlapping toxicity (Gale et al., 1976). Continuous infusion of 5-FU at 1 gm/m^2 for 4 or 5 days,

Table 16-6. Cisplatin + 5-Fluorouracil in Recurrent Disease

REFERENCE	DRUGS	NO. OF PATIENTS	RESPONSES	
			CR(%)	*PR(%)*
Kish (1984)	Cisplatin 5-fluorouracil	19	37	53
Rowland (1984)	Cisplatin 5-fluorouracil	21	24	48

with ciplatin as a 100 mg/m^2 bolus on day 1, has been effective and well tolerated (Table 16-6). A CR and PR rate of 90 percent was obtained in patients previously treated with surgery with or without radiation therapy or radiation therapy alone (Kish et al., 1984).

A response benefit was shown for recurrent local and regional diseases versus metastatic disease (89% vs. 36%). The overall median survival was 27 weeks; for all responders, the median survival was 36 weeks, and the average duration of CR was 11.3 months (Kish et al., 1984). In a similar study of 20 patients with recurrent disease, only five (25%) had "objective responses" of short duration; they experienced substantially more gastrointestinal and bone marrow toxicity (Creagen et al., 1984).

SEQUENTIAL DELIVERY OF 5-FLUOROURACIL AND METHOTREXATE

Sequential administration of MTX and 5-FU, responses rates based on biochemical data supporting the concept of sequence-dependent synergy produced superior response rates (Table 16-7) (Heppner et al., 1977; Bertino et al., 1977; Cadman et al., 1979; Pitman et al., 1980, 1983; Ringborg et al., 1983). A schedule of weekly MTX at 125 to 250 mg/m^2 plus leucovorin rescue, followed by 5-FU 1 hour later at 600 mg/m^2, elicited an overall response rate of 58.1 percent in patients with recurrent disease (Pitman et al., 1983; Ringborg et al., 1983). A third study employing the same schedule was only able to demonstrate a 16 percent response rate (Jacobs et al., 1982).

The conflicting reports on response and toxicity in these uncontrolled clinical studies cast doubt on the biochemical relevance of sequence-dependent synergy (Browman et al., 1984). In an attempt to substantiate the importance of the order in which the drugs were administered, a randomized trial of the 1-hour sequential versus simultaneous MTX plux 5-FU was performed (Browman et al., 1983). In patients with recurrent disease, the sequential delivery of MTX and 5-FU (43% CR plus PR rate) was not superior to simultaneous treatment (67% rate). The combined response rate was 56% in both groups, the duration of response was 5.5 months, and the median survival was 15 months for the responders (Browman et al., 1983).

Another group evaluated the effectiveness of reversing the order of MTX-5-FU administration, again in a randomized study (Coates et al., 1984). Although the trend of response

Table 16-7. Methotrexate and 5-Fluorouracil

REFERENCE	NO. OF PATIENTS	CR (%)	PR (%)	TOTAL (%)
Ringborg (1983)	21	14	33	48
Pitman (1983)	23	13	52	65
Jacobs (1982)	30	3	13	16
Browman (1983)				
Sequential	14	14	29	43
Simultaneous	18	28	39	67
Coates (1984)				
Methotrexate-5-fluorouracil	35	11	40	51
5-fluorouracil-methotrexate	35	6	34	40

and survival favored MTX first and 5-FU second, this superiority was not substantiated by multivariate analysis; thus, sequence may not be an important determinant of response.

Despite the overall response rates of 50 to 60 percent in these clinical studies, median-response durations were similar to those of single agents. The median survival in some circumstances, however, was prolonged (11 to 15 months) in responders.

We conclude that combination therapy with MTX and 5-FU is generally well tolerated, with acceptable side-effects. Survival may be prolonged (11 months vs. 3–4 months) over single-agent therapy, but the total number of patients reported in the literature is small and longer follow-up is required.

SEQUENTIAL METHOTREXATE/ 5-FLUOROURACIL PLUS CISPLATIN

We attempted to incorporate several novel ideas into our approach to recurrent head and neck cancer by using the sequential administration of MTX-5-FU and adding high-dose cisplatin (Dimery et al., 1984). Sequential MTX at 250 mg/m^2 on day 1 was followed at 1 and 24 hours a days 1 and 2 by 5-FU at 600 mg/m^2. Calcium leucovorin at 6 mg/m^2 was infused at 24 hours, then every 6 hours for four doses. High-dose cisplatin at 60 mg/m^2 (age $<$ 60 years, Zubrod performance status 0–1) or 50 mg/m^2 (age $>$ 60 years, Zubrod performance status 2–3) was administered in a randomized fashion. Cisplatin was given either in 300 ml of 3 percent saline over 3 hours on day 3 and 4, or with physiologic saline hydration plus conventional mannitol diuresis to evaluate the effect of these delivery methods of platinum on the development of nephrotoxicity.

Of 50 patients in this study, 47 patients were evaluable for response and toxicity. They had an overall response rate of 44.7% (8.5% CR and 36.2% PR) and a median overall survival of 7 months. Median survival for responders was 11.5 months compared with 5.7 months for nonresponders; the median overall duration of response was 23 weeks. Toxicity reactions were mucositis, nausea, and vomiting. Hematologic toxicity consisted of anemia and leukopenia. Patients receiving mannitol diuresis had a lower incidence of nephrotoxicity (serum creatinine $>$ 1.5 mg/dL) than the group receiving cisplatin in 3 percent saline. Although the rate of response and overall median survival of 7 months was not substantially superior to the single-agent results, the median length of survival of those responding (11.5 months) was more durable, and that in itself is an encouragement to continue the multiagent regimens.

High-Dose Cisplatin

Cisplatin at doses of 100 to 120 mg/m^2 is considered high-dose; there is little information on higher doses, whether as single-agent or combination therapy for head and neck tumors. Thus, there has been no evidence for a dose-response relationship above this level until recently. Additionally, the safety of higher doses was unknown. At the University of Michigan, 10 patients with recurrent disease were treated with 40 mg/m^2/day in 3 percent saline $\times$ 5 every 4 weeks, plus hydration and furosemide diuresis (Forastiere et al., 1984). A 70 percent response rate was obtained (all PR), with neurotoxicity and myelosuppression being dose-limiting. It appeared that cisplatin displayed a dose-response relationship.

A pilot study was conducted, combining cisplatin at 30 or 40 mg/m^2 (depending on the patient's age) given for 5 days with 1000 mg/m^2 of 5-FU by continuous infusion over 5 days (Legha et al., 1985). Because we were unable to prove that hypertonic saline protected kidney function, only vigorous hydration was used. Thirteen patients with recurrent, measurable disease were treated. Seven patients received cisplatin, 40 mg/m^2 ($<$ 60 years of age), whereas six received 30 mg/m^2 (age $>$ 60 years of age) plus 5-FU, 1 g/m^2 by continuous infusion daily for 5 days. There were two CRs and four PRs, for an overall response rate of 46 percent, with six of eight patients (75%) in the higher-dose group achieving an objective response. Two examples of response are shown in Figures 16–1 and 16–2. The dose-limiting toxicity was mucositis and severe myelosuppression, which all patients experienced. Neuropathy was severe in five patients who received three or more courses of cisplatin, whereas nephrotoxicity was not a problem even at cumulative dosages as high as 850 mg/m^2. Thus, the results of this study support a dose-response relationship, but undue toxicity prohibits routine use of concentrations of cisplatin greater than 30 $mg/m^2 \times 5$ days (Woods et al., 1981; Legha et al., 1984).

INVESTIGATIONAL AGENTS

New agents continue to be investigated for their antineoplastic activity. Activity found in broad, phase I trials may lead to the investigation of more tumor-specific use of the agent. Few drugs are useful in the treatment of head and neck cancer, so a thorough search for new agents is mandatory if progress is to be made in the treatment of this disease. Table 16–8 lists some of the recent results that have evolved from these trials. Early responses to the drugs used alone or in combination with more familiar drugs are promising, but more extensive evaluation is needed to confirm them.

Biologic Response Modifiers

Patients with head and neck cancer show some of the most profound derangements of immune function, which seem to be altered even further in those who undergo irradiation or develop recurrent disease (Lichtenstein et al., 1980). These derangements include a decrease in the lymphocyte count, E-rosette-forming cell count, and T-cell count.

Attempts at reconstituting the immune system with various adjuncts such as bacillus Calmette-Guerin (BCG), *Corynebacterium parvum*, or levamisole have thus far met with failure. The combination of chemotherapy plus immunorestorative agents has not definitely enhanced response or survival in randomized trials (Zighelboim et al., 1979; Woods et al., 1976; Medina, 1983; Taylor et al., 1983).

One group of biologic response modifiers that has shown some promise is the retinoids. Retinoids are both naturally occurring and synthetic analogs of vitamin A. They possess several properties that make them potentially beneficial in the treatment of cancer: they increase cell adhesiveness and humoral and cellular immunity, inhibit cell growth, and induce cell differentiation (Lotan et al., 1980).

The retinoids have shown antiproliferative activity against human malignant cell lines, and were therefore brought to clinical trial as chemopreventive agents and for the treatment of recurrent disease. In an ongoing study at the University of Arizona, patients with locally recurrent and metastatic squamous cell carcinoma of the head and neck were treated with 13-cis-retinoic acid at 3 mg/kg/day (Meyskens et al., 1982). In a recent update, of 19 patients treated, three achieved PR, all in the skin or local regional sites, with a response duration of 3 to 4 months (Meyskens, 1985). These early results encourage the development of larger trials to provide more precise response figures.

DISCUSSION

The successful treatment of recurrent and metastatic head and neck cancer remains our major goal, which we hope will not continue to be an elusive one. Much progress has been made in developing drugs and drug combinations effective in palliative treatment of patients who are incurable.

Methotrexate remains the drug against which all other agents are compared. Cisplatin has equal activity, whereas bleomycin and 5-FU are used in a variety of combinations and schedules in attempts to improve the antineoplastic activity. Although single-agent methotrexate is less expensive and easier to administer than combination chemotherapy, which often requires hospitalization, improved response and survival can be demonstrated in individuals who respond to combination chemotherapy treatment.

Because of the heterogeneity of the disease and the patient population that is treated, there is a need for a continuing effort to com-

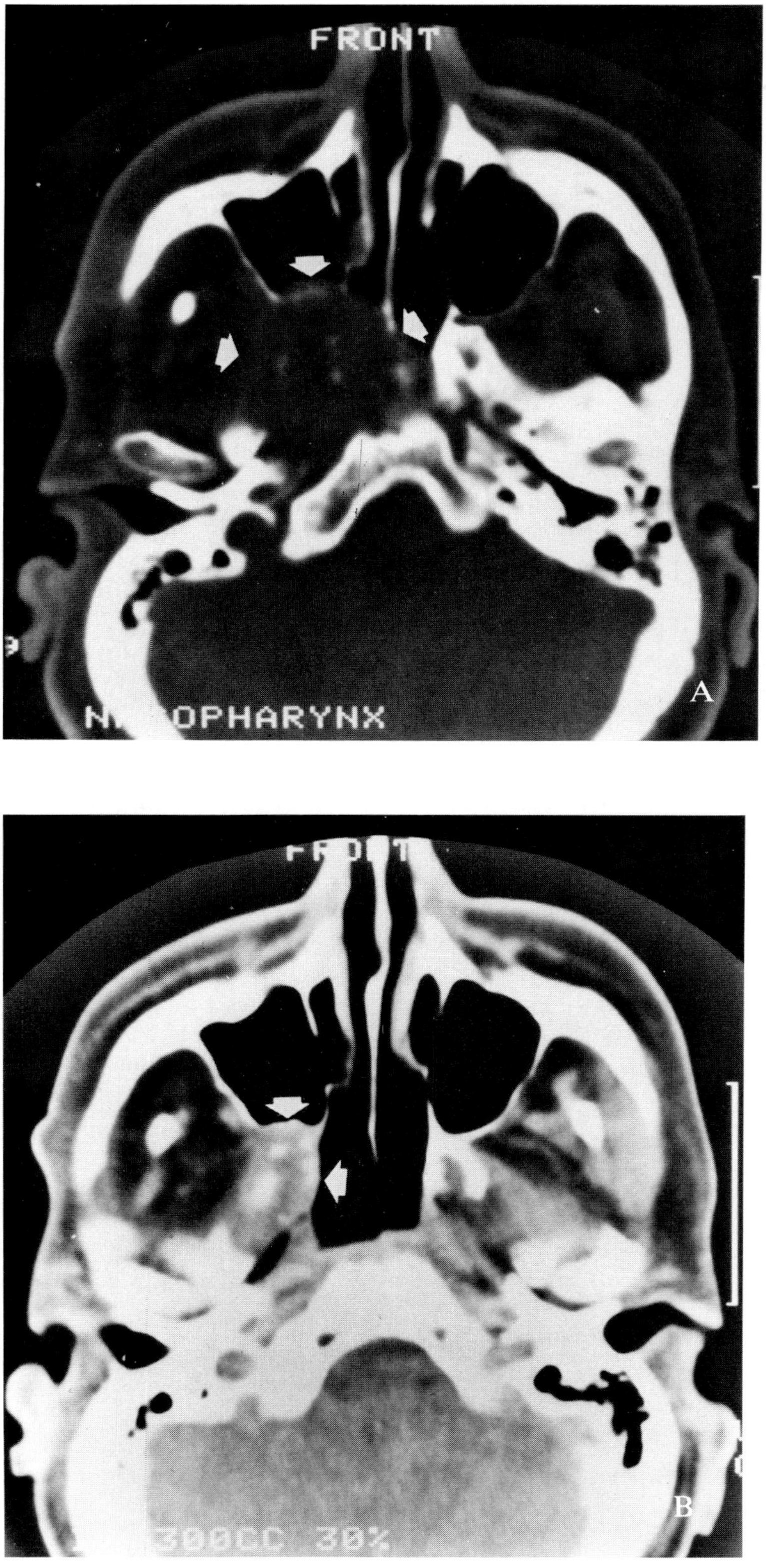

Figure 16–1. Locally recurrent nasopharyngeal carcinoma. (*A*) Prior to treatment. (*B*) After two courses of high-dose cisplatin and 5-FU.

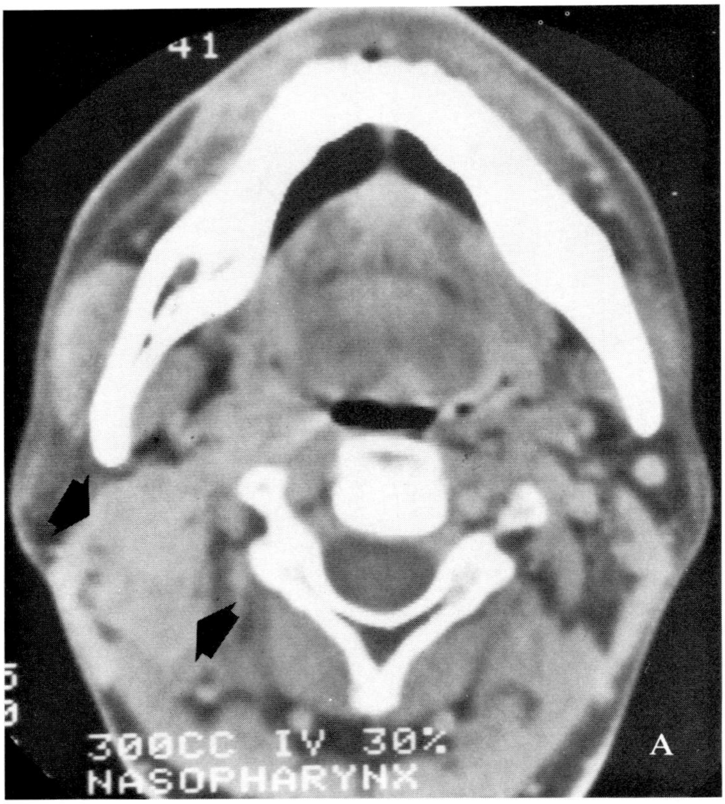

Figure 16-2. Regionally recurrent nasopharyngeal carcinoma. (*A*) Prior to treatment.

pare therapies in a randomized fashion and to stratify the entrants in terms of important prognostic factors such as performance status, previous therapy, and the presence or absence of distant metastasis. The choices of treatment available are unfortunately few for the patient with recurrent diseases. It is therefore imperative that newer chemotherapeutic agents be identified through broad phase I trials, and that specific activity in head and neck tumors be identified in phase II trials.

The activity of immunorestorative agents or

Table 16-8. New Agents in Head and Neck Cancer

AGENT	REFERENCE	RESPONDING	PATIENTS (%)
Prospidin	Frei et al. (1980)	4/15	26.6
Gallium nitrate	Creagan et al. (1985)	0/16	0
4′-epi-doxorubicin	Lichtenstein et al. (1980)	3/28 (PRs)	10.7
Diaziquone (AZQ)	Creagan et al. (1984)	0/28	0
Razoxane	Rowland et al. (1984)	2/21	9.5
Thioproline	Baccardo et al. (1982)	1/16	6.2
Mitoguazone (methyl-G)	Perry et al. (1983)	9/22 (2 CRs)	41
Vindesine	Popkin et al. (1980)	4/16 (1 CR)	25
Dichloromethotrexate + Cisplatin	Taylor et al. (1983)	13/24 (6 CRs)	54
PCNU	Dimery et al. (1984)	0/29	0
Homoharringtonine	Ajani, et al. (1985)	0/16	0

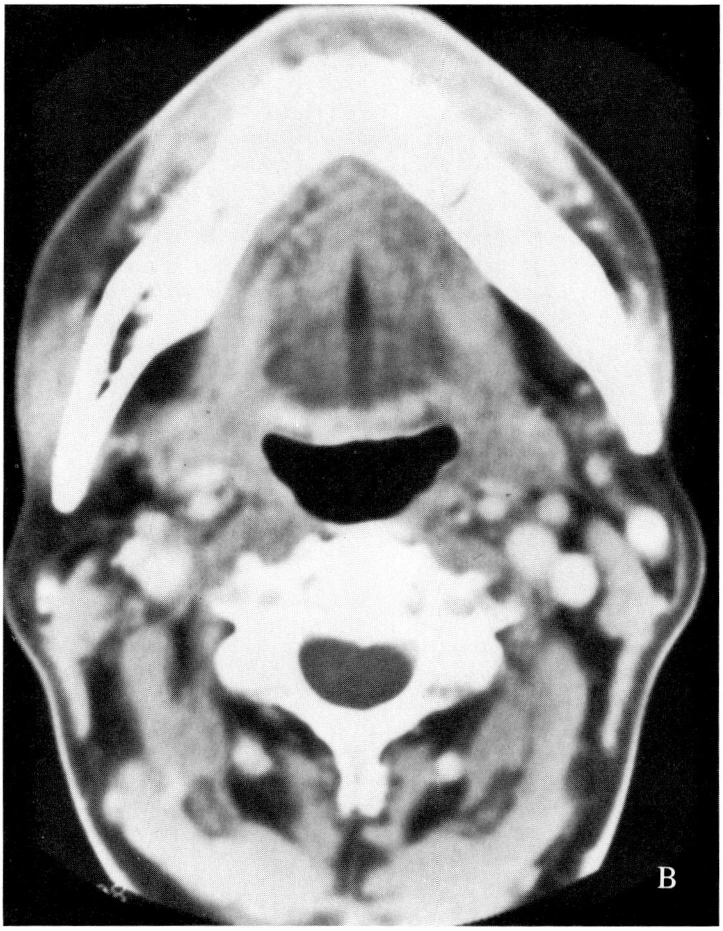

Figure 16–2 (cont.). (*B*) After two courses of high-dose cisplatin and 5-FU.

biologic response modifiers has not been adequately evaluated. Perhaps the combination of existing agents with newer agents or biologic response modifiers will improve results. Only with a continued intensive effort from clinicians and researchers are advances in this area likely to be made.

REFERENCES

Ajani, J. A., Dimery, I. W., Benjamin, R. S., Pinnamaneni, K. I., Legha, S. S., and Krakoff, I. H.: Phase II studies of homoharringtonine (NSC 141633) in patients with advanced malignant melanoma, sarcoma, head and neck carcinomas, breast, and colorectal carcinomas. Accepted in *Cancer Treat. Rep.*

Al-Sarraf, M.: Chemotherapy strategies in squamous cell carcinoma of the head and neck. *CRC Critical Reviews in Oncology/Hematology*, 1:323–54, 1984.

Amer, M. H., Al-Sarraf, M., and Vartkervicius, V. K.: Factors that affect response to chemotherapy and survival of patients with advanced head and neck cancer. *Cancer*, 43:2202–6, 1979.

Amrein, P. C., Fingert, H., and Wertzman, S. A.: Cisplatin-vincristine-bleomycin therapy in squamous cell carcinoma of the head and neck. *J. Clin. Oncol.*, 7:421–27, 1983.

Baker, L., and Al-Sarraf, M.: A comparative trial of cisplatinum (C), oncovin (O), and bleomycin (B) versus methotrexate (M) in patients with advanced epidermoid carcinoma of the head and neck (abstract). *Proc. Am. Assoc. Cancer Res. Am. Soc. Clin. Oncol*, 20:202, 1979.

Bertino, J. R., Boston, B., and Capizzi, R. L.: The role of chemotherapy in the management of cancer of the head and neck: a review. *Cancer*, 36:752–8, 1978.

Bertino, J. R., Mosher, M. D., and DeConti, R. C.: Chemotherapy of cancer of the head and neck. *Cancer*, 31:1141–49, 1973.

Bertino, J. R., Sawicki, W. L., and Linquist, C.: Schedule-dependent antitumor effect of methotrexate and 5-fluorouracil. *Cancer Res.*, 27:327–28, 1977.

Boccardo, F., Barbieri, A., Canobbiol, L., Guarneri, D., Merlano, M., and Rosso R.: Phase II trial of thioproline in advanced epidermoid head and neck tumors. *Cancer Treat. Rep.*, 3:585–86, 1982.

Bonadonna, G., DeLana, M., Monfardini, S., Bartoli, C., Bajetta, E., Baretta, G., and Fossati-Belani, F., Clinical trials with bleomycin in lymphomas and in solid tumors. *Eur. J. Cancer*, 8:205–15, 1972.

Browman, G. P.: Clinical applications of the concepts of methotrexate plus 5-FU sequence-dependent "synergy": how good is the evidence? *Cancer Treat Rep.* 68:465–69, 1984.

Browman, G. P., Archibald, S. D., Young, J. E. M., Hyryniuk, W. M., Russell, R., Kiehl, K., and Levine, M. N.: Prospective randomized trial of one-hour sequential versus simultaneous methotrexate plus 5-fluorouracil in advanced and recurrent squamous cell head and neck cancer. *J. Clin. Oncol.*, 12:787–92, 1983.

Cadman, E., Heimer, R., and Davis, L.: Enhanced 5-fluorouracil nucleotide formation after methotrexate administration: Explanation for drug syngergism. *Science*, 205:1135–37, 1979.

Capizzi, R. L., DeConti, R. C., Marsh, J. C., and Bertino, J. R.: Methotrexate therapy of head and neck cancer: improvement in therapeutic index by the use of leucovorin "rescue." *Cancer Res.*, 30:1782–88, 1970.

Caradonna, R., Paladine, W., Ruckdeschel, J. C., Goldstein, J. C., Olson, J. E., Jaski, J. W.; Silvers, S. A., Hillinger, S., and Horton, J.: Methotrexate, bleomycin, and high-dose cis-diamminedichloroplatinum (II) in the treatment of advanced epidermoid carcinoma of the head and neck. *Cancer Treat. Rep.*, 63:489–91, 1979.

Chuiten, D., Vogl, S. E., Kaplan, B. H., and Greenwald, E.: Effective outpatient combination chemotherapy for advanced cancer of the head and neck. *Surg. Gynecol. Obstet.*, 151:659–62, 1980.

Clinical Screening Cooperative Group of the European Organization for Research on Treatment of Cancer: Study of the clinical efficiency of bleomycin in human cancer. *Br. Med. J.*, 2:643–45, 1970.

Coates, A. S., Tattersall, M. H. N., Swanson, C., Hedley, D., Fox, R. M., and Raghavan, D.: Combination therapy with methotrexate and 5-fluorouracil: A prospective randomized clinical trial of order of administration. *J. Clin. Onc.*, 7:756–61, 1984.

Cortes, E. P., Kalra, J., Amin, V. C., Attie, J., Eisenbud, L., Khafif, R., Wolk, D., Aral, I., Sciubba, J., Akbiyik, N., and Heller, K.: Chemotherapy for head and neck cancer relapsing after radiotherapy. *Cancer*, 47: 1966–70, 1981.

Creagan, E. T., Ingle, J. N., Schutt, A. J., and O'Fallon, J. R.: A phase II study of cis-diamminedichloroplatinum and 5-fluorouracil in advanced upper aerodigestive neoplasms. *Head Neck Surg.*, 6:1010–23, 1984.

Creagan, E. T., O'Fallon, J. R., Woods, J. E., Ingle, J. N., Schutt, A. J., and Nichols, W. C.: Cis-diamminedichloroplatinum (II) administered by 24-hour infusion in the treatment of patients with advanced upper aerodigestive cancer. *Cancer*, 51:2020–23, 1983.

Creagan, E. T., Long, H. J., Kvols, L. K., Edmonson, J. H., and O'Fallon, J. R.: Phase II trial of diaziquone in advanced upper aerodigestive cancer. *Cancer Treat. Rep.*, 1:141, 1985.

Davis, S., and Kessler W.: Randomized comparison of cis-diamminedichloroplatinum versus cis-diamminedichloroplatinum, methotrexate, and bleomycin in recurrent squamous cell carcinoma of the head and neck. *Cancer Chemother. Pharmacol.*, 3:57–9, 1979.

Decker, D. A., Costanzi, J. J., McCracken, J. D., and Baker, L. H.: Evaluation of gallium nitrate in metastatic or locally recurrent squamous cell carcinoma of the head and neck: A southwest oncology group study. *Cancer Treat. Rep.*, 7/8:1047–48, 1984.

DeConti, R. C., and Schoenfeld, D.: A randomized prospective comparison of intermittent methotrexate, methotrexate with leucovorin, and a methotrexate combination in head and neck cancer. *Cancer*, 48: 1061–72, 1981.

Dimery, I., Legha, S., and Goepfert, H.: Phase II trial of MTX, 5-FU, and cisplatin in recurrent head and neck squamous carcinoma (HNSC). *Am. Soc. Clin. Oncol.*, 3:184, 1984.

Dimery, I. W., Legha, S. S., Murphy, W. K., Moran, M. E., Stewart, D. J., Goepfert, H., and Bodey, G. P.: Phase II study of PCNU in the treatment of head and neck carcinoma. *Cancer Treat. Rep.*, 68:437–38, 1984.

Drelichman, A., Cummings, G., and Al-Sarraf, M.: A randomized trial of the combination of cisplatinum, oncovin, and bleomycin (COB) versus methotrexate in patients with advanced squamous cell carcinoma of the head and neck. *Cancer*, 52:399–403, 1983.

Durkin, W. J., Pugh, R. P., Jacobs, E., Sadoff, L., Pajak, T., and Bateman, J. R.: Bleomycin (NSC-125066) therapy of responsive solid tumors. *Oncology*, 33:260–64, 1976.

Evans, W. E., Yee, G. C., Crom, W. R., Pratt, C. B., and Green, A. A.: Clinical pharmacology of bleomycin and cisplatin. *Head Neck Surg.*, 4:98–110, 1981.

Forastiere, A. A., Crain, S. M., Callahan, K., VanEcho, D., Mattox, D., VonHoff, D. D., and Wiernik, P. H.: Phase II trial of aziridnylbenzoquinone (AZQ) in head and neck cancer. *Cancer Treat. Rep.*, 12:2097–98, 1982.

Forastiere, A. A., Wolf, G. T., and Medvec, B. R.: Treatment of head and neck cancer with high-dose cisplatin in hypertonic saline. *Clin Res.* 32:765A, 1984.

Frei, E. III, Blum, R. H., and Pitman, S. W.: High-dose methotrexate with leucovorin rescue. Rationale and spectrum of antitumor activity. *Am. J. Med.* 68:370–76, 1980.

Gale, G. R., Atkins, L. M., Meischen, S. J., Smith, A. B., and Walker, E. M., Jr.: Combination chemotherapy of L1210 leukemia with platinum compound and cyclophosphamide plus other selected antineoplastic agents. *J. Nat. Cancer Inst.*, 57:1363–66, 1976.

Glick, J. H., Zehnegebot, L. M., and Taylor, S. G., IV: Chemotherapy for squamous cell carcinoma of the head and neck: A progress report. *Am. J. Otolaryngol.*, 1:306–23, 1980.

Grohn, P., Heinonem, E., Appelqvist, P., Hajba, A., Holopainen, E., Paavolainen, M., and Palva, T.: Prospidin chemotherapy in recurrent head and neck carcinoma: A phase II study. *Cancer Treat. Rep.*, 6:915–16, 1984.

Haas, C. D., Coltman, C. A., Jr., Gottlieb, J. A., Haut, A., Luce, J. K., Tally, R. W., Samal, B., Wilson, H. E., and Hoogstraten, B.: Phase II evaluation of bleomycin: A Southwest Oncology Group Study. *Cancer*, 30:8–12, 1976.

Halnan, K. E., Bleehen, N. M., Brewin, T. B., Deeley, T. J., Harrison, D. F. N., Howland, C., Kunkler, P. B., Ritchie, G. L., Wiltshaw, E., and Todd, I. D. H.: Early clinical experience with bleomycin in the United Kingdom in a series of 105 patients. *Brit. Med. J.*, 4:635–38, 1972.

Heidelberger, C.: Fluorinated pyrimidines and their nucleosides. Sartoreilli and Johns (eds.), In *Handbook of Experimental Pharmacology*, pp. 193–231. Springer-Verlag, New York, 1974.

Henderson, E. S., Adamson, R. H., and Olverio, V. T.: The metabolic fate of tritiated methotrexate-II. Absorption and excretion in man. *Cancer Res.*, 25:1018–24, 1965.

Heppner, G. H., and Calabresi P.: Effect of sequences of administration of methotrexate, leucovorin, and 5-fluorouracil on mammary tumor growth and survival in syngenic C3H mice. *Cancer Res.*, 37:4580–83, 1977.

Hill, B. T., Shaw, H. J., Dalley, V. M., and Price, L. A.: 24-hour combination chemotherapy without cisplatin in patients with recurrent or metastatic head and neck cancer. *Am. J. Clin. Oncol.*, (CCT) 7:335–40, 1984.

Hill, J. M., Loeb, E., and Maclellam, A.: Clinical studies of platinum coordination compounds in the treatment of various malignant diseases. *Cancer Chemother. Rep.* 59:647, 1979.

Holoye, P. Y., Byers, R. M., Gard, D. A., Goepfert, H., Guillamondequi, O. M., and Jesse, R. H.: Combination chemotherapy of head and neck cancer. *Cancer*, 42:1661–69, 1978.

Hong, W. K., Schaefer, S., Issel, B., Cummings, C., Luedke, D., Bromer, R., Fofonoff, S., D'Aoust, J., Shapshay, S., Welch, J., Levin, E., Vincent, M., Vaughan, C., and Strong, S.: A prospective randomized trial of methotrexate versus cisplatin in the treatment of recurrent squamous cell carcinoma of the head and neck. *Cancer*, 52:206–10, 1983.

Hong, W. K., Shapshay, S. M., Bhutani, R., Craft, M. L., Ucmakli, A., Yamaguchi, K. T., Vaughan, C. W., and Strong, M. S.: Induction chemotherapy in advanced squamous head and neck carcinoma with high-dose cisplatinum and bleomycin infusion. *Cancer*, 44:19–25, 1975.

Jacobs, C.: High dose methotrexate and cis-platinum in the treatment of recurrent head and neck cancer: Recent results. *Cancer Res.*, 76:290–95, 1981.

Jacobs, C.: Use of methotrexate and 5-FU for recurrent head and neck cancer. *Cancer Treat. Rep.* 66:1925–28, 1982.

Jacobs, C., Bertino, J. R., Goffinet, D. R., Fee, W. E., and Goods, R. L.: 24-hour infusion of cis-platinum in head and neck cancers. *Cancer*, 42:2135-40, 1978.

Jacobs, C., Meyers, F., Hendrickson, C., Kohler, M., and Carter, S.: A randomized phase III study of cisplatin with or without methotrexate for recurrent squamous cell carcinoma of the head and neck. *Cancer*, 52:1563–69, 1983.

Kaplan, B. H., Schoenfeld, D., and Vogl, S. E.: Treatment of recurrent or metastatic squamous cancer of the head and neck with methotrexate (M) plus corynebacterium parvum, or M plus bleomycin (B) plus diamminedichloroplatinum (D): A prospective randomized trial of the Eastern Cooperative Oncology Group (abstract). *Proc. Am. Assoc. Cancer Res. Am. Soc. Clin. Oncol.*, 22:532, 1981.

Kirkwood, J. M., Canellos, G., Pervin, T. J., Pitman, S. W., Weichselbaum, R., and Muller, D.: Increased therapeutic index using moderate dose methotrexate and leucovorin twice weekly versus weekly high dose methotrexate-leucovorin in patients with advanced squamous carcinoma of the head and neck. A safe new effective regimen. *Cancer*, 47:2414–21, 1981.

Kish, J. A., Weaver, A., Jacobs, J., Cummings, G., and Al-Sarraf, M.: Cisplatin and 5-Fluorouracil infusion in patients with recurrent and disseminated epidermoid cancer of the head and neck. *Cancer*, 53:1819–24, 1984.

Lane, M., Moore, J. E. III, Levin, H., and Smith, F. E.: Methotrexate therapy for squamous cell carcinoma of the head and neck. *J.A.M.A.*, 204:561–64, 1968.

Legha, S., and Dimery, I. W.: High dose cisplatin administration without hypertonic saline. Manuscript accepted, *J. Clin. Oncol.*

Leone, L. A., Albala, M. M., and Rege, V. B.: Treatment of carcinoma of the head and neck with intravenous methotrexate. *Cancer*, 21:828–37, 1968.

Levitt, M., Mosher, M. B., and DeConti, R. C.: Improved therapeutic index of methotrexate with "leucovorin rescue." *Cancer Res.*, 33:1729–34, 1973.

Lichtenstein, A., Zighelboim, J., Dorey, F., Brossman, S., and Fahen, J. L.: Comparison of immune derangements in patients with different malignancies. *Cancer* 45:2090–95, 1980.

Lotan, R.: Effects of vitamin A and its analogs (retinoids) on normal and neoplastic cells. *Biochim. Biophys. Acta*, pp. 33–91, 1980.

Magee, M. J., Howard, J., Bosl, G. J., and Wittes, R. E.: Phase II trial of 4'-epi-doxorubicin in advanced carcinoma of head and neck origin. *Cancer Treat. Rep.*, 1:125–6, 1985.

Mead, G. M., and Jacobs, C.: Changing role of chemotherapy in treatment of head and neck cancer. *Am. J. Med.*, 73:582–95, 1982.

Medina, J. E.: The controversial role of BCG in the treatment of squamous cell carcinoma of the head and neck (commentary). *Arch. Otolaryngol.*, 109:543, 1983.

Mesic, J. B., Fletcher, G. H., and Goepfert, H.: Megavoltage irradiation of epithelial tumors of the nasopharynx. *Int. J. Radiat. Oncol. Biol. Phys.*, 7:447–58, 1981.

Meyskens, F. L.: Experience with 13-cis-retinoic and as therapy for serious precancers and advanced cancers at the Arizona Cancer Center. Second International Conference on the Modulation and Mediation of Cancers by Vitamins and Micronutrients. February 10–13, 1985.

Meyskens, F. L., Gilmartin, E., Alberts, D. S., Levine, N. S., Brooks, R., Salmon, S. E., and Swivitt, E. A.: Activity of isotretinoin against squamous cell cancers and preneoplastic lesions. *Cancer Treat. Rep.*, 66: 1315–19, 1982.

Panethiere, F. J., Lehane, D., and Fletcher, W. J.: Cisplatinum therapy of previously treated head and neck cancer: The Southwest Oncology Group two-dose-per-month outpatient regimen. *Med. Pediatr. Oncol.*, 8: 221, 1980.

Papac, R. J., Jacobs, E. M., Foye, L. V., and Donohue, D. M.: Systemic therapy with amethopterin in squamous carcinoma of the head and neck. *Cancer Chemother. Rep.*, 32:47–54, 1963.

Peppard, S. B., Al-Sarraf, M., Powers, W. E., Loh, J. K., and Weaver, A. W.: Combination of cisplatin, oncovin, and bleomycin (COB) prior to surgery and/or radiotherapy in advanced untreated epidermoid cancer of the head and neck. *Laryngoscope*, 90:1273–80, 1980.

Perry, D. J., Crain, S. M., Weltz, M. D., Wilson, J. P., Davis, R. K., Woolley, P. V., Forastiere, A. A., Taylor, H. G., and Weiss, R. B.: Phase II trial of mitoguazone in patients with advanced squamous cell carcinoma of the head and neck. *Cancer Treat. Rep.*, 1:91–92, 1983.

Perry, D. J., Weltz, M. D., Broan, A. W. Jr., Henderson, R. L., Negha, W. J., and Berenberg, J. L.: Vinblastine, bleomycin, and cisplatin for recurrent or metastatic squamous cell carcinoma of the head and neck. *Cancer*, 50:2257–60, 1982.

Pitman, S. W., and Bertino, J. R.: Chemotherapy of squamous head and neck cancer. In van der Waal and Snow, G. B. (eds.): *Oral Oncology*, pp. 217–50, Martinus Nijhoff, Boston, 1984.

Pitman, S. W., Minor, D. R., Papac, R., Knopf, T., Lomenthal, I., Nystrom, S., and Bertino, J. R.: Sequential methotrexate, leucovorin (MTX-LCV), and cisplatinum in head and neck cancer. *Proc. Am. Assoc. Cancer Res. Proc. Am. Soc. Clin. Oncol.* 20:419, 1979.

Pitman, S. W., Kowal, C. D., Papac, R. J., and Bertino, J. R.: Sequential methotrexate-5-fluorouracil: A highly active drug combination in advanced squamous cell carcinoma of the head and neck. *Proc. of A.S.C.O.* 21:473, 1980.

Pitman, S. W., Kowal, C. D., and Bertino, J. R.: Methotrexate and 5-fluorouracil in sequence in squamous head and neck cancer. *Semin. Oncol.*, 10(2):15–9, 1983.

Popkin, J. D., Bromer, R. H., Vaughan, C. W., Byrne, R. E., Licciardello, J. T. W., Hoffer, S. M., Welch, J. M., Fofonoff, S. A., Strong, M. S., and Hong, W. K.: Continuous vindesine infusion in advanced head and neck cancer. *Am. J. Clin. Oncol.*, 6:301–4, 1983.

Price, L. A., Hill, B. T., Calvert, A. H., Dalley, M., Levene, A., Busby, E. R., Schacter, M., and Shaw, H. J.: Improved results in combination chemotherapy of head and neck cancer using a kinetically based approach: A randomized study with and without adriamycin. *Oncology*, 35:26–8, 1978.

Priestman, T. J.: Results in the 50 cases of advanced squamous cell carcinoma of the head and neck treatment by intravenous chemotherapy. *Br. J. Cancer*, 27:400–5, 1973.

Randolf, V. L., Vallejo, A., Spiro, R. H., Shah, J., Strong, E. W., Huvos, A. G., and Wittes, R. E.: Combination therapy of advanced head and neck cancer: Induction of remissions with diaminedichloroplatinum (II), bleomycin, and radiation therapy. *Cancer*, 41: 460–7,1978.

Randolf, V. L., and Wittes, R. E.: Weekly administration of cis-diammine-dichloroplatinum (II) without hydration or osmotic diuresis. *Eur. J. Cancer*, 14:753, 1978.

Ringborg, U., Ewert, G., Kunnman, J., Lundquist, P. G., and Straneler, H.: Methotrexate and 5-fluorouracil in head and cancer. *Semin. Oncol.*, 10(2):20–2, 1983.

Rowland, K. M., Taylor, S. G. IV, O'Donnell, M. R., Spiers, A., Stott, P. B., DiConti, R. C., and Milner, L.: Cisplatin/5-fluorouracil infusion chemotherapy in advanced recurrent cancer of the head and neck. An ECOG Pilot Study. *Proc. Am. Soc. Clin. Onc.*, 3:184, 1984.

Rozencweig, M., Dodion, P., Brumtsch, U., Crallmeier, W., Clavel, M., Gignoux, B., Funes, H. C., Cavalli, F., Kirkpatrick, A., Dalesio, O., and Rijmenant, M. V.: Combination chemotherapy with cisplatin, methotrexate, bleomycin, and vincristine (CABO) in advanced squamous cell carcinoma of the head and neck. *Cancer*, 54:1499–1503, 1984.

Sako, K., Razack, M. S., and Kalmus, I.: Chemotherapy for advanced and recurrent squamous cell carcinoma of the head and neck with high- and low-dose cis-diammine-dichloroplatinum. *Am. J. Surg.*, 136:529–33, 1978.

Shah, M. K., Engstrom, P. R., Catalaus, R. B., Paul, A. R., Bellet, R. E., and Creech, R. H.: Phase II trial of razoxane (ICRF-159) in patients with squamous cell carcinoma of the head and neck previously exposed to systemic chemotherapy. *Cancer Treat. Rep.*, 66:557–58, 1982.

Spaulding, M. B., Klotch, D., Grillo, J., et al.: Adjuvant chemotherapy in the treatment of advanced tumors of the head and neck. *Am. J. Surg.*, 140:538–42, 1980.

Stephens, R., Coltman, C., Rossof, A., et al.: Cis-dichlorodiammine-platinum (II) in adult patients: Southwest Oncology Group Studies. *Cancer Treat. Rep.*, 63:1609–10, 1979.

Taylor, S. G., McGuire, W. P., Hauck, W. W., Showel, J. L., and Lad, T. E.: A randomized comparison of high-dose infusion methotrexate versus standard-dose weekly therapy in head and neck squamous cancer. *J. Clin. Onc.*, 9(2):1006–11, 1984.

Taylor, S. G., Sisson, G. A., and Bytell, D. E.: A randomized trial of adjuvant BCG immunotherapy in head and neck cancer. *Arch. Otolaryngol.*, 109:544–49, 1983.

Vogl, S. E., and Kaplan, B. H.: Chemotherapy of advanced head and neck cancer with methotrexate, bleomycin, and cis-diamminedichloroplatinum (II) in an effective out-patient schedule. *Cancer*, 44:26–31, 1979.

Vogler, W. R., Jacobs, J., Moffitt, et al.: Methotrexate therapy with or without citrovorium factor in carcinoma of the head and neck, breast, and colon. *Cancer Clin. Trials*, 2:227–36, 1979.

Von Hoff, D. D., Alberts, D. S., Mattox, D. E., and Coulthard, S.: Combination chemotherapy with cisplatin, bleomycin, and methotrexate in patients with advanced head and neck cancer. *Cancer Clin. Trials*, 4:215–81, 1981.

Wheeler, R. H., Natale, R. B., Roshan, S. G., and Baker, S. R.: A phase I-II trial of cisplatin and dichloromethotrexate in squamous cell cancer of the head and neck. *J. Clin. Oncol.*, 7:831–35, 1984.

Williams, S. D., Einhorn, L. H., Velez-Garcia, E., Essessee, I., Ratkin, G., Birch, R., and Garrard, J.: Chemotherapy of head and neck cancer: Comparison of cisplatin and vinblastine and bleomycin (PVB) versus methotrexate (MTX). *Proc. Amer. Soc. Clin. Oncol.*, 1:202, 1982.

Wittes, R. E., Cvitkovic, E., Shah, J., Gerold, F., and Strong, E. W.: Cis-dischorodiammineplatinum (II) in the treatment of epidermoid carcinoma of the head and neck. *Cancer Treat. Rep.*, 61:359–66, 1977.

Wittes, R. E., Heller, K., Randolf, V., Howard, J., Vallejo, A., Farr, H., Harrold, C., Gerold, F., Shah, J., Spiro, R., and Strong, E.: Cis-dichlorodiammineplatinum (II)-based chemotherapy as initial treatment of advanced head and neck cancer. *Cancer Treat. Rep.*, 63:1533–38, 1979.

Woods, J. E.: Current status of chemotherapy in the treatment of head and neck cancer. *Arch. Surg.*, 111:1055, 1976.

Woods, R. L., Fox, R. M., and Tattersall, M. H. N.: Methotrexate treatment of squamous cell head and neck cancers: Dose response evaluation. *Br. Med. J.*, 282:600–2, 1981.

Yagoda, A., Mukhergi, B., Young, C., Etcubanas, E., Lamonte, C., Smith, J. R., Tan, C. T. C., and Krakoff, I. H.: Bleomycin: An antitumor antibiotic clinical experience of 247 patients. *Ann. Intern. Med.*, 77:861–80, 1972.

Zighelboim, J., Dorey, F., Parker, N. H., Calcaterra, T., Ward, P., and Fahey, J. L.: Immunologic evaluation of patients with advanced head and neck cancer receiving weekly chemoimmunotherapy. *Cancer*, 44:117–23, 1979.

Zwelling, L. A., and Kohn, K. W.: Mechanisms of action of cis-dichlorodiammineplatinum (II). *Cancer Treat. Rep.*, 63:1439–44, 1979.

PART SIX

MANAGEMENT OF THE NECK IN MELANOMA, THYROID, AND UNUSUAL TUMORS IN THE NECK

CHAPTER 17

Multifactorial Considerations in the Treatment of Melanoma of the Head and Neck

Marshall M. Urist, Seng-jaw Soong, and Charles M. Balch

EDITORS' COMMENT

In many respects, malignant melanoma is an unsettling disease. The clinician never feels very "comfortable" in treating melanoma of the head and neck because it has so many manifestations. The next three chapters deal with three vital parts of the larger picture of the definitive care of melanoma—retrospective analysis of presentation and treatment results (Urist), tumor immunology (Cassel), and innovative treatment modalities (Harwood). Hopefully, these workers and others will solve the complex puzzle we now only partially appreciate.

To understand the treatment and interpret the results, we must first view the environment in which we find melanoma. Dr. Urist, Dr. Soong, and Dr. Balch provide us with valuable information in this chapter to aid us in that understanding. The authors supply information based on evaluation of 534 patients from a combined study of the University of Alabama at Birmingham and the Sydney Melanoma Unit, Australia. Based on a median follow-up of 8.5 years, the authors identify the value of growth pattern, tumor thickness, ulceration, and anatomic site variation in determining the appropriate treatment of a given melanoma patient. They then address both the local and regional treatment based on these prognostic subgroups. Their conclusion, confirmed by others, is that a wide local excision (> 3 cm) is not desirable, necessary, or even possible in melanoma of the head and neck. This combined series also permitted evaluation of the role of elective lymphadenectomy: elective neck dissection for 1.5- to 3.99-mm tumor thickness correlates significantly with increased survival.

It is only by data collection and its analysis, such as that shown in this chapter, that the answer to melanoma will be found.

INTRODUCTION

Although the incidence of melanoma in the United States is steadily increasing, the outlook for patients with this disease continues to improve because of the increasing capacity for early detection (Balch et al., 1984). It is estimated that approximately 22,000 cases of melanoma will be diagnosed in the United States in 1985 (American Cancer Society, 1985). Approximately 15 to 25 percent of these melanomas will occur in the head and neck region. Fortunately, the proportion of head and neck melanomas to melanomas occurring at other sites is steadily decreasing (Donnellan et al., 1972). Effective treatment of patients with melanoma is based on an accurate estimation of the biologic potential for local recurrence and metastases in the lymph nodes and distant sites. This biologic potential can be measured by analyzing clinical and histologic factors.

DATA BASE

Much of the evidence provided in this discussion is derived from a recent analysis of records of 534 head and neck melanoma patients collected from the combined registries of the University of Alabama at Birmingham, Birmingham, Alabama, and the Sydney Melanoma Unit, Sydney, Australia (Urist et al., 1984). Details from the combined registries have been reported previously (Balch et al., 1982). The median follow-up time of both groups exceeds 8.5 years. The clinical and pathologic factors evaluated in this series include tumor location within the head and neck (neck, face, scalp, or ear), thickness (according to Breslow), level (according to Clark), growth pattern, pigmentation, ulceration, lymphocyte infiltration, and initial surgical treatment. The analysis only included patients with cutaneous melanomas. The pathologic definitions, surgical procedures, staging methods, and methods of statistical analysis have been summarized in previous reports (Balch et al., 1978; 1980; 1982; McGovern, 1977; McGovern et al., 1979; 1982; Urist et al., 1985). The majority of patients underwent standard radical lymph-node dissection. Parotidectomy or occipital neck dissections were performed when appropriate. Important characteristics of the patient population are listed in Table 17-1.

Table 17-1. Clinical and Pathologic Characteristics of 534 Head and Neck Melanoma Patients

CHARACTERISTICS	GROWTH PATTERN*	
	LMM	*SSM and NM*
Number of patients	81	453
Mean age	61	46
Sex		
Male (%)	44	58
Female (%)	56	42
Site		
Face (%)	70	43
Neck (%)	15	30
Scalp (%)	7	14
Ear (%)	7	13
Tumor thickness (mm)		
< 0.76 (%)	27	18
0.76–1.49 (%)	22	26
1.5–399 (%)	45	39
≥ 4.0 (%)	6	17
Ulceration present	25	27

Key: LMM = lentigo maligna melanoma, SSM = superficial spreading melanoma; NM = nodular melanoma.

SURVIVAL IN PROGNOSTIC SUBGROUPS

Growth Pattern

A preliminary analysis clearly demonstrated that lentigo maligna melanoma (LMM) was associated with a better prognosis than either superficial spreading melanoma (SSM) or nodular melanoma (NM). Survival curves for patients with these growth patterns are shown in Figure 17-1. The survival rates at 5 years were significantly different (LMM vs. SSM, $p = 0.032$; LMM vs. NM, $p = 0.00061$).

There is no clear consensus regarding the favorable prognostic value of LMM (Koh, 1984; Eldh et al., 1978; Drzewiecki and Andersen, 1982). McGovern et al. (1980) compared the survival rate of head and neck melanoma patients with LMM with the survival rate of a similar group of non-LMM patients, and showed that among patients with tumors greater than 1.5 mm in thickness there was a distinctly improved survival rate for LMM. In an effort to clarify this controversy, we have further analyzed the survival rate of 81 LMM patients, and compared it with the survival rate of 81 SSM and NM patients matched for important prognostic variables (see Table 17-2). Survival curves for these populations (see Figure 17-2) show that the differences in survival rate are significant 5 years later ($p = 0.051$) and 10 years ($p = 0.017$) later. The differences were also significant according to log-rank analysis ($p = 0.07$), which justified the separation of the two groups for subsequent analyses.

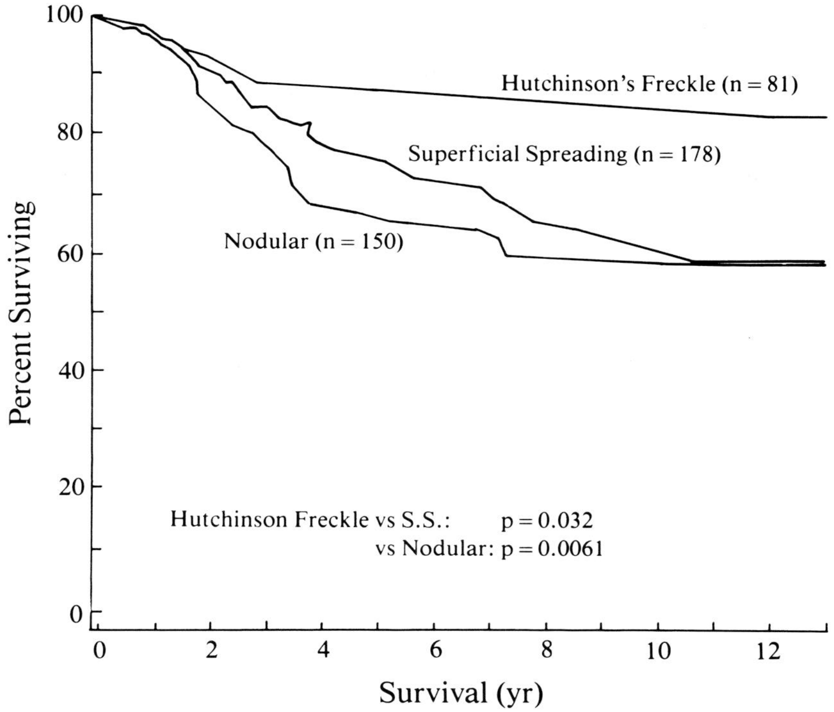

Figure 17-1. Survival rates for clinical stage I head and neck melonoma patients subgrouped according to growth pattern. Number of patients in each category is shown in parentheses. Patients with LLM (Hutchinson's freckle) had a better survival rate than those with SSM or NM. (Reproduced from Urist et al., 1984; used with permission of J.B. Lippincott.)

Tumor Thickness

As previously observed for the entire melanoma patient registry and for specific anatomic locations, survival rate was closely related to tumor thickness for patients with SSM and NM (see Figure 17-3). The thickness of LMM tumors also correlated with survival, and the outlook was better for LMM than SSM and NM in each category of tumor thickness.

Table 17-2. Clinical and Pathologic Characteristics of Matched Populations of Lentigo Maligna Melanoma and Superficial Spreading or Nodular Melanoma Patients

FACTOR	GROWTH PATTERN*	
	LMM *(n = 80)*	*SMM and NM* *(n = 81)*
Tumor thickness (mm)		
<.76	27	27
0.76–1.49	22	22
1.50–3.99	45	44
≥4.0	6	7
Ulceration	18	18
Site		
Ear (%)	7	10
Face (%)	70	67
Neck (%)	15	16
Scalp (%)	7	7
Initial treatment		
WLE + ELND†	26	30

*LMM = lentigo maligna melanoma; SMM = superficial spreading melonoma; NM = nodular melanoma.
†WLE = wide local excision; ELND = elective lymph-node dissection.

Ulceration

The presence of ulceration carried a poor prognosis for all growth-pattern groups (see Figure 17-3). Ulceration was also associated with decreased survival rates for all tumor-thickness categories. These findings were consistent with our previous observations of melanoma at other sites.

Anatomic Sites Within the Head and Neck Area

Analysis according to anatomic location within the head and neck of patients with SSM and NM tumors revealed that scalp tumors had a significantly worse prognosis than tu-

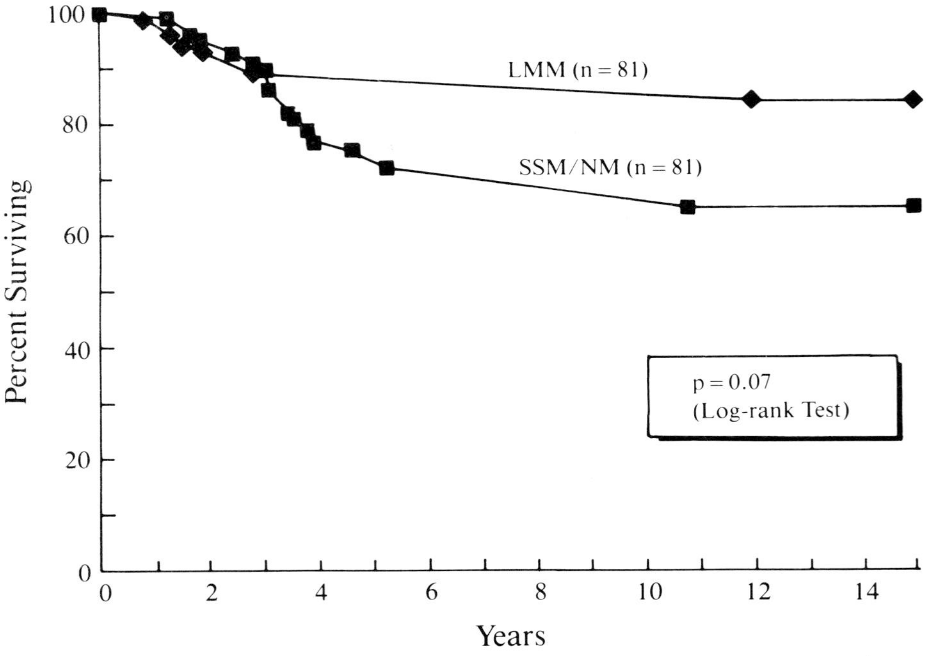

Figure 17–2. Survival rates for matched populations of LMM, and SSM and nodular NM patients. The survival rate of patients with LMM was significantly higher than in patients with SSM and NM ($p = 0.07$).

mors arising at other sites (see Figure 17–3). This observation was made in a previously reported series (Close et al., 1979). Lesions on the scalp were also thicker than lesions elsewhere, with a higher frequency of nodular growth pattern and ulceration. When different prognostic factors were matched by specific locations, scalp and neck melanomas still had less favorable prognoses.

Head and Neck Melanoma Versus Extremity Melanoma

Ten-year survival rates of patients with head and neck melanoma and patients with extremity melanoma were compared by major thickness category. Patients with extremity melanoma had a higher survival rate than those with head and neck melanoma; however, the difference in survival rates was statistically significant only for patients with tumors less than 1.5 mm in thickness. Other authors have suggested a lower survival rate for patients with head and neck melanomas than for those with extremity melanomas, but their analyses have not considered other risk factors.

OUTCOME OF SURGICAL TREATMENT

Surgical therapy for primary melanoma involves two controversial subjects: the optimal extent of wide local excision, and the value of regional or elective lymph-node dissection. Although a great deal of data are available about both modes of therapy, conclusive studies on the effect of such treatments on head and neck melanoma have not yet been performed.

Resecting a perimeter of normal skin around the melanoma biopsy site is designed to reduce the risk of local recurrence by excising microscopic tumor deposits. Tradition dictates that 3 to 5 cm must be resected around the biopsy site before the risk is reduced; however, surgeons must often substantially reduce these margins in the head and neck area because of the proximity of important structures. It is not clear whether the high local recurrence rates reported in the head and neck area are due to insufficient margins or the aggressive biologic properties of melanoma.

In this series, local recurrence was defined as regrowth of tumor under a skin graft or

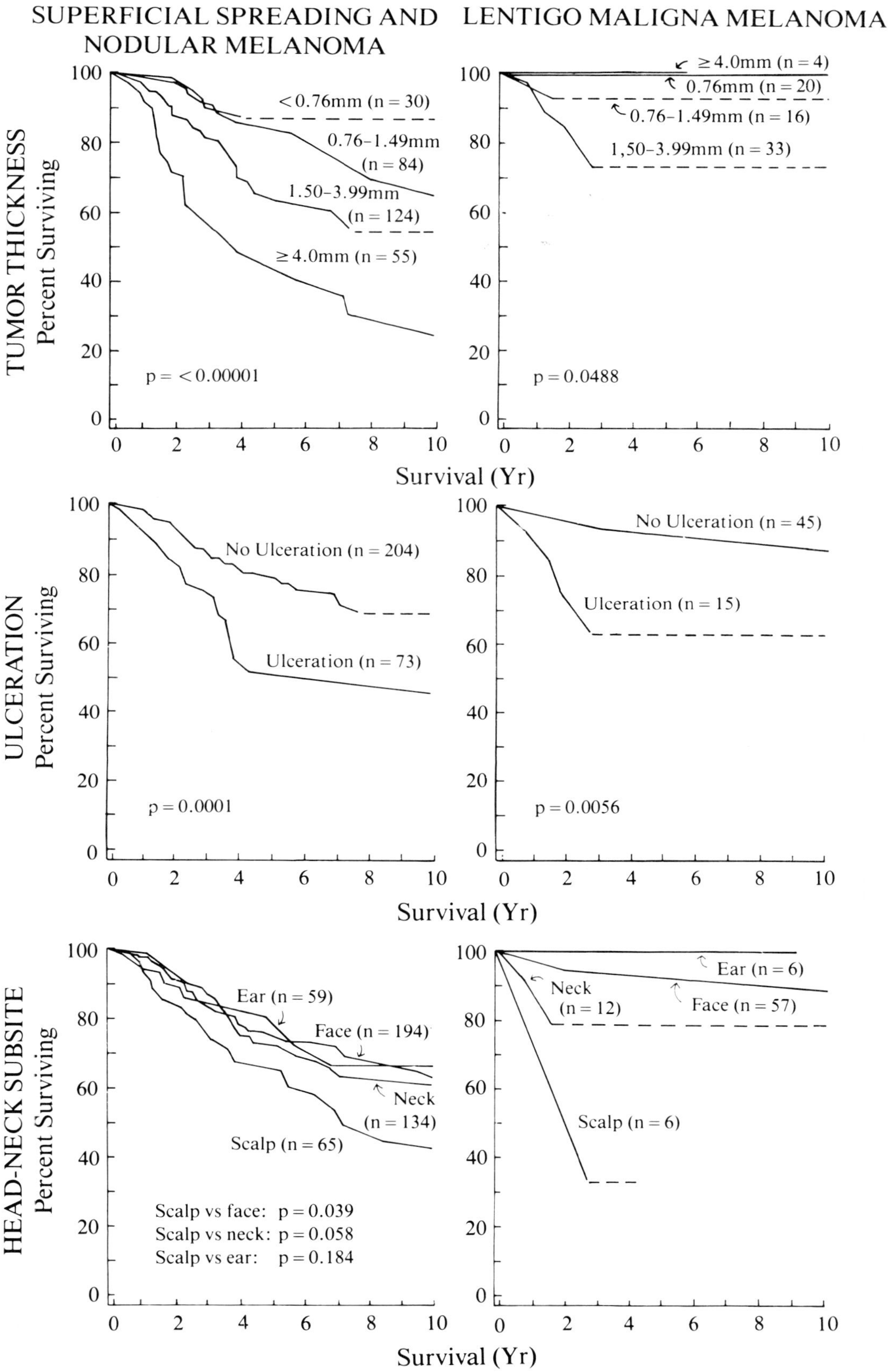

Figure 17-3. Survival rates for clinical stage I head and neck melanoma patients subgrouped, first, according to the growth pattern (SSM and NM versus LLM), then categorized according to tumor thickness, ulceration, and anatomic site. (From Urist et al., 1984; used with permission of J.B. Lippincott.)

within 3 cm of the scar from the wide local excision. An analysis of factors associated with local recurrence in the head and neck melanoma population showed that tumor thickness and ulceration were the most important factors to consider. Local recurrence rates were quite low (< 2.4%) when tumors were less than 2.5 mm in thickness and ulceration was absent (3.3%) instead of present (10.3%). Lentigo maligna melanoma tumors recurred locally less often than SSM or NM tumors, but the difference in recurrence was not statistically significant. The differences can be partially explained by the fact that SSM and NM tumors were slightly thicker; however, the incidence of ulceration was the same in both growth-pattern groups. The majority of LMM patients in this series underwent resection with margins of 1 cm or less because of the excellent prognosis associated with this type of melanoma.

Since the ideal margins of resection are subject to compromise more often in the head and neck area than at other sites, a higher rate of local recurrence might be expected with head and neck cancer than with other types of cancer, if the width of local excision is a critical factor. Our analysis demonstrated that local recurrence rates remained low in the head and neck area, suggesting that narrower local resections do not increase the risk of subsequent reappearance of melanoma. In fact, a report from the World Health Organization Melanoma Group found the same incidence of local recurrence in the head and neck area as we did, but in a larger patient population (Cascinelli et al., 1980). Recurrence rates reported in several other head and neck melanoma series have ranged between 4% and 15% (Storm and Eilber, 1982; Byers et al., 1980; Close et al., 1979; Roses et al., 1980). Recurrence rates reported in various series cannot be compared unless tumor thickness and ulceration have been taken into account.

Surgeons disagree considerably about the treatment of regional lymph nodes in head and neck melanoma patients. The size of the present series permitted evaluation of regional lymphadenectomy; it also allowed us to account for other important variables. The survival rates of SSM and NM patients undergoing wide local excision alone and those undergoing wide local excision plus elective lymph-node dissection were calculated for each tumor-thickness group (see Figure 17–4). No significant increase in survival rate relative to surgical treatment was observed for patients with tumors < 0.76 mm or ≥ 4.0 mm in thickness. A small increase in survival rate was observed for patients with tumors 0.76 to 1.49 mm thick who underwent wide local excision plus elective lymph-node dissection; however, a statistically significant increase in the survival rate of patients who underwent wide local excision plus elective lymph-node dissection was only seen for tumors 1.5 to 3.99 mm in thickness. These results also held up in the multifactorial analysis.

Proponents of elective lymph-node dissection base their position on the fact that melanoma frequently first metastasizes to regional lymph nodes (Balch et al., 1980; Ames et al., 1976; Close et al., 1979; Conley and Hamaker, 1977; Das Gupta, 1977). Their positive experience has been countered by others who have found no benefit from regional lymphadenectomy (Roses et al., 1980; Ballantyne, 1970; Polk and Bland, 1981). These conflicting reports may be a result of different prognostic factors in the two surgical treatment groups.

All of these trials have been retrospective analyses, and neither of the available prospective trials (Veronesi et al., 1978; Sim et al., 1978) have accounted for all prognostic variables or included patients with head and neck melanomas. The only retrospective trial that considered tumor thickness in relation to the results of surgical therapy showed that elective lymph-node dissection did result in an increase in survival rate for patients with tumors greater than 1.5 mm in thickness (Hansen and McCarten, 1974).

Lymphatic pathways within the head and neck region may differ greatly from patient to patient, so specific node-bearing regions should be defined before regional lymphadenectomy is performed. Cutaneous scanning with technetium-labeled antimony trisulfide colloid demonstrates the lymphatic flow pattern to specific areas (Logic and Balch, 1985). Studies examining the benefit of elective lymph-node dissection should define these

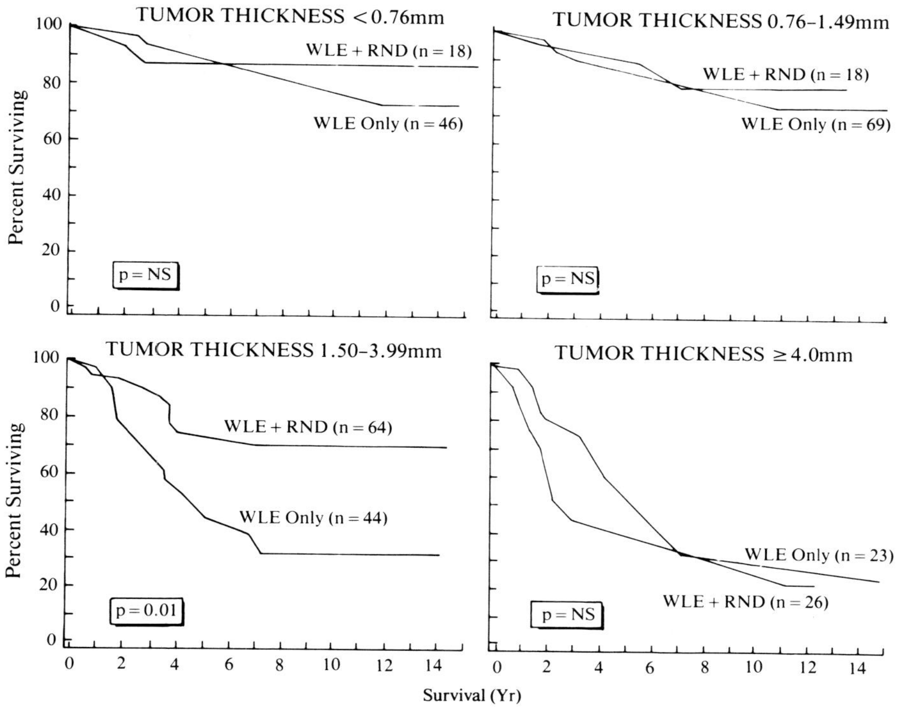

Figure 17–4. Survival rates for stage I patients with SSM and NM subgrouped according to tumor thickness and initial surgical treatment. There was a significant increase in the survival rate of patients who underwent elective lymph-node dissection (ELND) in addition to wide local excision (WLE) over the survival rate of those who underwent WLE alone, only in patients whose tumors were from 1.5- to 3.99-mm thick.

routes of lymphatic drainage to avoid missing any potential tumor-bearing nodes.

MULTIFACTORIAL ANALYSIS

To determine the relative values of the various prognostic factors related to survival, multifactorial analyses were performed separately for the LMM and the NM and SSM groups. Among SSM and NM patients, tumor thickness, anatomic location (scalp or neck versus face or ear), and ulceration were the strongest predictors of survival rate ($p < 0.00001$, $p = 0.0213$, and $p = 0.0289$, respectively). Elective lymph-node dissection did not improve the overall survival rate of the combined SSM and NM group.

This finding is quite logical, since little benefit is expected from elective lymph node dissection in patients who have either a low risk (tumor thickness < 0.76 mm) or a high risk (tumor thickness > 4.0 mm) of both regional and systemic disease. Patients with intermediate-thickness lesions have been shown to have a relatively high risk of regional disease and a low risk of distant disease, so they would theoretically benefit from resection of regional lymph nodes.

A multifactorial analysis was thus performed for patients in this category with tumor thicknesses of 1.5 to 3.99 mm because the category had been found to have a significantly better survival rate after elective lymph-node dissection in addition to wide local excision. Such an analysis was expected to detect whether the improved survival rate was related to an imbalance of other factors; however, surgical treatment remained a significant factor ($p = 0.035$), independently predictive of improved survival rates within this group.

Few of the patients who underwent elective lymph-node dissection had lymph nodes histologically positive for disease, but we postulate that the subgroup of patients benefits from the procedure because they have nodal disease undetectable by current routine lymph-node sampling techniques.

An ongoing national multiinstitutional trial of elective regional lymph-node dissection is stratified for prognostic factors including anatomic site, microstage, and patterns of lymph flow to nodes. Unfortunately, the results of this trial will not be available for several years.

DISCUSSION

Multiple clinical and pathologic factors in head and neck melanoma patients are predictive of survival rates, including growth pattern, thickness, ulceration, and anatomic location of the tumor within the head and neck area. An analysis of a large, nonrandomized series has shown that local recurrence within 3 cm of the wide local excision site is related to tumor thickness and ulceration. Results of surgical therapy indicate that elective lymph-node dissection is associated with significantly improved survival rates only in SSM and NM patients with tumors 1.5 to 3.99 mm thick. This observation was confirmed by a multifactorial analysis that simultaneously accounted for the effects of other important parameters. Our results are currently being tested in a prospective randomized trial. Until the results of that trial are available, treatment planning should be based on a careful analysis of those important clinical and pathologic parameters already known to be predictive of survival.

REFERENCES

American Cancer Society: Cancer Statistics 1985. *CA*, 35:19–56, 1985.

Ames, F. C., Sugarbaker, E. V., and Ballantyne, A. J.: Analysis of survival and disease control in stage 1 melanoma of the head and neck. *Am. J. Surg.*, 132:484–91, 1976.

Balch, C. M., Karakousis, C., Mettlin, C., Natarajan, N., Donegan, W. L., Smart, C. R., and Murphy, G. P.: Management of cutaneous melanoma in the United States. *Surg. Gynecol. Obstet.*, 158:311–18, 1984.

Balch, C. M., Murad, T. M., Soong, S-J., Ingalls, A. L., Halpern, N. B., and Maddox, W. A.: A multifactorial analysis of melanoma: Prognostic histopathological features comparing Clark's and Breslow's staging methods. *Ann. Surg.*, 188:732–42, 1978.

Balch, C. M., Soong, S-J., Milton, G. W., Shaw, H. M., McGovern, V. J., Murad, T. M., McCarthy, W. H., and Maddox, W. A.: A comparison of prognostic factors and surgical results in 1786 patients with localized (stage 1) melanoma treated in Alabama, USA, and New South Wales, Australia. *Ann. Surg.*, 196:677–84, 1982.

Balch, C. M., Wilkerson, J. A., Murad, T. M., Soong, S-J., Ingalls, A. L., and Maddox, W. A.: The prognostic significance of ulceration of cutaneous melanoma. *Cancer*, 45:3012–17, 1980.

Ballantyne, A. J.: Malignant melanoma of the skin of the head and neck: An analysis of 405 cases. *Am. J. Surg.*, 120:425–31, 1970.

Byers, R. M., Smith, J. L., Russell, N., and Rosenberg, V.: Malignant melanoma of the external ear: Review of 102 cases. *Am. J. Surg.*, 140:518–21, 1980.

Cascinelli, N., van der Esch, E. P., Breslow, A., Morabito, A., and Bufalino, R.: Stage 1 melanoma of the skin: The problem of resection margins. *Eur. J. Cancer*, 16:1079–85, 1980.

Close, L. G., Goepfert, H., Ballantyne, A. J., and Jesse, R. H.: Malignant melanoma of the scalp. *Laryngoscope*, 89:1189–96, 1979.

Conley, J., and Hamaker, R. C.: Melanoma of the head and neck. *Laryngoscope*, 87:760–64, 1977.

Das Gupta, T. K.: Results of treatment of 269 patients with primary cutaneous melanoma. A five-year prospective study. *Ann. Surg.*, 186:201–9, 1977.

Donnellan, M. J., Seemayer, T., Huvos, A. G., Mike, V., and Strong, E. W.: Clinicopathologic study of cutaneous melanoma of the head and neck. *Am. J. Surg.*, 124:450–55, 1972.

Drzewiecki, K. T., and Andersen, P. K.: Survival with malignant melanoma. A regression analysis of prognostic factors. *Cancer*, 49:2414–19, 1982.

Eldh, J., Boeryd, E., and Peterson, L. E.: Prognostic factors in cutaneous malignant melanoma in stage 1: A clinical, morphological, and multivariate analysis. *Scand. J. Plast. Reconstr. Surg.*, 12:243–55, 1978.

Hansen, M. G., and McCarten, A. B.: Tumor thickness and lymphocyte infiltration in malignant melanoma of the head and neck. *Am. J. Surg.*, 128:557–61, 1974.

Harris, T. J., and Hinckley, D. M.: Melanoma of the head and neck in Queensland. *Head Neck Surg.*, 5:197–203, 1983.

Koh, H. K., Michalik, E., Sober, A. J., Lew, R. A., Day, C. L., Clark, W., Mihm, M. C., Kopf, A. W., Blois, M. S., Fitzpatrick, T. B.: Lentigo maligna melanoma has no better prognosis than other types of melanoma. *J. Clin. Oncol.*, 2:994–1001, 1984.

Logic, J. R., and Balch, C. M.: Defining lymphatic drainage patterns with cutaneous lymphoscintigraphy. In Balch, C. M., Milton, G. W. (eds.): *Cutaneous Melanoma: Clinical Management and Treatment Results Worldwide*, pp. 159–70. J.B. Lippincott, Philadelphia 1985.

McGovern, V. J.: Etiology of melanoma; classification and histological reporting; spontaneous regression; frozen section diagnosis. In Milton, G. W. (ed): *Malignant Melanoma of the Skin and Mucous Membrane*, pp. 1–25. Churchill Livingstone, New York, 1977.

McGovern, V. J., Shaw, H. M., Milton, G. W., and Farago, G. A.: Prognostic significance of the histological features of malignant melanoma. *Histopathology*, 3:385–93, 1979.

McGovern, V. J., Shaw, H. M., Milton, G. W., and Farago, G. A.: Is malignant melanoma arising in a Hutchinson's melanotic freckle a separate disease entity? *Histopathology*, 4:235–42, 1980.

McGovern, V. J., Shaw, H. M., Milton, G. W., and McCarthy, W. H.: Ulceration and prognosis in cutaneous malignant melanoma. *Histopathology*, 6:399–407, 1982.

Olson, R. M., Woods, J. E., and Soule, E. H.: Regional lymph-node management and outcome in 100 patients with head and neck melanoma. *Am. J. Surg.*, 142:470–73, 1981.

Polk, H. C., Jr. and Bland, K. I.: Routine elective lymph dissection in melanoma—unnecessary treatment? In O'Connell, T. X. (ed): *Surgical Oncology: Controversies in Cancer Treatment*. G. K. Hall, Boston, 1981.

Roses, D. F., Harris, M. N., Grunberger, I., and Gumport, S. L.: Selective surgical management of cutaneous melanoma of the head and neck. *Ann. Surg.*, 192: 629–32, 1980.

Sim, F. H., Taylor, W. F., Ivins, J. C., Pritchard, D. J., and Soule, E. H.: A prospective randomized study of the efficacy of routine elective lymphadenectomy in management of malignant melanoma: Preliminary results. *Cancer*, 41:948–56, 1978.

Storm, F. K. and Eilber, F. R.: The value of lymphadenectomy in melanomas of the head and neck. In Kagan, A. R.; Miles, J. W. (eds): *Head and Neck Oncology: Controversies in Cancer Treatment*, pp. 127–138. G.K. Hall, Boston, 1982.

Urist, M. M., Balch, C. M., and Milton, G. W.: Surgical management of the primary melanoma. In Balch, C. M.; Milton, G. W. (eds): *Cutaneous Melanoma: Clinical Management Treatment Results Worldwide*, pp. 71–90. J.B. Lippincott, Philadelphia, 1985.

Urist, M. M., Balch, C. M., Soong, S-J., Shaw, H. M., Milton, G. W., and Maddox, W. A.: The influence of surgical margins and prognostic factors predicting the risk of local recurrence in 3445 patients with primary cutaneous melanoma. *Cancer*, 55:1398–402, 1985.

Urist, M. M., Balch, C. M., Soong, S-J., Milton, G. W., Shaw, H. M., McGovern, V. J., Murad, T. M., McCarthy, W. H., and Maddox, W. A.: Head and neck melanoma in 534 clinical stage 1 patients: A prognostic factors analysis and results of surgical treatment. *Ann. Surg.*, 200:769–75, 1984.

Veronesi, U., Adamus, J., Bandiera, D. C., Brennhovd, I. O., Caceres, E., Cascinelli, N., Cladiou, F., Ikonopisov, R. L., Javorskj, V. V., Kirov, S., Kulakowski, A., Lacour, J., Lejeune, F., Mechl, Z., Morabito, A., Rode, I., Sergeev, S., van Slooten, E., Szczguel, K., Trapeznikov, N. N., and Wagner, R. L.: Inefficacy of immediate node dissection in stage 1 melanoma of the limbs. *N. Engl. J. Med.*, 297:627–30, 1977.

CHAPTER 18

Viral Oncolysate in the Treatment of Regional Metastases of Melanoma

William A. Cassel and Douglas R. Murray

EDITORS' COMMENT

The importance of the immune system in the definitive treatment of all tumors is generally recognized, particularly so in melanoma. Dr. Cassel and Dr. Murray, from the Departments of Microbiology and Surgery at Emory University, Atlanta, have extensive experience in the apparently promising area of viral oncolysate. Dr. Cassel reviews the history of these tumor-destroying viruses and their rather patchy clinical application over the last three decades. This is supplemented with a most complete bibliography for those requiring more information.

The authors then cover their own experience with viral oncolysate treatment for melanoma. The rationales for the selection of melanoma and the Newcastle virus strain are noted by the authors, as is their 10-year experience in treating stage II and stage III melanoma patients safely and effectively. Dr. Cassel and Dr. Murray then focus on their impressive results with 32 patients, treated for at least 5 years, resulting in 72 percent having no evidence of disease. Results with a similar group followed less than 5 years appear equally impressive.

Attention is finally drawn to the authors' experience with head and neck stage II and stage III melanoma patients, which includes 21 patients. Their results, noted in Tables 18–1 and 18–2, appear as promising as those for the other anatomic sites previously noted. In conclusion, Dr. Cassel and Dr. Murray are appropriately cautious in recommending the widespread application of their viral oncolysate in the treatment of melanoma.

In their attack on melanoma, the authors have taken on one of the most formidable aspects of melanoma—regional metastases, which many clinicians automatically associate with systemic disease. It would seem only logical that a systemic treatment such as stimulation of the body's own natural defenses is proper. Dr. Cassel and Dr. Murray appear to be on the right track, but we must be cautious in accepting this modality until their results are confirmed by others.

INTRODUCTION

Events leading to the use of viral oncolysate in the management of malignant disease trace their origin to the observation that cancer patients sometimes showed regressions following viral disease or active immunization against viral disease. Eventually, tumor-destroying viruses were selected in the laboratory and directed toward application in humans (Webb and Smith, 1970). Some benefits were noted, but most of the applied viruses had the disadvantage of being neuropathic; reports of success in human studies with nonneuropathic mumps virus were exceptional (Asada, 1974; Okuno et al., 1978). By 1970, interest in the direct application of oncolytic viruses had largely faded.

In 1950, attention was drawn to a postoncolytic tumor immunity in chickens following tumor destruction by viruses (Sharpless et al., 1950). A similar observation was made in mice (Koprowski et al., 1957). Findings of this sort led to the use of viral oncolysates per se for the immunization of animals against transplantable tumors (Lindenmann and Klein, 1967). Viral oncolysate is produced by lysing cultured tumor cells through infection with a virus, which usually requires about 3 days. Possible mechanisms were proposed for the marked immunogenic action of viral oncolysates. Several studies provided substantial evidence suggesting a helper-antigen role for the virus in enhancing recognition of tumor antigens (Boone et al., 1974; Kobayashi et al., 1977; Svet-Moldavsky and Hamburg, 1967). Interferon and natural killer (NK) cell activation certainly might enter the picture (Byrne et al., 1983). The amount of virus released per cell and the occurrence of tumor-cross-reactive immunizing capacity in association with interferon, NK cells, and macrophages also merit consideration (Silagi et al., 1972; Silagi and Cavelli, 1982). Obviously, the overall immune response may include specific and nonspecific activities working in concert.

Occasional allusions have been made to the possible employment of viral oncolysates in the treatment of human malignancies. About 1970, the first step was taken in this direction (Sinkovics et al., 1974a; 1974b); ultraviolet-irradiated influenza virus lysates of sarcoma and malignant melanoma cells were employed. Our own studies were initiated independently late in 1971 (Cassel et al., 1977; Murray et al., 1977). Unsuccessful efforts to treat osteosarcoma with an influenza virus oncolysate were described (Green et al., 1976), along with a similar report on the attempted treatment of myelogenous leukemia with a fowl plague virus oncolysate (Sauter, 1976). The preparations of Green and Sauter contained formalin to inactivate the viruses, a step that probably damaged the antigenicity of the lysates.

Vaccinia virus oncolysates have been found to cause significant tumor-burden reductions in patients with various malignancies (Wallack et al., 1977; Wallack, 1981); further studies on malignant melanoma are in progress (personal communication, Dr. P. Hersey, 1984). Ultraviolet-irradiated influenza virus oncolysate has been applied to patients with vulvar carcinoma, with a reported doubling of the median recurrence time by comparison with controls (Freedman et al., 1980). Patients with squamous cell carcinoma of the uterine cervix who were treated with viral oncolysate showed a median survival time five times that of the control group (Freedman et al, 1983). Beneficial results have also been observed in oncolysate-treated cases of ovarian carcinoma (Lotzova et al., 1984), accompanied by a dramatic increase in NK cell activity in the ascitic fluids and regression of ascites-producing tumors.

Sinkovics used viral oncolysate always in conjunction with chemotherapy, bacillus Calmette-Guerin (BCG), or both (Sinkovics et al., 1982). Progression of metastatic sarcoma was slowed by the inclusion of oncolysate in the treatment program, and malignant melanoma patients evidenced benefits in the first few years of treatment. This effect then tended to disappear until the 5th year, when patients not receiving oncolysate began to show recurrences, whereas the lysate-treated patients did not.

Another application of viral oncolysate has been in testing for delayed cutaneous hypersensitivity to malignant cells. Eighty-five percent of malignant melanoma patients tested with a vesicular stomatitis virus lysate of melanoma cells showed a delayed skin response, compared with 10 percent in controls tested with a membrane extract of melanoma cells (Boone et al., 1978). Similar results were seen in tests with breast cancer (Austin et al., 1982). The degree of specificity in each of these two studies was statistically significant.

An excellent comprehensive review is available for readers who wish to pursue the subject of viral oncolysates in more detail (Austin and Boone, 1979).

MALIGNANT MELANOMA

Turning to our own studies, we selected malignant melanoma as a model for examining the possible clinical benefits of viral oncolysate treatment. This tumor appeared to offer several advantages: (1) Its antigenicity and related immunologic responses in humans have been recognized for many years (Lewis, 1977). Even the absence of a history of a primary lesion in about 15 percent of stage II cases suggests regression occurs through immune mechanisms. (2) The nature of the tumor usually allows us to obtain sterile tissue well-suited for cell culture. (3) The pathogenesis of the disease includes numerous parameters by which to follow its progress.

We selected a particular strain of Newcastle disease virus for our studies, one that seemed appropriate because the virus (1) can replicate in a wide variety of cells, (2) is a potent inducer of interferon in humans, (3) shows no neurovirulence in humans, and (4) is neutralized by a natural inhibitor present in human serum. To avoid deleterious alterations of antigens and to retain the maximal capacity for stimulating the immune system, no measure was taken to inactivate the virus in the final oncolysate.

Our first study (Cassel et al., 1977; Murray et al., 1977) was with terminal (stage III) patients, and established to our satisfaction that the oncolysate was a reasonably safe product that elicited favorable responses in some patients. Up to this time, we have administered almost 7000 doses (2.5 ml each) of oncolysate to 163 patients without obvious detrimental effects. Parenthetically, it is interesting to note that patient 5 in our initial study (Murray et al., 1977), who had been unresponsive to multiple courses of surgery and chemotherapy, is still alive and free of detectable disease more than 10 years beyond the time when oncolysate treatment was begun.

Most recently, we described 32 consecutively entered stage II cases of malignant melanoma (Cassel et al., 1983). All patients had palpable regional lymph-node disease, which was confirmed in the pathology laboratory following radical lymphadenectomy. The mean disease-free interval in the historical control group was 40 weeks. We selected four such intervals (160 weeks) as a target time at which to compare the treated and the untreated control groups of patients. At that point, 12 percent of the treated patients evidenced recurrent disseminated disease, compared with 90 percent in the control group, all of whom died. Although factual, the control figure is unusual, and most studies report a 70 to 80 percent recurrence rate at 160 weeks after surgery (Aranha et al., 1979; Camacho et al., 1981; Eilber et al., 1976; Gutterman et al., 1973; Hilal et al., 1981; Hill et al., 1981; Knost et al., 1982; Veronesi et al., 1982).

The consistency of the figures, covering 1973 to 1982, suggests that variables such as radiologic scanning accuracy, surgical procedure, and the natural history of malignant melanoma have not changed significantly in recent years. All patients in the group of 32 have been under treatment for over 5 years, some for 8 to 9 years, and 72 percent remain free of detectable disease. Meanwhile, another group, consisting of 51 patients with stage II disease, has been brought under study. Individual treatment times in this group vary from 1 year and 3 months to 5 years and 3 months. Half the cases have remained free of disseminated disease for over 3 years. The current incidence of recurrent disseminated disease among the 51 cases is 17 percent.

The measurement of various immunologic parameters was mentioned in our first report (Cassel et al., 1977). Since then, other tests have been implemented, including T-lymphocyte helper/suppressor ratio, effects of mitogens on lymphocytes, and NK cell determinations. The test results are still being scrutinized, but we have not been greatly impressed with their prognostic potentials. Although no single test was exceptionally helpful, we believe that some prognostic indication is derived by examining the combined information from T-lymphocyte counts and delayed cutaneous hypersensitivity to recall antigens and dinitrochlorobenzene (DNCB). The ultimate measurement, however, is how well the patient fares.

We have made a direct histologic observation that provides supportive evidence of immunologic enhancement by viral oncolysate. Five patients, two of whom had stage II disease, developed solitary cerebral metastases, thereby justifying surgical intervention. Intensive mononuclear cell responses were noted in and around these tumors. We have been unable to find any report describing such a marked response in cerebral metastases of malignant melanoma patients. Although we have seen sparse infiltration in an occasional control case, no control case has matched the intensity observed in the patients receiving viral oncolysate.

HEAD AND NECK CASES

This book's immediate concern is head and neck disease. The seriousness of malignant melanoma of the head and neck has been described in one report (Roses et al., 1980) as follows: "Regional node metastases with malignant melanoma of the head and neck is an almost certain indication of systemic disease." The 5-year survival (not necessarily disease free) of patients with head and neck melanoma has been reported to be close to either 10 percent (Conley and Pack, 1963; Day et al., 1981; Fitzpatrick et al., 1972; Gumport and Harris, 1974; Knutson et al., 1971; Roses et al., 1980) or 30 percent (Ames et al., 1976; Ballantyne, 1970; Knutson et al., 1972; Simons, 1972; Southwick et al., 1963).

Most of these reports consist of a mixture of cases, some with histologically positive lymph nodes determined after elective node dissection, and others with clinically positive lymph nodes. Reasons for the discrepancies in these reports probably will become evident as experience accumulates and stratification criteria are recognized and evaluated better.

Our studies include only 21 cases of head and neck disease, three of whom have not yet reached the targeted 160 weeks after surgery. The status of the 21 cases, divided between our two stage II groups, is presented in Table 18-1. Five (63%) of the eight cases of head and neck disease from our first group of 32 patients survived free of disseminated disease for over five years. Only patient 5 showed an early recurrence (at 38 weeks). Not all of the 13 cases from our second group of 51 patients have been under study long enough to permit the determination of a 5-year survival figure. The shortest study time among the 13 patients is 2 years, 24 weeks (patient 21), but it is evident that nine of the 13 patients (69%) maintained disease-free status for well over 29 months, the reference time used in Table 18-2.

In Table 18-2, a comparison of disease-free intervals is made between our findings and a report representative of the 30 percent figure mentioned earlier (University of Texas M.D. Anderson Hospital and Tumor Institute at Houston data for 1970 to 1979 provided by Dr. Robert M. Byers). In addition, Roses et al. (1980) reported a 3 percent (1/30) 29-month disease-free interval, but because nodal status was not reported, direct comparison with the other two studies is not possible. Comparisons are made at 29 months after surgery because this time is the cutoff point in Roses' study and represents the longest time common to all three studies under comparison. At 29 months after surgery, Roses et al. found four of 30 patients still surviving, but only one was free of detectable disease. The UTMDAH data, covering 1970-79, are similar to those in an earlier report from the same institution (Ballantyne, 1970): At 29 months after surgery, 25 percent of the patients remained free of detectable disease. The interpretation of our limited number of cases must be made with appropriate reservations. Nevertheless, the data in Table 18-2 show a distinct trend for oncolysate-treated patients to experience a disease-free interval considerably greater than those patients who have been treated by surgery

Table 18–1. Malignant Melanoma: Status of Stage II Head and Neck Cases Treated with Viral Oncolysate

PATIENT*	PRIMARY LESION	PALPABLE LYMPH NODES†	DISEASE-FREE SINCE SURGERY‡	SURVIVAL SINCE SURGERY‡	FIRST SITE OF RECURRENCE
1	Posterior neck	3	4 yr, 47 wk	6 yr, 32 wk	Brain
2	Ear lobe	1 (parotid)	6 yr, 46 wk	ONED§	
3	Ear rim	6 (1 parotid)	3 yr, 33 wk	4 yr, 29 wk	Lung
4	Zygomatic	8 (all parotid)	5 yr, 2 wk	5 yr, 33 wk	Mesentery
5	Temple	4 (1 parotid)	38 wk	2 yr, 6 wk	Brain
6	Posterior neck‖	2	5 yr, 24 wk	ONED	
7	Unknown	2 (1 parotid)	5 yr, 35 wk	ONED	
8	Posterior neck	1	5 yr, 22 wk	ONED	
9	Above ear	3	43 wk	2 yr, 4 wk	Liver
10	Eyebrow	3	1 yr, 41 wk	ONED# 5 yr, 17 wk	Brain
11	Cheek	9	4 yr, 48 wk	ONED	
12	Posterior neck	Several	4 yr, 2 wk	ONED 4 yr, 2 wk**	
13	Cheek	6	4 yr, 19 wk	ONED	
14	Posterior neck	>7	4 yr, 4 wk	ONED	
15	Ear canal	1	3 yr, 28 wk	ONED	
16	Temple (with satellite)	4 (all parotid)	1 yr, 15 wk	1 yr, 29 wk	Adrenal
17	Posterior neck	10	1 yr, 21 wk	1 yr, 44 wk	Lung
18	Ear rim	1 (parotid)	22 wk	1 yr, 4 wk	Lung
19	Forehead	3 (all parotid)	2 yr, 32 wk	ONED	
20	Ear rim	1	2 yr, 39 wk	ONED	
21	Posterior scalp	1	2 yr, 24 wk	ONED	

*Patients above line belong to the first group of 32. Patients below line belong to a second group of 52. Patients listed in order of entry.

†All had palpable nodes, which were confirmed in the pathology laboratory to contain malignant melanoma.

‡Each time interval is determined to March 8, 1985.

§ONED = ongoing, with no evidence of disseminated disease.

‖Patient had two palpable, positive axillary nodes removed (radical dissection) 12 weeks before the appearance of neck disease.

#Patient developed a solitary cerebral metastasis at 1 year, 41 weeks, and has continued disease-free since surgical removal of the tumor at that time.

**Patient died of cardiac failure.

alone, with 71 percent of the oncolysate-treated cases remaining disease free at 29 months.

BANS CASES

Evidence has been submitted for an increased risk among patients designated as BANS cases (Day and Lew, 1983; Sober et al., 1983), cases in which the primary lesion has occurred on the upper back, back of the upper arm, or posterior of the neck or scalp. Among our 32 patients described in an earlier report (Murray et al., 1977), 13 (42%) were BANS cases. The shortest observation period in this group is 5 years, 18 weeks, although some of these patients have been under observation for 9 years since surgery. Two patients have experienced recurrent disseminated disease. It is too early to make a firm statement about the second group of 51 patients we are studying. The minimum observation time in this group is 1 year, 14 weeks, and the maximum time is 5 years, 14 weeks. This group includes 20 BANS cases (39%), and so far two of these patients have recurrent disseminated disease. If BANS cases truly are exceptional risks, the patients we are treating are responding unusually well.

DISCUSSION

Viral oncolysate is not a fully standardized product, and certain aspects of its application remain empiric. In the face of encouraging reports from various sources, however, viral oncolysate treatment cannot be dismissed lightly, particularly in connection with stage II malignant melanoma, for which no effective con-

Table 18–2. Disease-Free Survival of Stage II Head and Neck Disease Patients at 29 Months After Surgery

	NUMBER OF POSITIVE LYMPH NODES			OVERALL DISEASE-FREE AT 29 MONTHS
	1–3	*4–5*	*Over 5*	
UTMDAH, 1985 (surgery only) DF* survivors/total	21/60 (35%)	1/13 (8%)	1/19 (5%)	23/92 (25%)
Cassel and Murray, 1985 (surgery and oncolysate) DF* survivors/total†	9/12 (75%)‡	1/3 (33%)§	5/6 (83%)	15/21 (71%)

*DF = free of detectable disseminated disease.

†All patients in this study had positive, palpable nodes. The other study (and Roses et al., 1980) consisted of some patients with occult (microscopically) positive nodes only, as well as patients with palpable nodes.

‡Actually, 10 of 12 patients were disease-free at this time, because patient 10, counted as a recurrence, had been operated on for a solitary brain metastasis at 1 year, 41 weeks after lymphadenectomy, but remained disease-free at 5 years, 17 weeks after lymphadenectomy.

§Considered to have at least four positive nodes (see Table 18–1).

ventional treatment can be offered after surgery.

The so-called blood-brain barrier presents a problem in immunotherapy and chemotherapy. Among patients in whom we have witnessed recurring disseminated disease, the central nervous system has been the first site of detectable involvement in 30 percent of them. The inflammatory responses noted in the cerebral metastases probably occurred after the solitary tumors developed to a point where they caused sufficient alteration in local conditions to allow entry of the cellular immune system, although at that point the tumor was too advanced to be contained by the immune system.

Another limiting aspect of immunotherapy is the probable requirement for what we call durational therapy, or repeated administration of oncolysate at close intervals over a period of years. We have developed a strong impression about the advisability of this approach for the management of melanoma, where the incidence of disseminated disease recurrence under conventional treatment may be expected to be close to 100 percent (Geelhoed et al., 1977). The schedule we are currently following is to administer oncolysate initially at weekly intervals for the first 4 weeks, then biweekly intervals until a year after surgery. A 3-week schedule is then followed until 120 weeks after surgery, at which time the treatment interval is extended to 6 weeks. At 5 years postsurgically, the interval is moved to 3 months and held there indefinitely.

The aggressiveness of a malignancy and how it relates to host defenses is almost unexplored. The balance between these two elements is, in some cases, undoubtedly delicate, and treatment failure as a result of increased tumor virulence, recurring immune deficiency, or both should not be surprising. Durational therapy may play an important role in this context. Obviously, some patients may be so immunologically compromised they cannot respond to any immunostimulant. The administration of immunosupplements, such as immunomodulators, immune cells, or antibodies, may be of value in these cases.

The intent of our studies has been to examine the potential value of viral oncolysate as an immunotherapeutic agent, employing malignant melanoma as a study model. The findings have not been disappointing, but we remain very cautious in our interpretations. It appears that if patients with stage II disease (1) have unilateral regional lymph node involvement, (2) are thoroughly screened and found to be free of detectable disseminated disease at the time of radical lymphadenectomy, (3) undergo adequate surgery, (4) have no other complicating serious disease process, and (5) are placed on viral oncolysate treatment about 4 weeks after lymphadenectomy, we may expect about 80 to 85 percent of them to remain free of recurrent disseminated disease for more than 3 years, with a possible disease-free survival rate at 5 years of about 70%.

Ideally, the preferred point of attack in malignant melanoma is patients with high-risk stage I disease. There appear to be enough supporting data to justify taking this step with viral oncolysate application.

REFERENCES

Ames, F. C., Sugarbaker, E. V., and Ballantyne, A. J.: Analysis of survival and disease control in stage I melanoma of the head and neck. *Am. J. Surg.*, 132:484–91. 1976.

Aranha, G. V., McKhann, C. F., Grace, T. B., Gunnarsson, A., and Simmons, R. L.: Adjuvant immunotherapy of malignant melanoma. *Cancer*, 43:1297–303, 1979.

Asada, T.: Treatment of human cancer with mumps virus. *Cancer*, 34:1907–28, 1974.

Austin, F. C., and Boone, C. W.: Virus augmentation of the antigenicity of tumor-cell extracts. *Adv. Cancer Res.*, 30:301–45, 1979.

Austin, F. C., Boone, C. W., Levin, D. L., et al.: Breast cancer skin test antigens of increased sensitivity prepared from vesicular stomatitis virus-infected tumor cells. *Cancer*, 49:2034–42.

Ballantyne, A. J.: Malignant melanoma of the skin of the head and neck: An analysis of 405 cases. *Am. J. Surg.*, 120:425–31, 1970.

Boone, C. W., Austin, F. C., Gail, M., Case, R., Oharm, M., and Klein, E.: Melanoma skin-test antigens of improved sensitivity prepared from vesicular stomatitis virus-infected tumor cells. *Cancer*, 41:1781–87. 1978.

Boone, C. W., Paranjpe, M., Orme, T., and Gillette, R.: Virus-augmented tumor transplantation antigens: Evidence for a helper antigen mechanism. *Int. J. Cancer*, 13:543–51, 1974.

Byrne, J. A., Soloski, M., and Holowczak, J. A.: Immune responses of DBA/2 mice bearing melanoma tumors: Cell-mediated immune responses after challenge with vaccinia virus. *Cancer Immunol. Innumother.*, 16:81–87, 1983.

Camacho, E. S., Pinsky, C. M., Braun, D. W., et al.: DNCB reactivity and prognosis in 419 patients with malignant melanoma. *Cancer*, 47:2446–50, 1981.

Cassel, W. A., and Garrett, R. E.: Newcastle disease virus as an antineoplastic agent. *Cancer*, 18:863–68, 1965.

Cassel, W. A., Murray, D. R., Torbin, A. H., Olkowski, Z. L., and Moore, M. E.: Viral oncolysate in the management of malignant melanoma: I. Preparation of the oncolysate and measurement of immunologic responses. *Cancer*, 40:672–79, 1977.

Cassel, W. A., Murray, D. R., and Phillips, H. S.: A phase II study on the postsurgical management of stage II malignant melanoma with a Newcastle disease virus oncolysate. *Cancer*, 52:856–60, 1983.

Conley, J. J., and Pack, G. T.: Melanoma of the head and neck. *Surg. Gynecol. Obstet.*, 116:15–28, 1963.

Day, C. L., Jr., and Lew, R. A.: Malignant melanoma prognostic factors 2: The subsite concept. *J. Dermatol. Surg. Oncol.*, 9:525–26, 1983.

Day, C. L., Jr., Sober, A. J., Lew, R. A., et al.: Malignant melanoma patients with positive nodes and relatively good prognosis. *Cancer*, 47:955–62, 1981.

Eilber, F. R., Morton, D. L., Holmes, E. C., Sparks, F. C., and Ramming, K. P.: Adjuvant immunotherapy with BCG in treatment of regional-lymph node metastases from malignant melanoma. *N. Engl. J. Med.*, 294:237–40, 1976.

Fitzpatrick, P. J., Brown, T. C., and Reid, J.: Malignant melanoma of the head and neck: A clinicopathologic study. *Can. J. Surg.*, 15:90–101, 1972.

Freedman, R. S., Bowen, J. M., Herson, J., Wharton, J. T., Rutledge, F. N., and Hamberger, A. D.: Virus-modified homologous tumor-cell extract in the treatment of vulvar carcinoma. *Cancer Immunol. Immunother.*, 8:33–8, 1980.

Freedman, R. S., Rutledge, F. M., Wharton, J. T., et al.: Adjunctive immunotherapy with VMTCE (virus-modified tumor cell extract) in patients with high-risk squamous carcinoma of the uterine cervix. *Am. J. Clin. Oncol.* 6:155–56, 1983.

Geelhoed, G. W., Breslow, A., and McCune, W. S.: Malignant melanoma: Correlation of long-term follow-up with clinical staging, level of invasion, and thickness of primary tumor. *Ann. Surg.*, 43:77–85, 1977.

Green, A. A., Pratt, C., Webster, R. G., and Smith, K.: Immunotherapy of osteosarcoma patients with virus-modified tumor cells. *Ann. N.Y. Acad. Sci.*, 277:396–411, 1976.

Gumport, S. L., and Harris, M. N.: Results of regional lymph-node dissection for melanoma. *Ann. Surg.* 179: 105–8, 1974.

Gutterman, J. U., McBride, C., Friereich, E. J., Mavligit, G., Frei, E. III, and Hersh, E. M.: Active immunotherapy with BCG for recurrent malignant melanoma. *Lancet*, 1:1208–12, 1973.

Harris, M. N., Roses, D. F., Culliford, A. T., and Gumport, S. L.: Melanoma of the head and neck. *Ann. Surg.*, 182:86–91, 1975.

Hilal, E. Y., Pinsky, C. M., Hirshaut, Y., et al.,: Surgical adjuvant therapy of malignant melanoma with *Corynebacterium parvum*. *Cancer*, 48:245–51, 1981.

Hill, C. J. II, Moss, S. E., Golomb, F. M., et al.: DTIC and combination therapy for melanoma: III, DTIC (NSC 45388) surgical adjuvant study COG PROTOCOL 7040. *Cancer*, 47:2556–62, 1981.

Knost, J. A., Reynolds, V., Greco, F. A., and Oldham, R. K.: Adjuvant chemoimmunotherapy stage I/II malignant melanoma. *J. Surg. Oncol.*, 19:165–70, 1982.

Knutson, C. D., Hori, J. M., and Spratt, J. S., Jr.: Melanoma. *Curr. Probl. Surg.*, pp. 3–55, Dec. 1971.

Knutson, C. D., Hori, J. M., and Watson, F. R.: Melanoma of the head and neck. *Am. Jr. Surg.*, 124:543–50, 1972.

Kobayshi, H., Kodama, T., and Gotha, E.: Xenogenization of tumor cells. *Hokkaido Univ. Med. Libr. Ser.*, 9:1–124, 1977.

Koprowski, H., Love, R., and Koprowska, I.: Enhancement of susceptibility to viruses in neoplastic tissues. *Tex. Rep. Biol. Med.*, 15:559–76, 1957.

Lewis, M. G.: Immunology and immunotherapy of malignant melanoma. In Milton, G. W.; McGovern, V. J.; Lewis, M. G. (eds.): *Malignant Melanoma of the Skin and Mucous Membranes*, pp. 102–151. Churchill-Livingston, New York, 1977.

Lindenmann, J., and Klein, P. A.: Viral oncolysis: Increased immunogenicity of host cell antigens associated with influenza virus. *J. Exp. Med.*, 126:93–108, 1967.

Lotzova, E., Savary, C. A., Freedman, R. S., and Bowen,

J. M.: Natural killer-cell cytotoxic potential of patients with ovarian carcinoma and its modulation with virus-modified tumor cell extract. *Cancer Immunol. Immunother.*,17:124–29, 1984.

Murray, D. R., Cassel, W. A., Torbin, A. H., Olkowski, Z. L., and Moore, M. E.: Viral oncolysate in the management of malignant melanoma. II. Clinical studies. *Cancer*, 40:680–86, 1977.

Okuno, Y., Asada, T., Yamanishi, K., et al.: Studies on the use of mumps virus for treatment of human cancer. *Biken J.*, 21:37–49, 1978.

Roses, D. F., Harris, M. N., Grunberger, I., et al.: Selective surgical management of cutaneous melanoma of the head and neck. *Ann. Surg.*, 192:629–32, 1980.

Sauter, C.: Viral oncolysis: Its application in maintenance treatment of acute myelogenous leukemia. In Terry, W. D., Windhorst, R. (eds.): *Progress in Cancer Research and Therapy*, Vol. 6, p. 25. Raven Press, New York, 1976.

Sharpless, G. R., Davies, M. C., and Cox, H. R.: Antagonistic action of certain neurotropic viruses toward a lymphoid tumor in chickens with resulting immunity. *Proc. Soc. Exp. Biol. Med.*, 78:270–75, 1950.

Silagi, S., Beju, D., Wrathall, J., and Deharven, E.: Tumorigenicity, immunogenicity, and virus production in mouse melanoma cells treated with 5-bromodeoxyuridine. *Proc. Natl. Acad. Sci. USA*, 69:3442–47, 1972.

Silagi, S., and Cavelli, T. A.: Relationship between rejection of several syngeneic tumors and retrovirus production by 5-bromodeoxyuridine-grown melanoma cells: Lack of protection in natural killer-deficient beige mice. *Cancer Res.*, 42:2562–66, 1982.

Simons, J. N.: Malignant melanoma of the head and neck. *Am. J. Surg.*, 124:485–88, 1972.

Sinkovics, J. G., Gonzalez, F., Campos, L. T., Kay, H. D., Shirato, E., and Gyorkey, F.: Immunology of human sarcomas. *Abstracts of the Annual Meeting of the American Society for Microbiology*, p. 206, 1974a.

Sinkovics, J. G., Papadoupoulos, N. E., and Plager, C.: Viral oncolysate for the immunotherapy of human tumors. In Yohn, D. S.; Blakeslee, J. R.; (eds.): *Advances in Comparative Leukemia Research*, International Symposium for Comparative Research on Leukemia and Related Diseases (10th: 1981), pp. 613–15. Elsevier-North Holland, New York, 1982.

Sinkovics, J. G., Thota, H., Kay, H. D., et al.: Intensification of immune reactions by immunotherapy: Attempts at measuring sarcoma-specific reactions in vitro. In Crispin, R. G. (ed.): *Neoplasm Immunity: Therapy and Application*, University of Illinois Medical Center, Chicago, 1974b.

Sober, A. J., Day, C. L., Jr., Fitzpatrick, T. B., Lew, R. A., Kopf, A. W., and Mihm, M. C.: Factors associated with death from melanoma from 2 to 5 years following diagnosis in stage I patients. *J. Invest. Dermatol.*, 80 (suppl 6):53s–55s, 1983.

Southwick, H. W., Slaughter, D. P., and Hinkemp, J. F.: Malignant melanoma of the head and neck. *Am. J. Surg.*, 106:852–55, 1963.

Svet-Moldavsky, G. J., and Hamburg, V. P.: An approach to the immunological treatment of tumors by artificial heterogenization. In Harris, J. C. (ed.): *Specific Tumor Antigens*, UICC Monograph Series, Vol. 2, pp. 323–27, Munksgaard, Copenhagen, 1967.

Veronesi, U., Adamus, J., Aubert, C., et al.: A randomized trial of adjuvant chemotherapy and immunotherapy in cutaneous melanoma. *N. Engl. J. Med.*, 307: 913–16, 1982.

Wallack, M. K.: Specific immunotherapy with vaccinia oncolysates. *Cancer Immunol. Immunother.*, 12:1–4, 1981.

Wallack, M. K., Steplewski, Z., Koprowski, H., et al.: A new approach in specific active immunotherapy. *Cancer*, 39:560–64, 1977.

Webb, H. E., and Smith, C. E. G.: Viruses in the treatment of cancer. *Lancet*, 1:1206–09, 1970.

CHAPTER 19

Role of Radiation Therapy in the Treatment of Melanoma

Andrew Ralph Harwood

EDITORS' COMMENT

Coming from the Princess Margaret Hospital in Toronto, an internationally recognized center in radiotherapy, Dr. Harwood introduces a concept that many clinicians may find unique in the treatment of regional metastasis of melanoma. Drawing from a 10-year experience, the author presents a historical and literature review of the topic. He acknowledges that melanoma has the reputation of being radioresistant, but as he notes "(these articles) . . . do not provide evidence for this frequently strongly held opinion." He then presents experimental and clinical evidence quite to the contrary, citing the importance of using larger-than-normal doses per fraction (> 270 cGy).

The experience at the Princess Margaret Hospital with 89 patients treated between 1975 and 1982 is presented. The technique involved the administration of 800 cGy three times—on days 0, 7, and 21 (a total of 2400 cGy in 3 weeks). The results of this regimen demonstrate a satisfactory regional control of microscopic residual disease in the neck, less so with gross residual disease (64% vs. 52%). The author notes an acceptable complication rate (< 6%), and speculates on the use of radiation therapy in the clinically negative neck. The University of Texas M.D. Anderson Hospital and Tumor Institute at Houston experience in the last 3 years in this clinical setting tends to support Dr. Harwood's speculation.

In summary, the author identifies the "good news" that radiation therapy appears to have a role in regional control, but also suggests the "bad news" that the overall survival and eventual death from distant metastasis appear to be only marginally improved. We do feel that radiation therapy will, in years to come, be demonstrated to be of value in the multidisciplinary approach to the control of melanoma; Dr. Harwood presents convincing evidence of this.

INTRODUCTION

Traditionally, malignant melanoma has been regarded as a radioresistant neoplasm (Jansen and Westbrook, 1981). It is only in recent years that this concept has been challenged. As a result, there is limited literature on experience with irradiation for treating neck node metastases.

Since 1975, we at the Princess Margaret

Hospital in Toronto have been exploring the use of large-dose-per-fraction radiotherapy for treating melanoma and, specifically, nodal metastases (Johanson et al., 1983). This has been an evolutionary process, and as we have become more experienced and confident of the results with large-dose-per-fraction irradiation, we have tended to use it more on patients with nodal diseases in earlier stages. Whereas we initially only treated patients who had advanced totally unresectable disease, we are now using large-dose-per-fraction radiotherapy as adjuvant therapy. We have not yet accumulated extensive experience, however, with the use of adjuvant irradiation in neck-node metastases specifically. The data presented in this chapter represent our total experience with the use of irradiation for all sites of nodal metastases (neck, axilla, supraclavicular fossa, and ileoinguinal areas). We do not believe that the site of nodal metastases has a major impact on the results of radiotherapy.

HISTORICAL AND LITERATURE REVIEW

Many articles in the literature state that melanoma is a radioresistant tumor; this implies that radiation therapy has little part to play in the treatment of the disease (Jansen and Westbrook, 1981). Generally, articles stating that melanoma is radioresistant either do not provide evidence supporting the contention, or they refer to data obtained more than 50 years ago, when primitive orthovoltage irradiation was used palliatively for patients unsuited for surgery (Harwood and Cummings, 1981).

We have recently undertaken a detailed historical literature review on the radiosensitivity of melanoma, and have documented how the myth of radioresistance arose (Harwood and Cummings, 1981). It is beyond the scope of this chapter to review all the recent evidence that has accumulated to refute this myth. It has been shown in work on experimental melanoma lines in cell cultures and on human melanoma cell lines grown in vitro that malignant melanoma is not an intrinsically radioresistant tumor and that melanoma cells have a large capacity to repair sublethal radiation damage (Harwood, 1984). It has been concluded that large-dose-per-fraction radiotherapy (more than 270 cGy per dose) is necessary to overcome this repair capacity of melanoma cells. The clinical experience at the Princess Margaret Hospital and the experience of others support the contention that large-dose-per-fraction irradiation is the preferred method of treating melanoma with irradiation.

Creagan et al. reported from the Mayo Clinic in 1979 the results of treating 31 patients with melanoma of the head and neck with conventional fractionated radiotherapy. Sixteen of these patients had gross residual tumor following surgery, and the other 15 were treated with adjuvant postoperative irradiation. A 28 percent 5-year survival rate was obtained. No difference was observed between the survival rates of patients with gross residual tumor and patients treated with adjuvant therapy.

In addition, the researchers at the Mayo Clinic carried out a randomized, controlled clinical trial in patients with nodal metastases from melanoma to determine if adjuvant postoperative irradiation was beneficial in terms of survival rates (Creagan et al., 1978). Less than 200 cGy per day of conventional fractionated irradiation was used. Fifty-six patients were randomized; 23 of these patients had only one node positive for disease in the surgical specimen taken. No difference was observed between the survival rates of irradiated patients and those not irradiated.

This study is the only randomized trial that tested whether adjuvant irradiation was of benefit in the treatment of nodal metastases from melanoma. Unfortunately, it is open to a number of criticisms. First, the number of patients randomized was small, and because of the small number of patients in the study it would not be possible to detect a difference in survival rates of less than 20 to 25 percent. Second, almost half the patients in the study had only one node involved by melanoma, and were therefore at low risk of developing recurrence. Finally, conventional fractionated radiotherapy, a technique we now believe to be less effective in treating melanoma than large-dose-per-fraction irradiation, was used to treat the patients in the study.

PRINCESS MARGARET HOSPITAL DATA

We have recently updated (February 1985) our experience with large-dose-per-fraction radiotherapy, and the analysis presented here is of the first 89 patients irradiated between 1975 and 1982.

Selection of Patients for Treatment

Two basic groups of patients were irradiated. The first group contained patients with gross residual or recurrent tumor within the lymph-node-bearing area following previous surgery. Generally, the residual tumor was unresectable. There were 48 patients in this group.

The other 41 patients included those who had had a complete excision of tumor by lymph-node biopsy or dissection, but who were believed to be at high risk of having microscopic residual diseases in the surgical field, and therefore at high risk (in excess of 30%) of relapse within the surgical field. This second group included patients who have had a lymph-node biopsy only (15 patients), or a lymph-node dissection because the melanoma was penetrating the lymph-node capsule (three patients); three or more nodes in the specimen were positive for disease (seven patients); the node size was greater than 3 cm (nine patients); or two or three of the last three factors were combined (seven patients). Patients with distant metastases at the time of irradiation were excluded from the analysis.

Irradiation Technique

The technique of irradiation employed has been described in detail elsewhere (Harwood, 1984; Johanson et al., 1983). It consisted of 800 cGy given on days 0, 7, and 21 (i.e., 2400 cGy in three fractions over 3 weeks). The choice of this fractionation regimen was purely empiric; it was based on the fact that it seemed to be an effective regimen for treating melanoma. In a small proportion of patients, dimethyltriazenoimidazole carboxamide (DTIC) was given prior to the first and third doses of radiation. The maximum dose was limited to 825 cGy per fraction to decrease the risk of delayed severe postirradiation fibrosis. The method of irradiation varied, but generally megavoltage irradiation was used. For patients with ipsilateral neck-node metastases, electron beam therapy techniques were frequently used. The radiation field usually extended at least one lymph node echelon beyond the known metastasis site. Care was taken to shield the brain, spinal cord, and eyes from stray x-rays when employing this fractionation regimen.

Survival Rate Data

The overall survival rate of all patients was 24 percent (see Figures 19-1 and 19-2). There is a statistically significant difference between the survival rates of the group of patients with gross residual or recurrent tumors (16%) and the group with microscopic residual tumor (35%) ($p = 0.001$). The survival rate in the group of patients with gross residual or recurrent tumors was found to be influenced by the size of the residual tumor. Twenty-nine patients had residual tumor more than 3 cm in size; these patients had a 13 percent 5-year actuarial survival rate, in contrast to those patients with residual disease less than 3 cm in size who had a 27 percent 5-year survival rate. Because of the small number of patients in this study, this difference is not statistically significant. The 5-year uncorrected actuarial survival rate for patients treated with lymph node biopsy and 0,7,21 irradiation was 48 percent, compared with 26 percent for those patients treated by lymph-node dissection and 0,7,21 irradiation (not statistically significant).

Regional Control Rate

The rate of tumor control after 5 years in the area where the irradiation was given (i.e., the lymph-node-bearing area) in the overall group of patients was 75 percent (see Figure

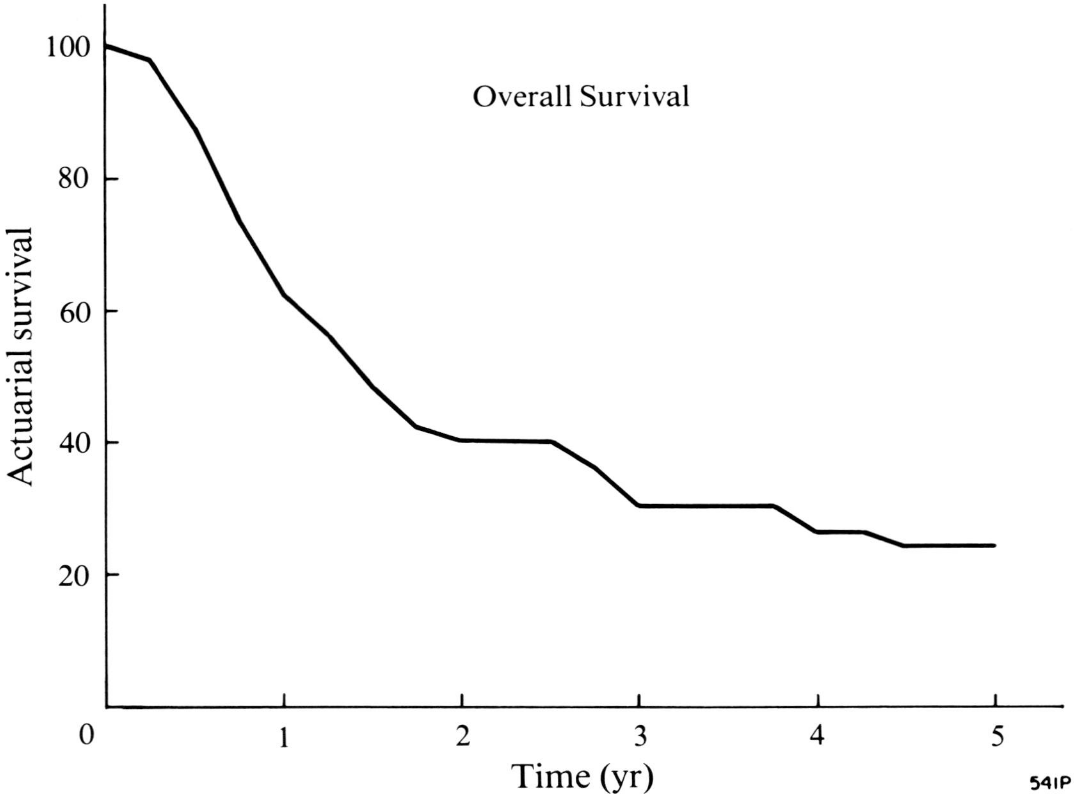

Figure 19–1. Uncorrected actuarial survival rate of entire group of patients.

19–3). There is a statistically significant difference between the regional tumor control in patients who had had all gross residual tumor removed (94%) and in those with gross residual or recurrent tumor (57%) ($p = 0.005$). Nevertheless, even patients with gross residual tumor have quite a high tumor-control rate 5 years after treatment, indicating the efficacy of this method of irradiation in controlling melanoma. The regional tumor-control rate for patients with residual disease less than 3 cm in size was 64 percent, compared with 52 percent in patients with residual disease larger than 3 cm ($p = 0.08$) (see Figure 19–4). The difference between the regional tumor-control rate in patients with microscopic residual tumor who had had a lymph-node biopsy (92%) and those who had had a lymph dissection (95%) in addition to 0,7,21 irradiation was not statistically significant. A small number of patients in the high-risk group who were not irradiated for a variety of reasons had a very high rate of recurrence within the surgical field.

Complications of Treatment

In general, the treatment was very well-tolerated. Eighty percent of the patients in the study had no complications. The maximum acute skin reaction occurred on day 14, and generally consisted of a dry desquamative reaction, which was rarely severe (14% of patients).

The most significant chronic complication of 0,7,21 irradiation was severe fibrosis, which in 2 percent of the study population led to nerve entrapment and significant neurologic complications. Severe fibrosis was observed in 4 patients, mainly those in whom the maximum dose exceeded 900 cGy per fraction. Because we have limited the maximum dose to 825 cGy per fraction, we have not observed these serious complications.

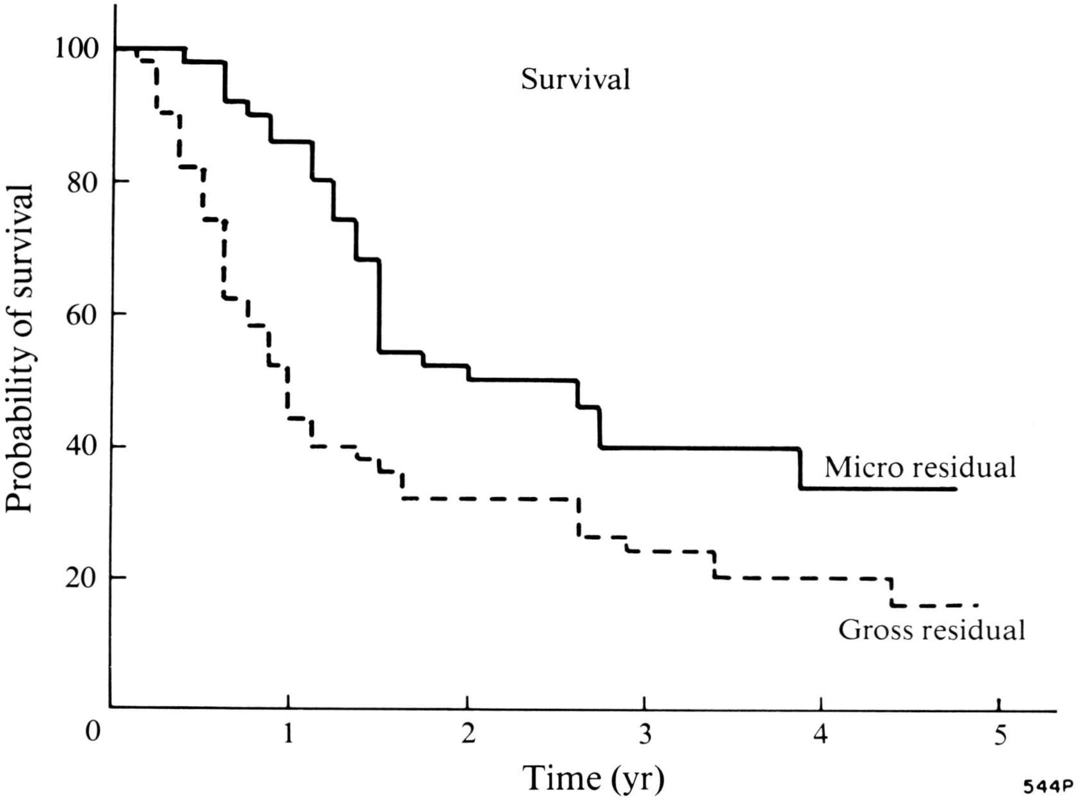

Figure 19–2. Uncorrected actuarial survival rates of the group of patients with residual or recurrent tumors and the group of patients with microscopic residual tumors.

These results emphasize that the amount of radiation employed in the 0,7,21 fractionation regimen is very close to the radiation tolerance level of the subcutaneous tissues, and that it would be hazardous to increase the dose. It is also important to note that this fractionation regimen is above the radiation tolerance level of the spinal cord, brain, and eye, and great care has to be taken to limit the dose to these structures when employing large-dose-per-fraction regimens.

Causes of Death

Twenty-seven of the 89 patients in the study group are alive, one with distant metastases. Three patients died of field recurrence, but the overwhelming cause of death was distant metastatic disease (59 patients). The most common sites of distant metastases were the brain, the liver, and the lung.

DISCUSSION

Patients with Gross Residual Tumor

The data document that melanoma is not a radioresistant tumor, that large-dose-per-fraction radiotherapy is an effective method of local palliative treatment for patients with melanoma in the lymph nodes, and that such treatment even has curative potential in a small proportion of patients with this disease.

It is important to debulk the tumor surgically as much as possible prior to irradiation, because irradiation is more effective regionally if the residual disease is less than 3 cm in diameter. (In this study, only a small proportion of patients with residual diseases more than 3 cm in diameter survived 5 years following irradiation.) In many patients, however, such surgery was not feasible because of the aggressiveness of the tumor; in fact, many pa-

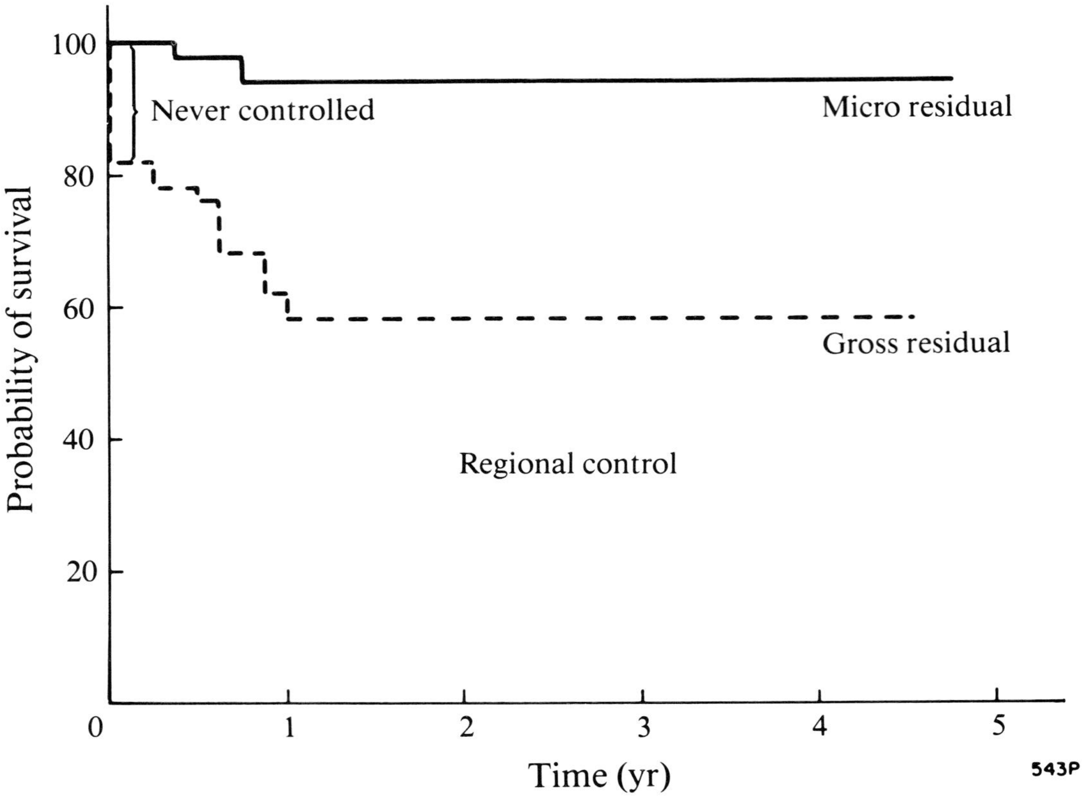

Figure 19–3. Actuarial 5-year regional tumor control rates for the group of patients with residual or recurrent tumors and the group with microscopic residual tumors.

tients die of distant metastases within the first year following treatment. The regional control rate 5 years after treatment and the response rates of the tumor to large-dose-per-fraction irradiation are clearly superior to those currently obtained with systemic chemotherapy (complete response rates in excess of 10 percent are rarely found with currently available drug combinations). Irradiation is therefore the treatment of choice for patients with regional disease that is residual or recurrent after prior surgery when distant metastases are not present.

Microscopic Residual Cases

In an effort to improve survival and reduce recurrence rates in patients undergoing lymph-node dissection, we explored the use of adjuvant 0,7,21 irradiation in patients at high risk of recurrence within the surgical field after lymph-node dissection. The criteria used to select patients who might benefit from postoperative irradiation were similar to those used to select such patients for postoperative irradiation following lymph-node dissection for squamous cell carcinoma—namely, capsular penetration, multiple nodal involvement, or total replacement of a single node with a tumor in excess of 3 cm in diameter.

We are not aware of any specific information in the literature that precisely estimates the risk of recurrence within the surgical field when the tumor is found on pathologic assessment to fit into the high-risk categories discussed. We estimate the risk of recurrence within the surgical field using these high-risk criteria to be in excess of 30 percent. The data presented here suggest that adjuvant irradiation significantly reduced the recurrence rate within the surgical field. It is unclear, however, whether the survival rate has been improved by such adjuvant therapy, because a large proportion of patients are dying of dis-

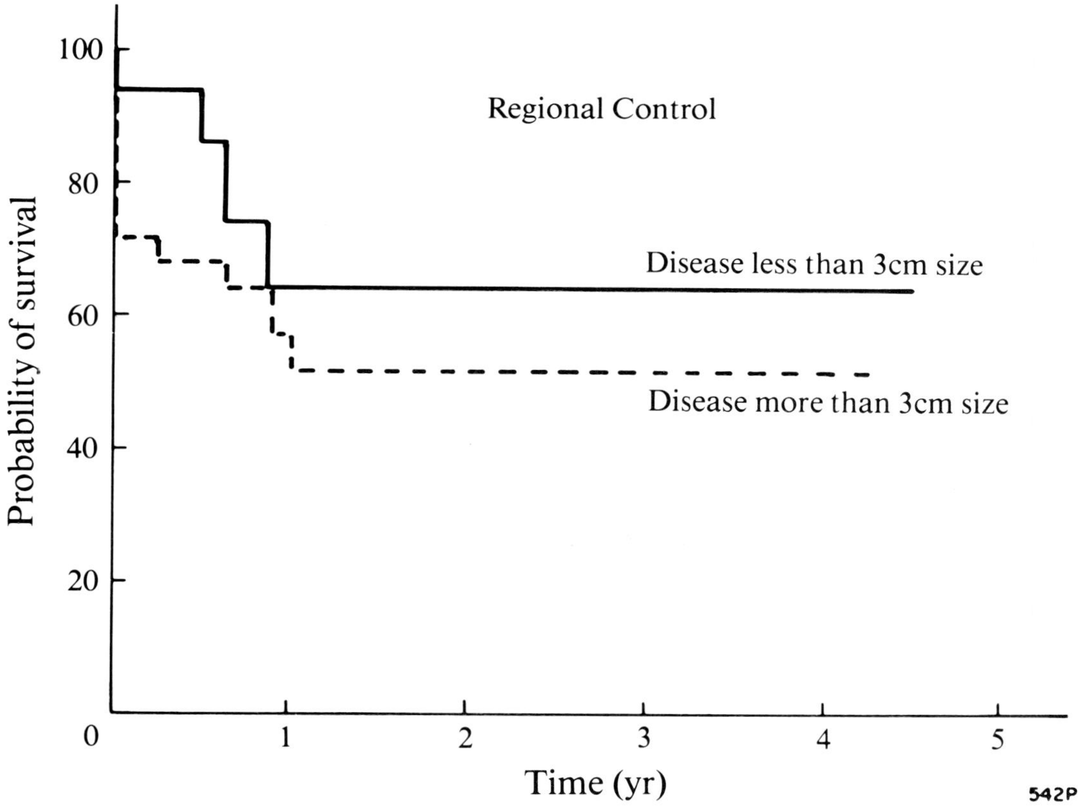

Figure 19–4. Actuarial 5-year regional tumor control rates for the group of patients with residual or recurrent tumors, compared by node size.

seminated disease. There is clearly a need for effective systemic adjuvant therapy in this patient group. The fact that lymph-node biopsy plus 0,7,21 irradiation is as effective as lymph-node dissection plus 0,7,21 irradiation indicates that patients at high risk of complications from lymph-node dissection may be adequately treated by the biopsy and irradiation method.

In view of the effectiveness of 0,7,21 irradiation in dealing with microscopic nodal metastases from melanoma, and also its low morbidity, it is interesting to speculate on the role of 0,7,21 irradiation delivered prophylactically to lymph nodes clinically negative for disease in patients with primary melanomas at high risk of developing microscopic lymph-node metastases (i.e., melanoma at Clarks's level 4 or 5, or with a Breslow thickness of more than 1.1 mm).

To definitely establish the role of adjuvant irradiation in patients with melanoma in the lymph nodes clearly requires a randomized, controlled clinical trial in which patients would be randomized to lymph-node dissection alone or to lymph-node dissection and adjuvant 0,7,21 radiotherapy. A third group in this trial would undergo lymph-node biopsy and 0,7,21 radiotherapy. In such a trial, which would require a minimum of 200 patients, 5-year regional control and survival rates would be evaluated.

ILLUSTRATIVE CLINICAL CASES

Case 1

A 54-year old man presented in August 1979 with a 4×2 cm superficial spreading melanoma on the posterior aspect of his right ear. It invaded to Clark's level 3. Primary irradiation was chosen as the treatment for this lesion, and 4500 cGy was delivered in 10 fractions over 2 weeks. The primary tumor responded completely to irradiation, and the patient had good cosmetic results. In July 1982, the patient developed a 3-cm node in the posterior triangle of the right side of his neck. A biopsy specimen was taken, and melanoma metastatic to the lymph node was diagnosed. A radical neck dissection was performed. Pathologic examination of the neck-dissection specimen revealed three nodes involved by melanoma; one node was more than 3 cm in size, and there was capsular penetration in the largest lymph node. In September 1982, the patient received adjuvant 0,7,21 irradition to the right side of his neck with electron beam therapy. In February 1985, the patient was alive and well.

The use of adjuvant irradiation in this case prevented recurrence in the neck.

Case 2

A woman presented in November 1977 with recurrent mucosal melanoma of the hard palate and bilateral neck-node metastases. The largest lymph node was 3cm in size and in the right side of her neck. A right radical neck dissection was undertaken to remove the largest node. Pathologic examination revealed melanoma invading the lymph-node capsule and sternomastoid muscle. In January 1978, the patient received 0,7,21 irradiation plus DTIC before the first and third doses of irradiation. The irradiation field included the primary site and both sides of the neck. The dose to the spinal cord was limited to 1600 cGy. The patient's disease completely disappeared with this therapy, and she was alive and well at her follow-up examination in June 1984.

This case illustrates the curative potential of 0,7,21 radiotherapy for mucosal melanoma with bilateral neck-node metastases.

Case 3

A man presented in January 1981 with Clark's level 5 lentigo maligna melanoma of the left ear. Primary irradiation was chosen to treat the primary tumor (Harwood, 1984), which was successfully controlled, but in December 1981, a lymph node metastasis developed in the left side of the neck. A lymph-node dissection was carried out, revealing that more than three nodes in the specimen were involved, one node was more than 3 cm in size. Adjuvant 0,7,21 irradiation was applied to the neck using electron beam therapy. In March 1982, with the primary tumor and neck metastases controlled, the patient developed lung metastases. In May 1983, the patient died of lung metastases.

This is the only patient of more than 70 with lentigo maligna or lentigo maligna melanoma who was primarily irradiated and developed lymph-node and distant metastases. This case illustrates the problem we have observed in many of our adjuvant high-risk patients—namely, the early development of distant metastases, about which little can be done.

CONCLUSION

Current indications for the use of 0,7,21 irradiation for lymph-node metastases from melanoma are gross or residual melanoma following attempted surgical excision of disease; lymph-node capsule penetration; multiple (three or more) nodes in the surgical specimen positive for disease; or a node totally replaced by melanoma or greater than 3 cm in size after lymph node dissection; and lymph-node biopsy confirming metastatic melanoma in patients who are unsuitable for lymph-node dissection. To definitively resolve the role of 0,7,21 radiotherapy as adjuvant treatment and to evaluate resultant survival and regional control rates, a randomized controlled clinical trial comparing three methods of treatment (lymph-node dissection alone, lymph-node dissection plus 0,7,21 radiation, and lymph-node biopsy plus 0,7,21 radiation) is necessary.

REFERENCES

Creagan, E. T., Woods, J. E., Cupps, R. E., and O'Fallon, J. R.: Radiation therapy for malignant melanoma of the head and neck. *Am. J. Surg*, 138:604–08, 1979.

Creagan, E. T., Cupps, R. E., Ivins, J. C., Pritchard, D. J., Sim, F. H., Soule, E. H., and O'Fallon, J. R.: Adjuvant radiation therapy for regional nodal metastases from malignant melanoma. *Cancer*, 42:2206–10, 1978.

Harwood, A. R., and Cummings, G. J.: Radiotherapy for malignant melanoma: A reappraisal. *Cancer Treat. Rev.*, 8:271–82, 1981.

Harwood, A. R.: Melanoma of the head and neck. In Millon R. R.; Cassisi, N. J. (eds.): *Management of Head and Neck Cancer. A Multidisciplinary Approach*, pp. 513–28. J. B. Lippincott, Philadelphia, 1984.

Jansen, G. T., and Westbrook, K. C.: Cancer of the skin. In Suen, J. Y. and Myers, E. N. (eds.): *Cancer of the Head and Neck*, p. 234. Churchill-Livingston, New York, 1981.

Johanson, C., Harwood, A. R., Cummings, B. J., and Quirt, I.: 0,7,21 radiotherapy in nodular melanoma. *Cancer*, 51:226–32, 1983.

CHAPTER 20

Management of Regional Metastasis in Salivary and Thyroid Cancer

Jatin P. Shah

EDITORS' COMMENT

Few question the value of neck dissection for clinically apparent nodes, but Dr. Shah provides us with an approach to management of the clinically negative neck for tumors of the salivary and thyroid glands. Reporting on the experience at Memorial Sloan-Kettering Hospital, New York City, Dr. Shah, a long-time member of the Section of Head and Neck Surgery there, gives us a unique look at the incidence and management of regional metastasis from both the salivary and thyroid glands. While concerning himself with the primary disease process, he outlines a logical approach to elective treatment of the neck based on the experience at Memorial Hospital.

The first half of the chapter deals with the salivary glands. After noting his use of the Foote and Frazell classification of salivary tumors, Dr. Shah reaffirms, by his data, a fact known to all—that the proportion of malignancy increases as the size of the gland decreases. He then notes the important prognostic value of the presence of clinically positive nodes in association with a salivary malignancy at the initial presentation (74% vs. 9% 5-year survival). By identification of the high-risk patient, we can better know which to treat adjunctively.

Dr. Shah then presents the Memorial Sloan-Kettering series (1939–1973) of patients with nodal metastasis from all salivary-gland tumors and their cell of origin. Aside from patients with N+ disease, he believes that elective treatment of the neck would be appropriate in patients who have high-grade tumors of any variety or in patients who have bulky primary disease. Dr. Shah also suggests adjunctive radiation therapy to both the primary and neck in these settings. This treatment, the author believes, would provide adequate local and regional control, although the impact on survival is not reported with this combined therapy.

The remainder of the chapter is devoted to the management of regional metastasis from the thyroid gland. Again, relying on the extensive Memorial Hospital experience, the author confirms the observations of others that the impact of clinically inapparent nodal metastasis from differentiated thyroid cancer probably has no bearing on the eventual clinical status of the patient. If the status of the nodes seems to have so little effect on the end result, it seems hard to justify a classical radical neck dissection in this clinical setting. The author then outlines his approach to neck treatment in a variety of primary thyroid tumors.

INTRODUCTION

A great deal has been written about salivary and thyroid tumors. Most authors deal with management of the primary tumor or a particular anatomic structure related to those glands, but few have identified the importance of the lymph nodes in the immediately adjacent area. There is general agreement that if the nodes are obviously involved with tumor, they should be removed—but with what type of lymphadenectomy? Should radiation therapy play a role? Does synchronous neck dissection really make a difference in the patient's survival? These and other questions the head and neck surgeon might have in dealing with salivary and thyroid glands are covered in this chapter.

THE SALIVARY GLANDS

The parotid gland is an unusual site for malignant tumors, and only 20 to 30 percent of all parotid tumors are malignant. On the other hand, nearly 50 percent of all tumors of the submandibular gland are malignant. The proportion of malignant tumors is highest (88%), however, when they arise in minor salivary glands (Spiro et al., 1975). Cancers of the salivary glands have a variable biologic course, and they do not follow the familiar pattern of squamous cell carcinomas of the upper aerodigestive tract. The great variance in diverse biologic behavior of these tumors is largely due to the different histologic nature of these neoplasms. The classic report of Foote and Frazell (1953) described the histopathogenesis of various salivary-gland tumors. Their histopathologic classification is widely accepted.

Although involvement of regional lymph nodes by metastases from malignant salivary tumors is infrequent, its impact on prognosis is profound (Table 20–1). For patients with previously untreated parotid cancers, a 5-year survival of 74 percent is obtained following surgical treatment if regional nodes are not involved. Only 9% of patients who have regional node involvement at the time of initial treatment, however, survive 5 years. Subsequent involvement of regional nodes also adversely affects survival, dropping it to only 17 percent. A similar adverse effect of regional lymph-node metastases is observed in patients with malignant tumors of the submandibular gland.

Although treatment of clinically apparent neck-node metastases from salivary-gland tumors by neck dissection with or without postoperative radiotherapy is generally accepted, the success of such treatment leaves much to be desired. A question must therefore be raised about the role of elective treatment of the regional lymph nodes, in the hope of improving survival for patients with malignant salivary gland tumors. We must also make an attempt to define the high-risk group where such elective treatment may have the maximum potential of benefit.

In analyzing factors influencing the prognosis in tumors of the major salivary glands, Spiro et al. (1975; 1976) concluded that the histologic type of primary tumor, its grade, and the stage of disease, including cervical-node metastases and facial-nerve function, were the most important predictors. It is important, therefore, to review the incidence of regional node involvement in relation to the histologic type and grade of primary malignant tumors of salivary origin.

Data from review of the records of patients

Table 20–1. Influence of Nodal Status on Five-Year Cure in Malignant Tumors of Major Salivary Glands

TIME OF APPEARANCE OF CERVICAL NODE METASTASIS	PAROTID CARCINOMA			SUBMANDIBULAR GLAND CARCINOMA		
	No. of patients	*NED*	*%*	*No. of patients*	*NED*	*%*
Never documented	213	157	74	68	28	41
Present on admission	57	5	9	32	3	9
Appeared later	18	3	17	4	1	25

NED = no evidence of disease.
Adapted from Spiro et al., 1975; 1976.

Table 20-2. Involvement of Cervical Lymph Nodes by Metastatic Disease from Primary Carcinomas of Parotid, Submandibular, and Minor Salivary Glands

TIME OF APPEARANCE	PAROTID (%) (N = 623)	SUBMANDIBULAR (%) (N = 129)	MINOR (%) (N = 526)
Initially	20	33	13
Subsequently	5	4	9
Total	25	37	22

with salivary gland cancers treated by the Head and Neck Service of Memorial Sloan-Kettering Cancer Center from 1939 to 1973 are presented. Twenty percent of patients with parotid cancer, 33 percent of those with submandibular gland carcinoma, and 13 percent of patients with primary carcinomas of minor salivary origin presented with cervical lymph-node metastases (Table 20–2). On the other hand, only 5 percent, 4 percent and 9 percent of patients with cancers of the parotid, submandibular gland, and minor salivary glands, respectively, later developed neck-node metastases. The breakdown of initial and subsequent involvement of cervical lymph nodes by histologic type of cancer for parotid, submandibular, and minor salivary glands is shown in Tables 20–3, 20–4, and 20–5.

None of the patients with low-grade mucoepidermoid carcinomas in all three sites developed regional lymph-node metastasis. The highest frequency of involvement of cervical lymph nodes occurred either initially or subsequently in patients with squamous carcinoma of major salivary glands, high-grade mucoepidermoid carcinomas, or high-grade adenocarcinomas, and in some patients with malignant mixed tumors. The incidence of neck node metastases from primary acinic cell carcinomas and adenoid cystic carcinomas was low. Thus, it appears that patients who are clinically negative for neck disease at presentation but have a high-staged, high-grade squamous carcinoma, mucoepidermoid carcinoma, adenocarcinoma, anaplastic carcinoma, or malignant mixed tumor are candidates for elective treatment of the neck. Neck dissection is indicated if the primary tumor is bulky, or metastases are confirmed at the time of surgery. The long-term benefit from elective treatment of the neck still remains to be proved.

All patients undergoing neck dissection for metastatic disease in the nodes should have postoperative radiotherapy to the primary site and the site of dissection. Although increased local or regional control can be expected, improvement in survival is not reported with combined therapy.

THE THYROID GLAND

There is no uniform agreement on the management of regional lymph nodes in patients with differentiated thyroid carcinoma. The thyroid gland contains an abundant intraglandular lymphatic network that anastomoses frequently through the thyroid capsule with periglandular lymph nodes and lymphatics, then with paratracheal and pretracheal lymph nodes, and finally with upper mediastinal and lateral cervical lymph nodes. A significant

Table 20-3. Involvement of Cervical Lymph Node by Metastatic Carcinoma from Primary Parotid Carcinomas

HISTOLOGY	NO. OF PATIENTS	TIME OF APPEARANCE		TOTAL (%)
		Initially	*Subsequently*	
Squamous Carcinoma	45	19	2	21 (47)
Adenocarcinoma	62	14	4	18 (29)
Mucoepidermoid	272	66	7	73 (27)
Malignant mixed	107	18	9	27 (25)
Other	8	2	0	2 (25)
Acinic	75	6	5	11 (15)
Adenoid cystic	54	2	5	7 (13)
Total	623	127 (20%)	32 (5%)	159 (25%)

Table 20–4. Involvement of Cervical Lymph Nodes by Metastatic Carcinoma from Primary Submandibular Gland Carcinomas

HISTOLOGY	NO. OF PATIENTS	TIME OF APPEARANCE		TOTAL (%)
		Initially	*Subsequently*	
Squamous Carcinoma	8	3	0	3 (37)
Adenocarcinoma	9	4	0	4 (44)
Mucoepidermoid	37	20	2	22 (59)
Malignant-mixed	24	4	0	4 (17)
Other	4	3	0	3 (75)
Acinic	2	0	0	0
Adenoid cystic	45	9	3	12 (27)
Total	129	43 (33%)	5 (4%)	48 (37%)

number of patients will present with clinically apparent cervical lymph-node metastasis at the time of initial diagnosis and treatment of papillary carcinoma of the thyroid gland. The prognostic significance of cervical lymph-node metastasis in differentiated thyroid cancer, however, is controversial. Involvement of cervical lymph nodes alone does not necessarily influence the prognosis of patients with papillary carcinoma of the thyroid gland.

In our own experience, 55 percent of the patients with papillary carcinoma of the thyroid gland presented with clinically apparent cervical lymph node metastasis (Table 20–6). Of the 376 previously untreated patients with papillary carcinoma of the thyroid treated by us, 293 underwent neck dissection as an integral part of the initial surgical treatment. Thirty-five of them had bilateral neck dissections, with histologic confirmation of metastatic cancer in all of them. One hundred and seventy patients underwent ipsilateral neck dissection, with histologic confirmation of metastatic carcinoma obtained in 166 (98%).

In contrast, 88 underwent elective neck dissection though they were clinically negative for neck disease, and 47 percent of them had histologic confirmation of metastastic cancer in the excised cervical lymph nodes. Thus, the detection rate for occult metastatic carcinoma from a primary papillary cancer of the thyroid was 47 percent. One could then cite this figure as an argument for considering elective treatment of the neck as an integral part of initial surgical treatment. The impact of these microscopic metastases in the cervical lymph nodes of patients who have nonpalpable lymph nodes, however, is very small. Few, if any, patients die of well-differentiated thyroid carcinoma metastatic to lateral cervical lymph nodes in the absence of local recurrence or distant metastasis.

The prognosis of cervical lymph-node metastasis from papillary carcinoma does not depend on the bulk of nodal metastatic disease. In our series of determinate cases involving radical neck dissection for gross metastases and elective neck dissection for occult metastasis, there was no survival difference at 5 years. Whether the metastatic disease was unilateral or bilateral did not seem to influence curability.

Although surgical removal of clinically involved cervical lymph nodes is well accepted,

Table 20–5. Involvement of Cervical Lymph Nodes by Metastatic Carcinoma from Primary Minor Salivary Gland Carcinomas

HISTOLOGY	NO. OF PATIENTS	TIME OF APPEARANCE		TOTAL (%)
		Initially	*Subsequently*	
Adenocarcinoma	154	18	16	34 (22)
Mucoepidermoid	130	20	15	35 (27)
Malignant-mixed	30	5	1	6 (20)
Other	23	8	5	13 (57)
Acinic	7	0	0	0
Adenoid cystic	182	16	10	26 (14)
Total	526	67 (13%)	47 (9%)	114 (22%)

Table 20-6. Cervical Lymph-Node Metastases in Carcinoma of the Thyroid

HISTOLOGY	NO. OF PATIENTS	NO. PRESENTING WITH POSITIVE NODES (%)*	NO. WITH OCCULT METASTASES IN ELECTIVE NECK DISSECTIONS (%)
Papillary	376	208 (55)	41/88 (47)
Follicular	69	18 (26)	3/14 (21)
Hurthle cell	35	3 (9)	1/7 (14)
Medullary	30	14 (47)	0/2 (0)

*Palpable nodes

such procedures have varied from simple local excisions to a classical radical neck dissection. Classical radical neck dissection is effective, but less disabling or deforming (and probably equally effective) dissection methods that spare the spinal accessory nerve and sternocleidomastoid muscle (and sometimes the internal jugular vein) are currently popular. No clear-cut superiority of the classical dissection over the modified radical neck dissection in the eradication of metastatic, well-differentiated thyroid cancer has been reported. The modified procedure is a more tedious and time-consuming operation. The cosmetic and functional advantages are obvious, but all potentially or actually involved lymph nodes in the pre- and paratracheal areas, superior mediastinum, and lateral aspects of the neck must be meticulously removed.

The Role of Neck Dissection

Patients with papillary thyroid carcinoma without clinical evidence of neck-node metastasis are candidates for observation until the surgical treatment of their neck nodes becomes necessary. Thus, a neck dissection can be deferred until the nodes become clinically palpable without apparently jeopardizing the prognosis. Hutter et al. (1970) reported a study of patients with papillary carcinoma and clinically uninvolved lateral cervical lymph nodes. The patients were divided into two equal groups—those who underwent elective neck dissection and those in whom dissection was delayed until nodes became clinically positive. There was no statistically significant difference between the two groups in the subsequent mortality from thyroid cancer or in prognosis. In fact, subsequent tumors in the delayed-dissection group were not confined to, or chiefly in, the cervical lymph nodes.

In our study, it would have been necessary to perform 88 neck dissections to prevent the subsequent cervical metastasis in eight patients, most of whom had successful local eradication of cervical disease by therapeutic neck dissection at the time of its appearance. Although no specific class of patients could be positively identified as benefiting from elective neck dissection, men over 40 years old whose tumors exceeded 5 cm in diameter had the poorest prognosis, and thus may have the most to gain from elective treatment of the neck. At present, we recommend neck dissection only for patients with clinically or pathologically documented lateral cervical lymph-node metastasis. Other authors have reached similar conclusions (Buckwalter and Thomas, 1972; Clark et al., 1966; Cline and Shingleton, 1968; Marchetta et al., 1970; Mustard, 1970; Woolner et al., 1961).

Treatment of Papillary Carcinoma of the Thyroid

Our current treatment approach for papillary carcinomas of the thyroid gland is as follows. If clinically apparent cervical lymph-node metastases are found at initial presentation, then we perform a modified neck dissection that preserves the sternomastoid muscle, accessary nerve, and the jugular vein. Meticulous clearance of tumor tissue from the tracheoesophageal groove lymph nodes, superior mediastinal lymph nodes, and lateral aspect of the neck is undertaken. If the neck is clinically negative for metastasis, then thyroidectomy is performed, its extent depending on the extension of the primary tumor. Once the diagnosis of papillary carcinoma is confirmed, usually by frozen section examination, then clearance of nodes from the tracheoesophageal groove and medial compartment of the neck on that side is performed immediately. Elective neck dissection is not undertaken, but a neck dissection is done if gross metastases are documented, either in the central compartment or the lateral compartment of the neck, during thyroid surgery.

Treatment of Other Thyroid Tumors

The incidence of cervical lymph-node involvement by primary follicular and Hurthle cell carcinomas of the thyroid gland is low. Therapeutic neck dissection is indicated in patients who present with clinically palpable cervical lymph-node metastases. Elective neck dissection is not necessary. Nearly half the patients with primary medullary carcinoma of the thyroid gland present with clinically apparent cervical lymph-node metastases. In these patients, a classical radical neck dissection is recommended because metastatic medullary carcinoma of the thyroid gland is more aggressive than differentiated thyroid cancer. Clearance of lateral neck and central compartment, as well as superior mediastinal lymph nodes, is mandatory for medullary carcinoma of the thyroid gland. The role of elective radical neck dissection in the management of medullary carcinoma of the thyroid gland is still not clear. In the absence of histologically confirmed metastatic nodes it has no impact on the prognosis.

DISCUSSION

Though uncommon, regional metastases from salivary and thyroid glands have very different prognostic values. In the former, nodal involvement carries a grave prognosis and seems to demand adjunctive treatment. In the latter, for the most common, differentiated cases, regional involvement has little impact. Regardless, it is most important for the surgeon to have a logical approach to the correct management of the regional lymph nodes for the expected, or unexpected, finding of metastasis from a salivary or thyroid primary tumor.

REFERENCES

Buckwalter, J. A., and Thomas, C. G., Jr.: Selection of surgical treatment for well-differentiated thyroid carcinomas. *Ann. Surg.*; 176:565–69, 1972.

Clark, R. L., Ibanez, M. L., and White, E. E.: What constitutes an adequate operation for carcinoma of the thyroid? *Arch. Surg.*, 92:23–26, 1966.

Cline, R. W., and Shingleton, W. W.: Long-term results in the treatment of carcinoma of the thyroid. *Am. J. Surg.*, 115:545–51, 1968.

Foote, F. W., Jr., and Frazell, E. L.: Tumors of the major salivary glands. *Cancer*, 6:1065–1133, 1953.

Hutter, R. V. P., Frazell, E. L., and Foote, F. W.: Elective radical neck dissection. An assessment of its use in the management of papillary thyroid cancer. *CA*, 20:87–93, 1970.

Marchetta, F. C., Sako, K., and Matsuara, H.: Modified neck dissection from carcinoma of the thyroid gland. *Am. J. Surg.*, 129:4452–55, 1970.

Mustard, R. A.: Treatment of papillary carcinoma of the thyroid with emphasis on conservation neck dissection. *Am. J. Surg.*, 120:697–703, 1970.

Spiro, R. H., Hajdu, S. I., and Strong, E. W.: Tumors of the submaxillary gland. *Am. J. Surg.*, 132:463–68, 1976.

Spiro, R. H., Huvos, A. G., and Strong, E. W.: Cancer of the parotid gland. *Am. J. Surg.*, 30:452–59, 1975.

Spiro, R. H., Koss, L. G., Hajdu, S. I., and Strong, E. W.: Tumors of minor salivary origin. *Cancer*, 32:117–29, 1975.

Woolner, L. B., Beahrs, O. H., Black, B. M., McConahey, W. M., and Keating, F. R., Jr.: Classification and prognosis of thyroid carcinoma. *Am. J. Surg.*, 102: 354–59, 1961.

CHAPTER 21

Treatment of Uncommon Tumors of the Neck: Sarcoma and Lymphoma

Robert D. Lindberg

EDITORS' COMMENT

Dr. Robert Lindberg, is recognized as one of the most knowledgeable radiotherapists in head and neck cancer. In this chapter, he brings us an uncommonly thorough review of two tumor types that present in the neck often enough to warrant a hasty literature review when unexpectedly found at operation.

After a historical review of the treatment and classification of lymphoma, the author stresses the importance of adequate biopsy by the surgeon, then outlines the typical workup once the diagnosis is made. The results of treatment of both Hodgkin's and non-Hodgkin's lymphoma are presented succinctly, in addition to the complications of radiation therapy of these entities.

Sarcomas most commonly arise in the extremities, but have the ability to originate from any type of connective tissue above the clavicles. The diagnosis of sarcoma in the neck is usually made at the "open biopsy" stage of an unknown primary evaluation. Because these tumors rarely metastasize to regional nodes, the clinician must decide the need for adjunctive therapy based on the local aggressiveness of the tumor and the adequacy of the resection. Regardless, long-term follow-up is essential because the most common site of spread is the lungs. Most patients, in Dr. Lindberg's experience, *do* receive radiation therapy for local control. He notes that massive neck disease should probably receive preoperative radiation therapy to facilitate a planned surgical resection. To date, no one has enough clinical data to determine the benefit of chemotherapy of sarcomas in the neck.

Though sarcomas are uncommon as primary tumors of the head and neck, when they are seen in a clinical setting the physician should have an up-to-date reference available on the evaluation, treatment, and long-term results of lymphoma and sarcoma management. Dr. Lindberg has provided us with that reference, in conjunction with an extensive bibliography for those requiring more information on the subject.

INTRODUCTION

The most common malignant tumor in the neck is metastatic squamous cell carcinoma from a primary head and neck site. The incidence of primary malignant tumors arising in the neck is very low; therefore, diagnosis of a primary neck tumor is usually based on the exclusion of metastatic cancer. A variety of benign and malignant tumors usually occur in the neck (see Table 21-1). Occasionally, the patient's medical history and the location of a palpable mass lead the investigator to suspect a primary tumor arising in the neck. Examples of such symptoms are slow-growing masses of long-standing duration in the submaxillary triangle (submaxillary gland tumors), masses arising in the bifurcation of the carotid artery (carotid body tumors), and masses arising in the thyroid gland.

Some primary tumors, such as soft tissue sarcomas and localized lymphoma, may not even be considered in the differential diagnosis. This discussion covers stage I lymphomas limited to the neck, and localized primary cervical soft tissue sarcomas in adults.

Table 21-1. Uncommon Tumors of the Neck

TYPE	NAME	DESCRIPTION
Benign	Teratomas	Usually present at birth
	Cysts	Bronchial cleft
		Thymic
		Thyroglossal duct
	Carotid body tumors	
	Thyroid gland	
	Submaxillary gland	
	Parathyroid	
Malignant	Skin	Squamous cell carcinoma
		Basal cell carcinoma
		Melanoma
	Lymphoma	Hodgkin's disease
		Non-Hodgkin's lymphoma
	Soft tissue sarcomas	
	Thyroid gland	
	Submaxillary gland	
	Parathyroid	

LYMPHOMA

Lymphomas are currently divided into two basic types: Hodgkin's and non-Hodgkin's lymphoma. The pathologic criteria for diagnosis of Hodgkin's disease are well-recognized, whereas the histologic classification continues to change in non-Hodgkin's lymphoma (Carbone et al., 1971; NCI, 1982) (see Table 21-2). This constant change in classification criteria causes numerous problems for the clinician in understanding the similarities and differences among the classification systems and in properly accessing the published results.

The biologic behaviors of Hodgkin's disease and non-Hodgkin's lymphoma are considerably different. Hodgkin's disease mainly affects the cervical lymph nodes (Fierstein and Thawley, 1978) with predictable patterns of spread, whereas patients with non-Hodgkin's lymphoma usually present with diseases in advanced stages of generalized involvement of both nodal and extranodal sites (Fuller et al., 1976; Johnson et al., 1974; Peters et al., 1968; Wong et al., 1975). The majority of extranodal sites are limited to the head and neck region (Plantenga et al., 1981; Wong et al., 1976).

The approach to treating lymphomas has changed dramatically in the past 25 years; the role of radiotherapy in particular has become more important over the past 40 years. In 1939, Gilbert laid the foundation for the principles of modern radiotherapy for Hodgkin's disease. In 1950, Peters reported the curability of Hodgkin's disease with radiotherapy, and Easson and Russell in 1963 showed that radiation therapy also cured non-Hodgkin's lymphoma. Subsequently, the Stanford group has published studies on the systematic use of aggressive radiation therapy and chemotherapy in lymphoma (Kaplan, 1980). Since then, there have been many studies on lymphomas reported from single institutions and cooperative groups, stressing the use of single or multimodality treatment depending on the stage of the disease.

Defining the extent of the disease is crucial in the treatment of lymphomas. First, there

Table 21–2. Working Formulation of Non-Hodgkin's Lymphoma

GRADE	NAME	DESCRIPTION
Low	Malignant lymphoma	Small lymphocytic; consistent with chronic lymphocytic leukemia
	Malignant lymphoma, follicular	Predominantly small cleaved cell; sclerosis
Intermediate	Malignant lymphoma, follicular	Predominantly large cell; diffuse areas; sclerosis
	Malignant lymphoma, diffuse	Small cleaved cell; sclerosis
	Malignant lymphoma, diffuse	Mixed, small and large cell; sclerosis; epithelioid cell component
	Malignant lymphoma, diffuse	Large cell; cleaved cell; noncleaved cell; sclerosis
High	Malignant lymphoma	Large cell, immunoblastic; plasmacytoid; clear cell; polymorphous; epithelioid cell component
	Malignant lymphoma	Lymphoblastic; convoluted cell; nonconvoluted cell
	Malignant lymphoma	Small noncleaved cell; Burkitt's lymphoma; follicular areas
Miscellaneous	Composite	
	Mycosis fungoides	
	Histiocytic	
	Extramedullary plasmacytoma	
	Unclassifiable	
	Other	

must be an adequate biopsy to properly define the histologic subtypes. The staging system used for Hodgkin's disease and non-Hodgkin's lymphoma is the Ann Arbor Staging Classification (Carbone et al., 1971). In addition to the routine studies—complete blood count, blood chemistry, and chest x-ray examinations—the workup of Hodgkin's disease includes a lymphangiogram or a computerized tomography (CT) scan of the abdomen and a bone-marrow biopsy. Other tests, such as a CT scan of the chest, an intravenous pyelogram, or a bone scan, may be indicated. An exploratory laparotomy should be considered on all patients with clinical stage I, II, or III disease if the findings alter the treatment approach. The workup is similar for non-Hodgkin's lymphoma, except that more emphasis is placed on the CT scan of the abdomen than on the lymphangiography. CT scans should be done on patients with non-Hodgkin's lymphoma, and lymphangiograms on patients with Hodgkin's disease. A bone marrow biopsy is indicated in all patients. Patients with clinical stage I or II non-Hodgkin's lymphoma should be considered for laparotomy.

TREATMENT AND RESULTS

Hodgkin's Disease

Patients with Hodgkin's disease may be cured by radiotherapy alone, by chemotherapy alone, or by a combination of both. In general, patients with stage I neck disease are treated by radiation therapy alone. Thar et al. (1979) recommended 3500 cGy in 150- to 170-cGy fractions for lesions less than 6 cm in diameter. The in-field recurrence rate of such lesions is 7 percent. Tumors larger than 6 cm in diameter may require doses up to 4000 cGy. Doses of more than 4000 cGy have not been shown to improve the survival rate significantly, but may increase the complication rate (Thar et al., 1979). The actual treatment of a particular patient depends on a number of factors.

Results of treatment for Hodgkin's disease are usually presented according to the stage rather than the anatomic location of the disease. Helman and Mauch (1982) reported an 80 percent 10-year relapse-free survival time in stage IA and IIA patients, with a 95 percent overall survival rate. The Stanford group showed that total nodal irradiation of patients with stages IA and IIA Hodgkin's disease improved the relapse-free survival time more than involved-field irradiation did, but not the overall survival rate. Thus, in patients with stage I Hodgkin's disease, total nodal irradiation is not necessary (Helman and Mauch, 1982).

Non-Hodgkin's Lymphoma

Although extranodal non-Hodgkin's lymphoma is common in the head and neck area, less than 10 percent of the patients have disease limited to the neck. The most common site of presentation in the head and neck region is Waldeyer's tonsillar ring (Mill et al., 1980; Plantenga et al., 1981; Wong et al., 1975). The two major sites of solitary neck involvement by this lymphoma are the thyroid and the submaxillary glands (Mill et al., 1980; Plantenga et al., 1981; Wong et al., 1975). One of the highest incidences of cervical node disease—16 percent—was reported by Fierstein and Thawley in 1978.

The treatment of choice for stage I non-Hodgkin's lymphoma is radiation therapy. There is still a debate as to which radiotherapy technique—involved- or extended-field—gives the better cure rate. For treatment purposes, non-Hodgkin's lymphoma can be divided into favorable and nonfavorable histiologic subtypes (Mill et al., 1980; Thar, 1984). The "favorable" lymphomas include nodular lymphomas (except for nodular histocytic lymphoma) and diffuse well-differentiated lymphocytic types. The remaining histologic subtypes, including diffuse histiocytic, diffuse poorly differentiated lymphocytic, nodular histiocytic, and diffuse undifferentiated lymphoma, are in the unfavorable group. The dose recommended for the favorable group is 3000 cGy in 150- to 170-cGy fractions, compared with 4500 to 5500 cGy in 180-cGy fractions for the unfavorable group. The radiotherapy techniques used to treat non-Hodgkin's lymphoma limited to the neck are similar to those used for squamous cell carcinomas.

Wong et al. (1975) used an anterior field to cover the neck and upper mediastinum to treat cancer presenting in the thyroid. A posterior field was used to augment the tumor dose calculated to the midplane of the mediastinum. They reported a 58 percent 5-year disease-free survival rate in patients with stage I head and neck disease. Since dissemination is common for extranodal stage I and stage II diffuse lymphomas, Wong et al. (1975) recommended a staging celiotomy and a clinical trial using multiagent chemotherapy in addition to the radiation therapy.

In 1980, Reddy et al. reported a 77 percent 5-year recurrence-free survival rate for stage I extranodal non-Hodgkin's lymphoma. They, too, recommended prospective trials with multiagent chemotherapy and radiation therapy in stage II extranodular non-Hodgkin's lymphoma. In patients with stages I and II extranodal presentation, Mill et al. (1980) reported a 5-year survival rate of 100 percent in the favorable group and 52 percent in the unfavorable group. The overall disease-free survival rate for stage I at 5 years was 49 percent.

The major problem in non-Hodgkin's lymphoma is not local control of the tumor but eradication of the occult disseminated disease. Between July 1951 and August 1975, 24 patients with diffuse histiocytic lymphoma of the thyroid were seen at The University of Texas M.D. Anderson Hospital and Tumor Institute at Houston (UTMDAH). All patients had presented with a mass in the neck, and the clinical diagnosis was primary thyroid malignancy; malignant lymphoma was never suspected. Twelve patients received radiation therapy using an anterior ^{60}Co field to cover the entire neck and mediastinum, which received a 5000-cGy dose over 5 weeks. A posterior mediastinal field was used to increase the tumor dose to the midmediastinum to 4000 cGy. None of the patients developed further manifestation of lymphoma. Five patients are living free of disease at 18, 30, 36, 52, and 54 months. Five patients have died because of intercurrent disease; two of the five lived more than 10 years without disease. The remaining two patients died of unknown causes.

In 1978, Fierstein and Thawley reported that of 88 patients with non-Hodgkin's lymphoma of the head and neck area, 55 had stage I disease, 12 of whom presented with disease in nodal sites. In general, patients with stage I disease were treated by radiation therapy alone, and received 4000 to 5500 cGy tumor dose. The failure rate was two of 43 patients with extranodal disease, compared with five of 12 patients with nodal stage I disease. Their's is one of two reports showing that patients presenting with nodal disease have a poor prognosis compared with those with disease in extranodal sites. Fierstein and Thawley also recommended combined chemotherapy and radiation in all patients except those with stage I disease. Thus, the consensus is that stage I non-Hodgkin's lymphoma can be adequately treated by radiation therapy alone, whereas in more advanced disease a combination of chemotherapy and radiotherapy should be used.

The late sequelae are minimal because the tumor dose is limited to 3000 to 5000 cGy in 180-cGy fractions or less. When the entire neck is treated, however, patients must be made aware of potential dental complications. Many of the dental problems can be prevented with proper care—i.e., proper cleaning and topical fluoride applications. Irradiation of the neck may cause some degree of xerostomia, especially if the patient is at rest, because most of the saliva produced at rest is produced by the submaxillary glands. Occasionally, some patients show fibrosis of the cervical muscles. The disability secondary to fibrosis can be minimized by proper exercises. Patients are also at risk for hypothyroidism. Although hypothyroidism is not usually manifested clinically, proper testing with free thyroxine and thyroid-stimulating hormone determinations may detect the disease. Although there is a risk of spinal cord damage by irradiation, its incidence is very rare when the radiation dose to the spinal cord is less than 4500 cGy over 5 weeks.

SOFT-TISSUE SARCOMAS

Soft-tissue sarcomas are relatively rare malignant tumors that arise from the connective tissues, and thus occur throughout the body. There are approximately 5000 new cases of soft-tissue sarcoma per year, according to American Cancer Society statistics (1985). The majority of the cases arise in the extremities (55%), especially the lower extremities (40%). The male-to-female ratio is almost 1:1 (53% vs. 47%, respectively), and the average patient age is 45 years. Most soft-tissue sarcomas are named for their tissue of origin. The most common histologic types are fibrosarcoma, liposarcoma, neurofibrosarcoma, and malignant fibrohistiocytoma (Hajdu, 1979).

The treatment of soft-tissue sarcomas has changed over the past two to three decades. Twenty-five years ago, the only treatment that had a significant cure rate was radical surgery. Because most soft-tissue sarcomas tend to be locally invasive, the incidence of local recurrence varied with the type of surgical procedure: 80 to 100 percent after local excision (Cadman et al., 1957; Shieber and Graham, 1962); approximately 40 percent after wide excision (Sheiber and Graham, 1962); 25 to 28 percent after en bloc resection (Castro et al., 1973; Shiu et al., 1979); and 7 to 18 percent after amputation (Cantin et al., 1968; Simon et al., 1979). Once the clinical behavior of the soft-tissue sarcomas was better understood, the overall incidence of local recurrence decreased from 30 percent in the 1960s (Cantin et al., 1969; Martin et al., 1965) to 20 percent by 1980 (Shiu et al., 1979; Simon et al., 1979).

Historically, soft-tissue sarcomas were considered radioresistant (Rostock, 1928). Recently, extremity lesions have been treated with a multimodality approach that includes limb-sparing surgery and usually radiation therapy, with or without chemotherapy (Eilber et al., 1980; Lindberg et al., 1981; 1983; Rosenberg et at. 1982; Suit et al., 1981). In 1982, Rosenberg et al. reported a prospective randomized trial from the National Cancer Institute showing no statistically significant difference between the survival and disease-free survival rates of patients treated by amputation or limb-sparing surgery plus radiation therapy. These conservative procedures are now being applied to soft tissue sarcomas arising in the head and neck region.

Since a cervical mass is usually considered metastatic squamous cell carcinoma, the workup is basically that used for an unknown primary. The diagnosis of a primary soft tissue sarcoma arising in the neck is one of exclusion. When the workup does not show any obvious primary tumor, the diagnosis of soft tissue sarcoma may be made by a core biopsy; more commonly, an excisional biopsy is performed. Once the diagnosis has been established, the next step is to assess the extent of disease.

The American Joint Committee (AJC) staging system (Russell et al., 1977) incorporates the grade of the lesion in addition to the tumor, node, metastasis system. Although some investigators have used the AJC staging system, pathologists have recently questioned the reproducibility of grading soft tissue sarcomas (Ayala, personal communication). Fewer than 5 percent of soft tissue sarcomas metastasize to lymph nodes (Weingard and Rosenberg, 1978).

The major question in staging is the presence or absence of distant metastasis. Pulmonary metastasis is the initial site of spread in approximately 90 percent of patients with soft tissue sarcomas. Some investigators recommend the routine use of whole-lung tomograms or CT scan, whereas others believe that routine chest x-ray examinations are adequate. Tomograms or CT scans of the lung are not indicated in well-differentiated or low-grade lesions since the incidence of metastasis is less than 10 percent. Liver and bone scans have been advocated as part of the routine workup (Rosenberg et al., 1982), but the diagnostic yield is so low that they are not worthwhile screening procedures.

Treatment and Results

The treatment approach for soft-tissue sarcomas arising in the neck is multimodal. Small to moderately sized lesions may be widely excised with minimal functional defect. Because of the invasiveness of soft-tissue sarcoma and the anatomic limitations of dissection, postoperative radiation therapy should be given. The volume irradiated varies with the anatomic location of the lesion in the neck. The techniques are similar to those used for metastatic squamous cell carcinoma. The irradiated volume covers the entire surgical bed, and increases in size with the increasing grade of the tumor. Usually, the entire ipsilateral side of the neck is irradiated from the mandible to the clavicle. The recommended dose is 6000 cGy delivered over 6 weeks for low-grade lesions, and 6500 cGy over 6.5 weeks for intermediate- and high-grade lesions, with a field reduction after 5000 cGy.

Occasionally, patients may present with massive disease in the neck. Based on experience with soft-tissue sarcoma in the extremities (Martin et al., 1977), the recommended therapy is irradiation followed by surgical excision. Usually a 5000 cGy tumor dose is delivered over 5 weeks using a technique that delivers a uniform dose. Surgical resection is performed 4 to 6 weeks after completion of the radiation therapy.

Occasionally, unresectable lesions have been treated by radiation therapy alone. According to data for other sites, the chance of local control by radiation therapy alone is low (37%) (Lindberg, 1973). The role of adjuvant chemotherapy in treatment of localized soft tissue sarcoma is undecided. There have been conflicting reports in the literature (Lindberg et al., 1977; Rosenberg et al., 1983), so any recommendation on adjuvant chemotherapy must await further clarification.

Because of the rarity of soft-tissue sarcomas arising in the neck, there are few reports in the literature with which to properly evaluate the different treatment approaches. One exception, however, is the report from Memorial Sloan-Kettering Cancer Center by Farr (1981) on 285 patients with soft tissue sarcomas of the head and neck region. Farr reported an overall 5-year absolute disease-free survival rate of 32 percent. If children are eliminated from the study population, however, the cure rate increases to 50 percent. The 5-year disease-free survival rate of patients with the four more common tumors (fibrosarcoma, neurofibrosarcoma, liposarcoma, and leiomyosarcoma) is 59.2 percent (58 of 98 patients). An unusually high proportion of the lesions—30 of 98—arose in the neck. Unfortunately, Farr did not give separate cure rates for the subset of patients.

Between 1963 and 1982, 550 patients with localized soft tissue sarcomas were treated at UTMDAH by radiotherapy alone or in addition to surgery. Only 13 (2.4%) of the patients had lesions that arose in the neck. Eight of them were treated by surgery and postoperative radiation therapy, and four of the eight are living free of disease 24 to 69 months later; one died 11 months later with recurrence in the neck; the remaining three patients died of distant metastasis. Three other patients received preoperative radiation therapy, and all three died of distant metastasis within 2 years (one also had uncontrolled disease in the neck). The remaining two patients were treated by radiation therapy alone. The first had massive unresectable fibrosarcoma and is living free of disease 16 years later. The second had stage IVA disease and died 10 months after treatment, with uncontrolled disease in the neck.

Although there have been no complications and only two local recurrences, there are too few patients in this study to draw any significant conclusions.

REFERENCES

American Cancer Society: Cancer statistics 1985. *CA*, 35:26.

Cadman, J., Soule, F. H., and Kelly, J. P.: Synovial sarcoma: An analysis of 134 patients. *Cancer*, 18:613–17, 1957.

Cantin, J., McNeer, G. B., Chu, F. C., and Booker, R. J.: The problem of local recurrence after treatment of soft tissue sarcomas. *Ann. Surg.*, 168:47–53, 1968.

Carbone, P. P., Kaplan, H. S., Musshoff, K., Smithers, D. W., and Tubiana, M.: Report of the Committee on Hodgkin's Disease Staging Classification. *Cancer Res.*, 31:1860–61, 1971.

Castro, E. B., Hajdu, S. I., and Fortner, J. G.: Surgical therapy of fibrosarcoma of extremities. *Arch. Surg.*, 107:284–91, 1973.

Easson, E. C., and Russell, M. H.: The cure of Hodgkin's disease. *Br. Med. J.*, 1:1704–8, 1963.

Eilber, F. R., Mirra, J. J., Grant, T. T., Weisenburger, T., and Morton, D.: Is amputation necessary for sarcoma? A seven year experience with limb salvage. *Ann Surg.*, 192:43–48, 1980.

Farr, H. W.: Soft tissue sarcomas of the head and neck. *Semin Oncol.*, 8:185–89, 1981.

Fierstein, J. T., and Thawley, S. E.: Lymphoma of the head and neck. *Laryngoscope*, 88:582–93, 1978.

Fuller, L. M., Banker, F. L., Butler, J. J., and Gamble, J. F.: Natural history of non-Hodgkin's lymphoma stage I and II. *Br. J. Radiol.*, 31(suppl 2):270–75, 1975.

Gilbert, G.: Radiotherapy in Hodgkin's disease (malignant granulomatosis) anatomic and clinical foundations: Governing principles: Results. *A.J.R.* 41:198–205, 1939.

Hajdu, S.I.: *Pathology of Soft Tissue Sarcomas*. Lea & Febiger, Philadelphia, 1979.

Helman, S., and Mauch, P.: Role of radiation therapy in the treatment of Hodgkin's disease. *Cancer Treat. Rep.*, 66:915–21, 1982.

Johnson, R. E., Chretien, P. B., O'Conor, G. T., Devita, V. J., and Thomas, L. B.: Radiotherapy implications of prospective staging in non-Hodgkin's lymphoma. *Radiology*, 110:655–70, 1974.

Kaplan, H. S.: *Hodgkin's Disease*. 2nd ed., Harvard University Press, Cambridge, MA, 1980.

Lindberg, R. D.: The role of radiation therapy in the treatment of soft tissue sarcoma in adults. In *Proceedings of the Seventh National Cancer Conference*, pp. 883–88. J.B. Lippincott, Philadelphia, 1973.

Lindberg, R. D., Martin, R. G., Romsdahl, M. M., and Barkley, H. T.: Conservative surgery in postoperative radiation therapy in 300 adults with soft tissue sarcomas. *Cancer*, 47:2391–97, 1981.

Lindberg, R. D., Murphy, W. K., Benjamin, R. S., Sinkovics, J. G., Martin, R. G., Romsdahl, M. M., Jesse, R. H., and Russell, W. D.: Adjuvant chemotherapy in the treatment of primary soft tissue sarcomas: A preliminary report. In *Management of Primary Bone and Soft-Tissue Tumors*, pp. 343–52. Yearbook Medical Publishers, Chicago, 1977.

Martin, R. G., Butler, J. J., and Albores-Saavadra, J.: Soft tissue tumors: Surgical treatment and results. In *Tumors of Bone and Soft Tissue*, pp. 333–47. Yearbook Medical Publishers, Chicago, 1965.

Martin, R. G., Lindberg, R. D., and Russell, W. O.: Preoperative radiotherapy and surgery in the management of soft-tissue sarcoma. In *Management of Primary Bone and Soft Tissue Tumors*, pp. 229–307. Yearbook Medical Publishers, Chicago, 1977.

Mill, W. B., Lee, F. A., and Franssila, K. O.: Radiation therapy treatment of stage I and II extranodal non-Hodgkin's lymphoma of the head and neck. *Cancer*, 45:653–61, 1980.

National Cancer Institute sponsored study of classification of non-Hogkins' lymphomas. Summary and description of a working formulation for clinical usage. *Cancer*, 49:2112–35, 1982.

Plantenga, K. F., Hart, G., van Heerde, P., and Tierie, A. H.: Non-Hodgkin's malignant lymphomas of the upper digestive and respiratory tracts. *Am. J. Radiat. Oncol. Biol. Phys.*, 7:1419–27, 1981.

Peters, M. V.: A study of survival of Hodgkin's disease treated radiologically. *A.J.R.* 63:299–311, 1950.

Peters, M. V., Hasselback, R., and Brown, R. C.: Natural history of lymphoma related to clinical classification. In Zarafonetis, C. (ed): *Proceedings of the International Conference on Leukemia Lymphoma*. Lea & Febiger, Philadelphia, 1968.

Reddy, S., Bellettiere, E., Saxena, V., and Hendrickson, F. R.: Extranodal non-Hodgkin's lymphoma. *Cancer*, 46:1925–31, 1980.

Rosenberg, S. A., Tepper, J., Glatstein, E., Costa, J., Young, R., Baker, A., Brennan, M., deMoss, E. V.,

Seipp, C., Sindelar, W. F., Sugarbaker, P., and Wesley, R.: Prospective randomized evaluation of adjuvant chemotherapy in adults with soft tissue sarcomas of the extremities. *Cancer*, 52:424–34, 1983.

Rosenberg, S. A., Tepper, J., Glatstein, E., Costa, J., Baker, A., Brennan, M., deMoss, E. V., Slipp, C., Sindelar, W. F., Sugarbaker, P., and Wesley, R.: The treatment of soft-tissue sarcomas of the extremities. Prospective randomized evaluations of (1) limb-sparing surgery plus radiation therapy compared with amputation, and (2) the role of adjuvant chemotherapy. *Am. J. Surg.*, 196:305–15, 1982.

Rostock, R.: Indikationsstelking und Dauerefoid der Rontgenbestrahlung bei Sarkomen. *Fartschr. D. Therap.*, 4:241–44, 1928.

Russell, W. O., Cohn, J., Enzinger, F., Hajdu, S. I., Heise, H., Martin, R. G., Meissner, W., Miller, W. T., Schmitz, R. L., and Suit, H. D.: A clinical and pathological staging for soft tissue sarcomas. *Cancer*, 40:1562–70, 1977.

Shieber, W., and Graham, P.: An experience with sarcoma of soft tissue in adults. *Surgery*, 52:295–98, 1962.

Shiu, M. H., Castro, E. B., Hajdu, S. I., and Fortner, J. G.: Surgical treatment of 297 soft tissue sarcomas in extremities. *Ann. Surg.*, 182:597–602, 1979.

Simon, M. A., Spanier, S. S., and Enneking, W. F.: Management of adult soft tissue sarcomas in extremities. *Ann. Surg.*, 11:363–402, 1979.

Suit, H. D., Proppe, K. H., Mankin, H. J., and Wood, W. C.: Preoperative radiation therapy for sarcoma of soft tissue. *Cancer*, 47:2269–74, 1981.

Thar, T. L., Million, R. R., Hausner, R. J., and McKetty, M. H. B.: Hodgkin's disease stage I, II: Relationship of recurrence to size of disease, radiation dose, and number of sites involved. *Cancer*, 43:1101–5, 1979.

Thar, T. L.: Lymphomas and related diseases presenting in the head and neck. In Million, R. R., and Cassisi, N. (eds.): *Management of Head and Neck Cancer*, pp. 635–46. J.B. Lippincott, Philadelphia, 1984.

Weingard, D. N., and Rosenberg, S. A.: Early lymphatic spread of osteogenic and soft tissue sarcomas. *Surgery*, 84:231–40, 1978.

Wong, D. S., Fuller, L. M., Butler, J. J., and Shullenberger, C. C.: Extranodal non-Hodgkin's lymphomas of the head and neck. *A.J.R.* 123:471–81. 1975.

Index

A

Page numbers in **boldface** *refer to main discussions of topics.*

B

C

D

E

F

G

H

I

J

K

L

M

N

O

P

R

S

U

V